METHODS IN MOLECULAR BIOLOGY

Series Editor
John M. Walker
School of Life and Medical Sciences
University of Hertfordshire
Hatfield, Hertfordshire, AL10 9AB, UK

For further volumes:
http://www.springer.com/series/7651

Cancer Cytogenetics

Methods and Protocols

Edited by

Thomas S.K. Wan

Haematology Division, Department of Anatomical and Cellular Pathology, The Chinese University of Hong Kong, Prince of Wales Hospital, Shatin, Hong Kong, China

Humana Press

Editor
Thomas S.K. Wan
Haematology Division
Department of Anatomical and Cellular Pathology
The Chinese University of Hong Kong
Prince of Wales Hospital
Shatin, Hong Kong, China

ISSN 1064-3745 ISSN 1940-6029 (electronic)
Methods in Molecular Biology
ISBN 978-1-4939-8278-3 ISBN 978-1-4939-6703-2 (eBook)
DOI 10.1007/978-1-4939-6703-2

Printed on acid-free paper

This Humana Press imprint is published by Springer Nature
The registered company is Springer Science+Business Media LLC
The registered company address is: 233 Spring Street, New York, NY 10013, U.S.A.

Preface

The discovery of the Philadelphia chromosome in 1960 ushered the field of cancer cytogenetics study into a new era. The development of fluorescence in situ hybridization (FISH) in 1980 helped to overcome many of the drawbacks in the assessment of genetic alterations in cancer cells by karyotyping. Subsequent methodological advances in molecular cytogenetics that were initiated in the early 1990s based on the principle of FISH have greatly enhanced the efficiency and accuracy of karyotype analysis by marrying conventional cytogenetics with molecular technologies. All of these molecular cytogenetic techniques add colors to the monotonous world of conventional chromosome banding. Currently, both karyotyping and FISH studies have emerged as indispensable tools for both basic and clinical research, which parallel their clinical diagnostic application in leukemia and cancers. The development, current utilization, detailed hands-on protocols, data interpretation, and technical pitfalls of these approaches used for cancer diagnosis and research will be included in this volume of book.

This volume *Cancer Cytogenetics: Methods and Protocols* of the Springer Methods in Molecular Biology series provides the readers with detailed protocols covering the main cancer cytogenetics techniques needed for clinical utilization and research purposes. Updated reviews on the recurrent chromosomal abnormalities in hematological malignancies provide an excellent, helpful benchmarking guide for cytogenetics data interpretation and specific malignant diseases correlation. All chapters were precisely written by professionally experienced cytogeneticists and/or pathologists working proactively in this specialized field. I have been very fortunate to have gathered a group of 52 experts from 15 countries or cities, including Australia, Canada, China, France, Germany, Hong Kong, Italy, Korea, the Netherlands, Poland, Russia, Singapore, Thailand, the United Kingdom, and the United States of America, in a short period of time to share their experiences empathetically and interactively. Although the circle of cancer cytogeneticists is relatively small, its task is notably significant, fostering worldwide contribution and collaboration. I would like to thank all of them for their generous contributions to this volume of book. In addition to the step-by-step description of every technique, much emphasis is placed on the pitfalls that accompany all testing procedures.

This book is intended for use by the novice in cytogenetics, providing helpful guiding protocols to them as well as deeper insights to those who are already engaged in the field, yet looking for some technical hints.

I am grateful to all colleagues in Cytogenetics Laboratory, Division of Haematology, Department of Anatomical and Cellular Pathology, The Chinese University of Hong Kong, Prince of Wales Hospital, under whose auspices this book was written. I would also like to thank Professor Ka-Fai To and Professor Margaret H. L. Ng for their continued encouragement. Last but not the least, I wish to express my thankful indebtedness to my wife, Mary, and my two sons, Conan and Eden, for their support and patience.

Hong Kong, China *Thomas S.K. Wan, PhD, FRCPath, FFSc(RCPA)*

Contents

Contributors

ETIENNE DE BRAEKELEER • *Haematological Cancer Genetics and Stem Cell Genetics, Wellcome Trust Sanger Institute, Hinxton, Cambridge, UK*
ELIZA CERVEIRA • *The Jackson Laboratory for Genomic Medicine, Farmington, CT, USA*
NELSON CHUN NGAI CHAN • *Department of Anatomical and Cellular Pathology, Prince of Wales Hospital, Shatin, Hong Kong, China*
NATALIE PUI HA CHAN • *Department of Anatomical and Cellular Pathology, Prince of Wales Hospital, Shatin, Hong Kong, China*
JIADI CHEN • *Fujian Institute of Hematology, Fujian Medical University Affiliated Union Hospital, Fuzhou, People's Republic of China*
PHILIPPE DESSEN • *UMR 1170 INSERM, Gustave Roussy, Villejuif, France*
PATRICIA K. DOWLING • *Cytogenetics, Pathline-Emerge Pathology Services, Ramsey, NJ, USA*
HANS G. DREXLER • *Department of Human and Animal Cell Lines, German Collection of Microorganisms and Cell Cultures, Leibniz Institute – DSMZ, Braunschweig, Germany*
AGATA A. FILIP • *Department of Cancer Genetics, Medical University of Lublin, Lublin, Poland*
TAMIZH GNANA-SEKARAN • *PROCyTOX Commissariat à l'Energie Atomique et aux Energies Alternatives (CEA), Fontenay-aux-Roses and Université Paris-Saclay, Fontenay-aux-Roses Cedex, France*
JUN GU • *Cytogenetic Technology Program, School of Health Professions, UT MD Anderson Cancer Center, Houston, TX, USA*
ROSALIND J. HASTINGS • *Cytogenetic External Quality Assessment, Women's Centre, John Radcliffe Hospital, Oxford University Hospitals NHS Foundation Trust, Oxford, UK*
HENRY H. HENG • *Center for Molecular Medicine and Genetics, Wayne State University School of Medicine, Detroit, MI, USA; Department of Pathology, Wayne State University School of Medicine, Detroit, MI, USA; Karmanos Cancer Institute, Detroit, MI, USA*
HUIFANG HUANG • *Central Laboratory, Fujian Medical University Affiliated Union Hospital, Fuzhou, People's Republic of China*
ELEANOR K.C. HUI • *Haematology Division, Department of Anatomical and Cellular Pathology, Prince of Wales Hospital, Shatin, Hong Kong, China*
JEAN-LOUP HURET • *Medical Genetics, Department of Medical Information, University Hospital, Poitiers, France*
IVAN Y. IOUROV • *Mental Health Research Center, Moscow, Russia; Separated Structural Unit "Clinical Research Institute of Pediatrics" named after Y.E. Veltishev, Russian National Research Medical University named after N.I. Pirogov, Ministry of Health of Russian Federation, Moscow, Russia; Moscow State University of Psychology and Education, Moscow, Russia*
MAREN E. KAUFMANN • *Department of Human and Animal Cell Lines, German Collection of Microorganisms and Cell Cultures, Leibniz Institute – DSMZ, Braunschweig, Germany*

DOROTA KOCZKODAJ • *Department of Cancer Genetics, Medical University of Lublin, Lublin, Poland*
THOMAS LIEHR • *Jena University Hospital, Friedrich Schiller University, Institute of Human Genetics, Jena, Germany*
ALVIN S.T. LIM • *Cytogenetics Laboratory, Department of Molecular Pathology, Singapore General Hospital, Singapore, Singapore*
TSE HUI LIM • *Cytogenetics Laboratory, Department of Molecular Pathology, Singapore General Hospital, Singapore, Singapore*
EDMOND S.K. MA • *Department of Pathology, Hong Kong Sanatorium and Hospital, Happy Valley, Hong Kong, China*
RODERICK A.F. MACLEOD • *Department of Human and Animal Cell Lines, German Collection of Microorganisms and Cell Cultures, Leibniz Institute – DSMZ, Braunschweig, Germany*
SARAH MOORE • *Genetics and Molecular Pathology, SA Pathology, Adelaide, South Australia, Australia*
HOSSAIN MOSSAFA • *Laboratoire CERBA, Saint Ouen l'Aumone, France*
MARGARET H.L. NG • *Haematology Division, Department of Anatomical and Cellular Pathology, The Chinese University of Hong Kong, Prince of Wales Hospital, Hong Kong, China*
MARIO NICOLA • *Genetics and Molecular Pathology, SA Pathology, Adelaide, Australia*
MONEEB A.K. OTHMAN • *Jena University Hospital, Friedrich Schiller University, Institute of Human Genetics, Jena, Germany*
TAE SUNG PARK • *Department of Laboratory Medicine, School of Medicine, Kyung Hee University, Seoul, South Korea*
LAURE PIQUERET-STEPHAN • *PROCyTOX Commissariat à l'Energie Atomique et aux Energies Alternatives (CEA), Fontenay-aux-Roses and Université Paris-Saclay, Fontenay-aux-Roses Cedex, France*
KATRINA RACK • *Cytogenetic External Quality Assessment, Women's Centre, John Radcliffe Hospital, Oxford University Hospitals NHS Foundation Trust, Oxford, UK*
MICHELLE RICOUL • *PROCyTOX Commissariat à l'Energie Atomique et aux Energies Alternatives (CEA), Fontenay-aux-Roses and Université Paris-Saclay, Fontenay-aux-Roses Cedex, France*
KATHARINA RITTSCHER • *Jena University Hospital, Institute of Human Genetics, Friedrich Schiller University, Jena, Germany*
MARIANO ROCCHI • *Department of Biology, University of Bari, Bari, Italy*
MALLORY ROMANOVITCH • *The Jackson Laboratory for Genomic Medicine, Farmington, CT, USA*
LAURE SABATIER • *PROCyTOX Commissariat à l'Energie Atomique et aux Energies Alternatives (CEA), Fontenay-aux-Roses and Université Paris-Saclay, Fontenay-aux-Roses Cedex, France*
MARY SHAGO • *Department of Paediatric Laboratory Medicine, The Hospital for Sick Children, Toronto, ON, Canada; Department of Laboratory Medicine and Pathobiology, University of Toronto, Toronto, ON, Canada*
ANNET SIMONS • *Department of Human Genetics, Radboud University Medical Center, Nijmegen, The Netherlands*
JANICE L. SMITH • *Cytogenetics/FISH Division, Baylor Genetics Laboratories, Department of Molecular and Human Genetics, Baylor College of Medicine, Houston, TX, USA*

Roscoe R. Stanyon • *Laboratory of Anthropology, Department of Animal Biology and Genetics, University of Florence, Florence, Italy*

Marian Stevens-Kroef • *Department of Human Genetics, Radboud University Medical Center, Nijmegen, The Netherlands*

Jeffrey M. Suttle • *Genetics and Molecular Pathology, SA Pathology, Adelaide, South Australia, Australia*

John Swansbury • *Clinical Cytogenetics Laboratory, The Royal Marsden Hospital, Sutton, Surrey, UK*

Montakarn Tansatit • *Unit of Medical Genetics, Medical Cytogenetics Laboratory, Department of Anatomy, Faculty of Medicine, King Chulalongkorn Memorial Hospital, Chulalongkorn University, Bangkok, Thailand*

Doron Tolomeo • *Department of Biology, University of Bari, Bari, Italy*

Meaghan Wall • *Victorian Cancer Cytogenetics Service, St. Vincent's Hospital, Melbourne, Australia; Department of Medicine, St. Vincent's Hospital, The University of Melbourne, Melbourne, Australia*

Thomas S.K. Wan • *Haematology Division, Department of Anatomical and Cellular Pathology, The Chinese University of Hong Kong, Prince of Wales Hospital, Hong Kong, Shatin, China*

John J. Yang • *Department of Laboratory Medicine, School of Medicine, Kyung Hee University, Seoul, South Korea*

Christine J. Ye • *The Division of Hematology/Oncology, Department of Internal Medicine, University of Michigan, Ann Arbor, MI, USA*

Chengsheng Zhang • *The Jackson Laboratory for Genomic Medicine, Farmington, CT, USA*

Qihui Zhu • *The Jackson Laboratory for Genomic Medicine, Farmington, CT, USA*

Chapter 1

Cancer Cytogenetics: An Introduction

Thomas S.K. Wan

Abstract

The Philadelphia chromosome was the first chromosomal abnormality discovered in cancer using the cytogenetics technique in 1960, and was consistently associated with chronic myeloid leukemia. Over the past five decades, innovative technical advances in the field of cancer cytogenetics have greatly enhanced the detection ability of chromosomal alterations, and have facilitated the research and diagnostic potential of chromosomal studies in neoplasms. These developments notwithstanding, chromosome analysis of a single cell is still the easiest way to delineate and understand the relationship between clonal evolution and disease progression of cancer cells. The use of advanced fluorescence in situ hybridization (FISH) techniques allows for the further identification of chromosomal alterations that are unresolved by the karyotyping method. It overcame many of the drawbacks of assessing the genetic alterations in cancer cells by karyotyping. Subsequently, the development of DNA microarray technologies provides a high-resolution view of the whole genome, which may add massive amounts of new information and opens the field of cancer cytogenomics. Strikingly, cancer cytogenetics does not only provide key information to improve the care of patients with malignancies, but also acts as a guide to identify the genes responsible for the development of these neoplastic states and has led to the emergence of molecularly targeted therapies in the field of personalized medicine.

Key words Cancer cytogenetics, FISH, Karyotyping, Molecular cytogenetics, Review

1 Introduction

It is widely acknowledged that human cytogenetics began in 1955, with the discovery by Tjio and Levan that normal human cells contain 46 chromosomes [1]. Subsequently, discovery of a minute abnormal chromosome, the Philadelphia (Ph) chromosome, as a hallmark of chronic myeloid leukemia (CML) in 1960 by Peter Nowell and David Hungerford, showed for the first time that cancer resulted from a specific genetic abnormality [2]. As chromosome preparation techniques improved, Janet Rowley demonstrated that the Ph chromosome was the result of a translocation between the long arms of chromosome 9 and 22 in 1973 [3]. Subsequent work revealed that this translocation resulted in a new fusion oncogenic protein (BCR-ABL1) overexpressing an aberrant tyrosine

Thomas S.K. Wan (ed.), *Cancer Cytogenetics: Methods and Protocols*, Methods in Molecular Biology, vol. 1541,
DOI 10.1007/978-1-4939-6703-2_1, © Springer Science+Business Media LLC 2017

kinase in leukemia cells of virtually every patient with CML, thus providing strong evidence of its pathogenetic role [4]. Strikingly, the description of the Ph chromosome ushered in a new era of cancer genetic diagnosis and that the remarkable success of imatinib for the treatment of Ph-positive CML has led to the emergence of molecularly targeted therapies, a field now known as personalized medicine. Over the past five decades, strong evidence has accumulated that genetic data are intimately associated with the diagnosis and prognosis of many cancers, thereby moving cancer cytogenetics studies from the bench to clinical practice. In 2008, the World Health Organization has further categorized four unique acute myeloid leukemia (AML) subtypes according to cytogenetics based on the association between specific cytogenetic abnormalities, certain cytological morphology, and clinical features [5]. Therefore, karyotyping of neoplastic cells is currently a mandatory investigation for all newly diagnosed leukemias, owing to its usefulness in diagnosis, classification, and prognostication. Furthermore, karyotyping of cancer cells remains the gold standard for understanding the relationship between clonal evolution and disease progression, since it provides a global analysis of the abnormalities in the entire genome of a single cell.

Fluorescence in situ hybridization (FISH) assay relies on the ability of single stranded DNA to hybridize to complementary DNA sequence. It is applicable to map gene loci on specific chromosomes [6], detect both structural and numerical chromosomal abnormalities, and reveal cryptic abnormalities. It has overcome many of the drawbacks of chromosome analysis, such as poor quality metaphases of cancer cells, low mitotic index, low specimen cell yield, and other unpredictable technical difficulties. Recently, FISH remains an indispensable and powerful tool in modern genetic laboratories. It is widely used for the detection of structural rearrangements such as translocations, inversions, insertions, and microdeletions, and for the delineation of unidentified (or marker) chromosomes and chromosomal breakpoint regions of genetic abnormalities [7, 8]. Of note, FISH has greatly enhanced the efficiency and accuracy of karyotype analysis by supplementing the technical pitfalls of karyotyping and molecular genetic technologies.

2 Conventional Cytogenetics

Chromosomal studies of malignancies even up to the present still pose a particular technical challenge in a clinical cytogenetics laboratory. As the chromosomal preparation results are so unpredictable, no single technique guarantees to work consistently and reliably. Therefore, every laboratory should adopt a slight variation of the standard operational protocol. Under optimal conditions, in most cases of neoplasm, clonal cytogenetic abnormalities with or without clonal evolution can be delineated by using this simple method. In general, chromosome analysis requires five principal steps: (1) cell culture of malignant cells, (2) harvest of metaphase chromosomes, (3) spreading of chromosomes on a microscopic slide, (4) banding and staining using an appropriate special chromosome banding protocol, and (5) analysis of chromosomes by light microscopy or karyotype assisted computer analysis [9] (Fig. 1). The discovery of colchicine (or colcemid) pretreatment that resulted in the destruction of the mitotic spindle apparatus allows accumulation of dividing cells in metaphase. Treatment of the mitotic cells with hypotonic solution swells the cell membrane, disperses the chromosomes, and improves the quality of metaphase spreads on the microscopic slide. As a result, enumeration and analysis of the structure of individual chromosomes in human cells are then possible. Chromosome analysis provides an overview of entire chromosomal aberrations in a single tumor cell and the relationship between clonal evolution and disease progression can be easily determined.

The duration of the cell cycle in malignant cells varies greatly among patients and different cell types. Therefore, one of the most significant factors in obtaining a successful result is setting

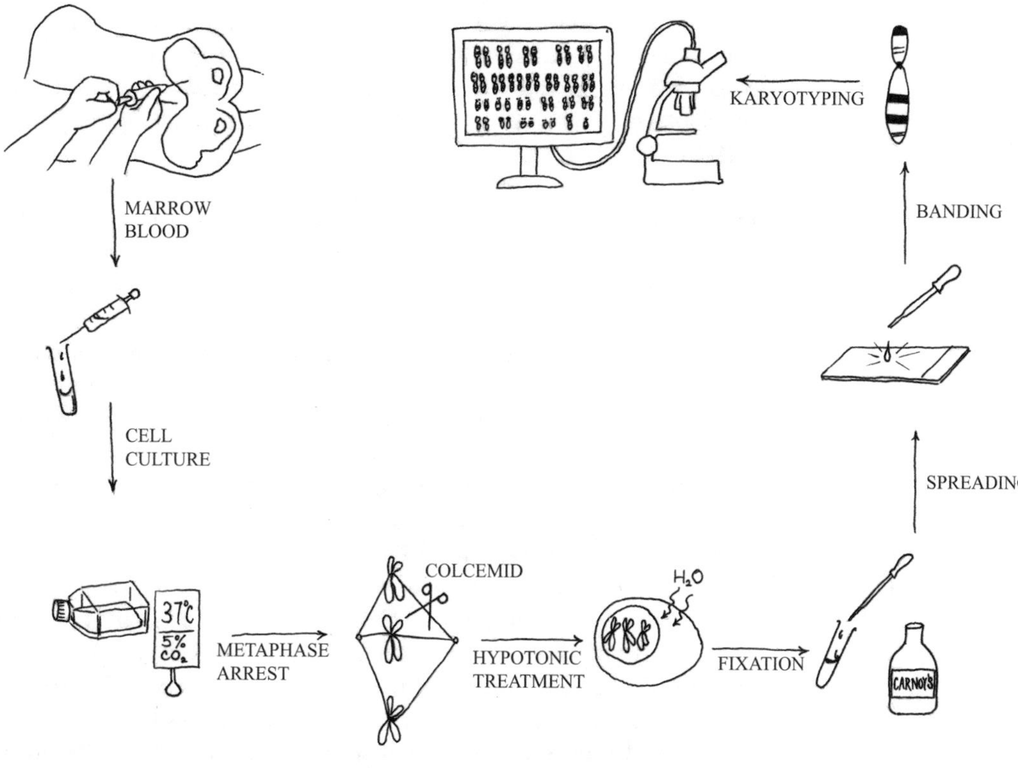

Fig. 1 Protocol for the preparation of a karyotype from a leukemic patient. (Reproduced from [9] with permission from Annals of Laboratory Medicine.)

up multiple condition cultures to maximize the chances of obtaining optimal malignant cell divisions. These conditions are: (1) direct harvest of neoplastic cells when the specimen is received, (2) overnight short-term culture in only culture medium, and (3) overnight culture with synchronization of the cell cycle (by blocking at S-phase of the cell cycle) of dividing malignant cells. The detailed protocols for setting up cultures for myeloid malignancies, acute lymphoblastic leukemia (ALL), chronic lymphoid malignancies, and solid tumors are described in Chaps. 2–5 respectively.

High-resolution banding of long chromosomes with good morphology in pro-metaphase or even prophase can be achieved by applying synchronization techniques in some cell types [10]. It enables greater precision in the identification of subtle structural chromosome abnormalities that are commonly found in malignant cells. However, it has been reported that fluorodeoxyuridine synchronization cultures are inferior to short-term cultures for chromosome analysis in ALL [11]. Obviously, ALL is a frustrating disease for most clinical cytogeneticists, as it has several technical challenges, including frequent low mitotic index, poor chromosome morphology, and samples that have a marked tendency to clot during harvest.

Standard cytogenetic harvesting techniques have not changed significantly in recent years. More importantly, optimized temperature, humidity, and airflow are three major factors to ensure chromosomes can spread well onto a microscopic slide by minimizing overlapping of chromosomes and therefore to obtain good chromosome morphology.

Chromosome banding techniques produce a series of consistent landmarks along the length of metaphase chromosomes that allow for both recognition of individual chromosomes within a genome and identification of specific segments of individual chromosomes (*see* Chaps. 6–7). Therefore, breakpoints and constituent chromosomes involved in chromosome translocations could be accurately identified, and deletions within a chromosome could be more specifically named and annotated. Currently, Giemsa banding (G-banding) and Reserve banding (R-banding) are two most common routinely used banding techniques for chromosome identification in clinical cytogenetic laboratory. Furthermore, C-banding is specifically useful in human cytogenetics to stain the centromeric chromosome regions and other regions containing constitutive heterochromatin. Heterochromatin is tightly packed and repetitive DNA, and is secondary constrictions of human chromosomes 1, 9, 16, and the distal segment of the Y chromosome long arm. The size of these C-bands differs between individuals and homologous chromosomes. Chromosome harvesting procedures and different banding techniques are described in Chaps. 2–6.

3 Molecular Cytogenetics

FISH was developed by biomedical researchers in the early 1980s. Molecular cytogenetics involves the use of a series of FISH and FISH-based techniques, in which DNA probes are labeled with different colored fluorophores to visualize one or more specific regions of the genome. It is used as a rapid, sensitive test for the detection of cryptic or subtle chromosomal changes. Furthermore, it can be used to detect genetic alterations in living cells, nondividing cell populations (interphase nuclei), metaphase spread, archived formalin-fixed paraffin-embedded (FFPE) tissue sections, fresh tissue sections, and cytology preparations. Recently, with the continuous isolation of commercially available DNA probes specific to a particular chromosome region, it is a convenient method to support the practice of personalized medicine. However, FISH assays are still hampered by reagent costs, which prevent its adoption by large-scale oncological screening. In view of this, home-brew FISH probes for specific chromosome loci are also widely used in cancer research nowadays (*see* Chap. 9).

Over the past decade, FISH techniques enjoyed a tremendous impact on molecular cytogenetic diagnosis by providing a better understanding of the role of both numerical and structural aberrations in neoplasms, in particular with the use of interphase FISH for the detection of known genes involved in chromosomal aberrations in leukemia. FISH is widely used today in clinical practice to help in the diagnosis, prognosis, management, and selection of appropriate treatments for patients with hematologic cancers (*see* Chap. 8) and solid tumors (*see* Chap. 11). It is particularly indispensable when karyotypic analysis may be difficult in the largely quiescent cells of certain hematologic malignancies such as the chronic lymphoid disorders. In addition, FISH can also be used for investigating the origin and progression of hematologic malignancies, and to establish which hematopoietic compartments are involved in neoplastic processes (*see* Chap. 12).

The standard FISH protocol is illustrated in Fig. 2 [9] and includes five main steps: (1) sample pretreatment using proteolytic enzymes to enhance sufficient probe penetration for efficient hybridization; (2) denaturation of the double stranded DNA of probe and sample to single stranded DNA; (3) hybridization of single stranded DNA probe to complementary DNA sequence of target cells or metaphase spreads (annealing); (4) post-hybridization washing to wash out the unbounded and not perfectly matched probe; and (5) detection using a simple epifluorescence microscope with appropriate filter sets (Fig. 2). When a new FISH test is implemented in a cancer genetic laboratory, the assay performance validation should include sensitivity, accuracy, precision, and specificity [12]. The upper cutoff for normal results in a FISH assay

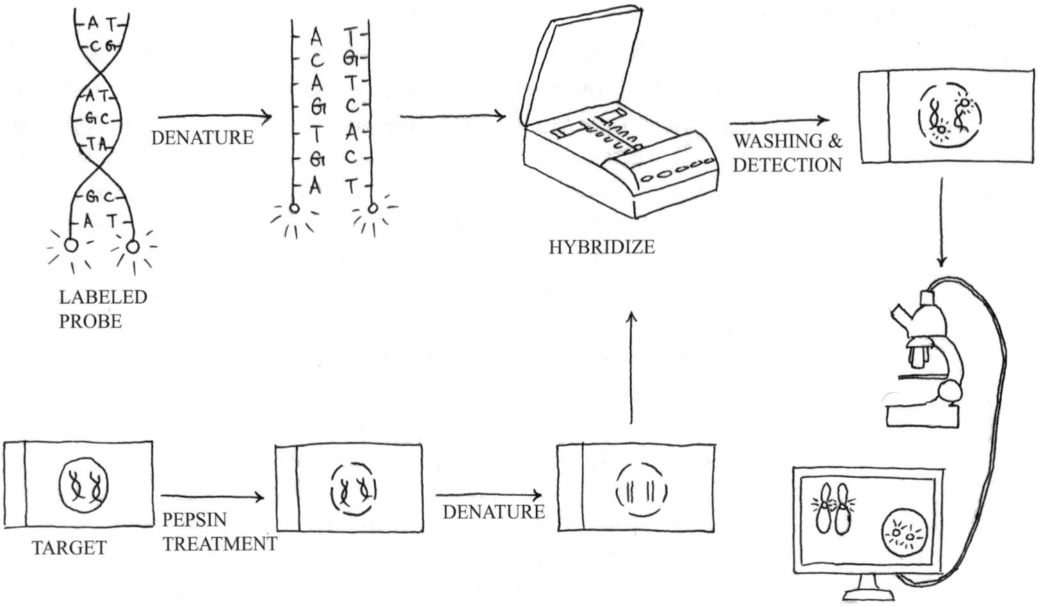

Fig. 2 FISH standard protocol. It includes sample pretreatment, denaturation of probe and sample, hybridization, post-hybridization washing, and fluorescent signal detection. (Reproduced from [9] with permission from Annals of Laboratory Medicine.)

should be established to ensure that FISH results are clear and interpretable (*see* Chap. 10). Furthermore, ongoing monitoring of inter-observer reproducibility, accomplished in part by having two laboratory personnel read in every case, can help detect changes in assay performance or loss of consistency in applying scoring criteria.

The impetus for many of these FISH technology innovations has been the direct result of an increased understanding of the sequence, structure, and function of the human genome, which has highlighted the intricate marvel of the DNA architectural blueprint housed within our chromosomes. Numerous methodological advances in FISH-based technology were developed in the early 1990s, including comparative genomic hybridization (CGH) [13], array CGH (aCGH) (*see* Chap. 15) [14], spectral karyotyping (SKY) [15], multicolor FISH (mFISH) (*see* Chap. 16) [16], and multicolor banding (mBAND) (*see* Chap. 16) [17]. Interestingly, all of these molecular cytogenetic techniques add colors to the monotonous world of conventional chromosome banding.

The CGH is based on quantitative dual-color FISH along each chromosome [13]. CGH can be used to detect genetic imbalances in test genomes, and to determine the chromosomal map positions of gains and losses of entire chromosomes or chromosomal subregions present in normal reference metaphase preparations. A distinct advantage of CGH is that tumor DNA is the only requirement for this analysis, and therefore archived, formalin-fixed and paraffin-embedded tissues can be used as well. CGH is useful for cancer research, especially for determining the low mitotic index of malignant cells with poor chromosome morphology and resolution [18–20]. The concept and methodology of aCGH is essentially the same as its traditional predecessor except that the template against which the genomic comparison performed is no longer a normal metaphase spread. The aCGH greatly improves the resolution of the technique by substituting the hybridization targets with genomic segments spotted in an array format in a microscopic slide.

Two multicolor fluorescence technologies, mFISH [16] and SKY [15], have been introduced in 1996. These technologies are based on simultaneous hybridization of 24 chromosome-specific composite probes. This technique is very useful for the identification of cryptic chromosomal abnormalities, unidentified (marker) chromosome, and unbalanced chromosomal translocation. Subsequently, mBAND has been developed to facilitate the identification of intrachromosomal rearrangements and to map the exact breakpoint by using human overlapping microdissection libraries that are differentially labeled [17]. The unique color band sequences have great value for delineating intrachromosomal exchanges, such as inversions, deletions, duplications, and insertions [7].

The main goal of the cancer cytogenetic laboratory is to select appropriate FISH techniques that are most useful and informative for a particular study and perform thorough analyses to arrive at an interpretation that is useful for research and diagnostic purposes. The telomere length of an individual human chromosome can be measured by quantitative FISH (Q-FISH) using peptide nucleic acids (PNA) probe [21] (*see* Chap. 13). Absence or low numbers of telomere repeats at junctions of dicentric chromosomes of viral immortalized human cells have first quantitatively been documented using Q-FISH technique [21]. Furthermore, the dicentric chromosome assay is the international gold-standard method for biological dosimetry and classification of genotoxic agents. The most recent introduction of telomere and centromere (TC) staining using PNA FISH probes offers the potential to render dicentric scoring more efficient and robust (*see* Chap. 17). The use of TC staining has permitted a reevaluation of the dose–response curve and the highly efficient automation of the scoring process, marking a new step in the management and follow-up of populations exposed to genotoxic agents including ionizing radiation. For gene mapping, high-resolution FISH on deproteinized, stretched DNA prepared by in situ extraction of whole cells immobilized on microscopic glass slides allows the visualization of individual genes or other small DNA elements on chromosomes with a resolution of approximate 1000 base pairs (*see* Chap. 14). This technique is useful for the determination of the number of repetitive genes and to establish the physical order of cloned DNA fragments along continuous sections of individual chromosomes.

4 Cancer Cytogenetic/Cytogenomic Resources and Information

Over the past five decades, innovative technical advances in the field of cancer cytogenetics have greatly enhanced the detection of chromosomal alterations and have facilitated the research and diagnostic potential of chromosomal studies in malignancies. The Mitelman Database of Chromosome Aberrations and Gene Fusions in Cancer (http://cgap.nci.nih.gov/Chromosomes/Mitelman) complies thousands of tumor cases including 66,517 published clonal cytogenetic aberrations. The database was further updated in May 2016 to include 10,256 chimeric fusion genes [22]. A steadily increasing number of specific abnormalities are found to be associated with particular malignancies or disease subgroups. The majority of malignant solid tumors, however, exhibit a complex pattern of chromosomal abnormalities, rarely showing any direct association with specific morphological or prognostic subgroups. In hematological neoplasms, certain abnormalities are often strongly associated with specific diagnostic entities, as is described in detail in Chaps. 18–23.

Cytogenetic resources available on the Internet are quite varied and overlapping. Currently, the two most commonly used cancer cytogenetics database are: (1) the Mitelman Database of Chromosome Aberrations and Gene Fusions in Cancer (http://cgap.nci.nih.gov/Chromosomes/Mitelman) [22], and (2) the Atlas of Genetics and Cytogenetics in Oncology and Haematology (http://atlasgeneticsoncology.org/) [23]. The Mitelman's database includes a comprehensive database of all published neoplasia-associated karyotypes and their corresponding gene fusions. The available information on chromosome abnormalities in human neoplasias has steadily increased over the past three decades. The Atlas of Genetics and Cytogenetics in Oncology and Haematology, which was established in 1997, is a peer-reviewed, open access, online journal, encyclopedia, and database that is devoted to genes, cytogenetics, and clinical entities in cancer and cancer-prone diseases. Approximately 3216 authors have contributed to the Atlas up to May 2016, making 30,519 documents and 32,554 images available (*Dr. Jean-Loup Huret, personal communication*). The use of cytogenetic/cytogenomic resources and information in Internet is described in Chap. 25.

In the clinical cytogenetics community, interpretation and scientific communication is often facilitated by universally accepted nomenclature with precisely defined terms and syntax conventions that minimize complexity and add precision to the process. Cytogenetic nomenclature is based on the reports of an international committee that was established in 1960, known as the International System for Human Cytogenetic Nomenclature (ISCN) [24]. The nomenclature is updated periodically. The most recently used ISCN 2016 [25] version offers standard nomenclature that is used to describe any genomic rearrangement identified by techniques ranging from karyotyping to FISH, microarray, various region-specific assays, and DNA sequencing. The title was renamed to the International System for Human *Cytogenomic* Nomenclature (ISCN) in 2016. However, whether two cells with the same loss of a single chromosome or one cell with a gain of a single chromosome in a composite karyotype should be counted and included in the size of the clone is still contradictory among different laboratories all over the world since then [9]. The ISCN standing committee should continue to discuss such discrepancies and make efforts to align the reporting system used by cancer cytogenetic laboratories [26]. The cytogenetic nomenclature and reporting system is described in Chap. 24.

5 Concluding Remarks

Conventional cytogenetics using regular banded chromosomal analysis remains a simple and popular technique to get an overview of the human genome. It is still the easiest way to understand the relationship between clonal evolution and disease progression of neoplasms. Karyotyping analysis can now be combined with FISH and other molecular techniques, leading to precise detection of genetic alterations in cancer. Therefore, techniques of cytogenetics are bound to continue to be indispensable tools for diagnosing genetic disorders and indicating possible treatment and management. Taken together, the morphologic, karyotyping, FISH, and molecular features should all be considered to obtain accurate diagnoses of malignancies, especially leukemias. This highlights the clinical importance of a combined modality approach for the accurate diagnosis and classification of cancers.

Acknowledgment

The author thanks Eden Wan for drawing Figs. 1 and 2.

References

1. Tjio JH, Levan A (1956) The chromosome number in man. Hereditas 42:1–6
2. Nowell PC, Hungerford DA (1960) A minute chromosome in human chronic granulocytic leukemia. Science 132:1497
3. Rowley JD (1973) A new consistent chromosomal abnormality in chronic myelogeneous leukaemia identified by quinacrine fluorescence and Giemsa staining. Nature 243:290–293
4. Konopka JB, Watanabe SM, Singer JW et al (1985) Cell lines and clinical isolates derived from Ph'-positive chronic myelogeneous leukemia patients express c-abl proteins with a common structural alteration. Proc Natl Acad Sci U S A 82:1810–1814
5. Vardiman JW, Thiele J, Arber DA et al (2009) The 2008 revision of the World Health Organization (WHO) classification of myeloid

neoplasm and acute leukemia: rationale and important changes. Blood 114:937–951
6. Manuelidis L, Langer-Safer PR, Ward DC (1982) High-resolution mapping of satellite DNA using biotin-labeled DNA probes. J Cell Biol 95:619–625
7. Wan TS, Ma ES (2012) Molecular cytogenetics: an indispensable tool for cancer diagnosis. Chang Gung Med J 35:96–110
8. Wan TS, Ma ES (2012) The role of FISH in hematologic cancer. Int J Hematol Oncol 1:71–86
9. Wan TS (2014) Cancer cytogenetics: methodology revisited. Ann Lab Med 34:413–425
10. Yunis JJ (1982) Comparative analysis of high-resolution chromosome techniques for leukemic bone marrows. Cancer Genet Cytogenet 7:43–50
11. Garipidou V, Secker-Walker LM (1991) The use of fluorodeoxyuridine synchronization for cytogenetic investigation of acute lymphoblastic leukemia. Cancer Genet Cytogenet 52:107–111
12. Saxe DF, Persons DL, Wolff DJ, Cytogenetics Resource Committee of the College of American Pathologists et al (2012) Validation of fluorescence in situ hybridization using an analyste-specific reagent for detection of abnormalities involving the mixed lineage leukemia gene. Arch Pathol Lab Med 136:47–52
13. Kallioniemi A, Kallioniemi OP, Sudar D et al (1992) Compararive genomic hybridization for molecular cytogenetic analysis of solid tumors. Science 258:818–821
14. Pinkel D, Segraves R, Sudar D et al (1998) High resolution analysis of DNA copy number variation using comparative genomic hybridization to microarrays. Nat Genet 20:207–211
15. Schröck E, du Manoir S, Veldman T et al (1996) Multicolor spectral karyotyping of human chromosomes. Science 273:494–497
16. Speicher MR, Gwyn Ballard S, Ward DC (1996) Karyotyping human chromosomes by combinatorial multi-fluor FISH. Nat Genet 12:368–375
17. Chudoba I, Plesch A, Lörch T et al (1999) High resolution multicolor-banding: a new technique for refine FISH analysis of human chromosomes. Cytogenet Cell Genet 84:156–160
18. Tsao SW, Wong N, Wang X et al (2001) Nonrandom chromosomal imbalances in human ovarian surface epithelial cells immortalized by HPV16-E6E7 viral oncogenes. Cancer Genet Cytogenet 130:141–149
19. Hu YC, Lam KY, Law SY et al (2002) Establishment, characterization, karyotyping, and comparative genomic hybridization analysis of HKESC-2 and HKESC-3, two newly established human esophageal squamous cell carcinoma cell lines. Cancer Genet Cytogenet 135:120–127
20. Wong MP, Fung LF, Wang E et al (2003) Chromosomal aberrations of primary lung adenocarcinomas in nonsmokers. Cancer 97:1263–1270
21. Wan TS, Martens UM, Poon SS et al (1999) Absence or low number of telomere repeats at junctions of dicentric chromosomes. Genes Chromosomes Cancer 24:83–86
22. Mitelman F, Johansson B, Mertens F (eds) Mitelman database of chromosome aberrations in cancer. http://cgap.nci.nih.gov/Chromosomes/Mitelman (Updated on May 4, 2016)
23. Atlas of genetics and cytogenetics in oncology and haematology. http://AtlasGeneticsOncology.org
24. Shaffer LG, Tommerup N (eds) (2005) ISCN (2005): an international system for human cytogenetic nomenclature. S. Karger, Basel
25. McGowan-Jordan J, Simons A, Schmid M (eds) (2016) An international system for human cytogenomic nomenclature. S. Karger, Basel. [Reprint of Cytogenet Genome Res 149(1–2)]
26. Mitelman F, Rowley JD (2007) ISCN (2005) is not acceptable for describing clonal evolution in cancer. Genes Chromosomes Cancer 46:213–214

Chapter 2

Chromosome Preparation for Myeloid Malignancies

Eleanor K.C. Hui, Thomas S.K. Wan, and Margaret H.L. Ng

Abstract

Many cases of myeloid malignancies are associated with recurring cytogenetic aberrations. Chromosomal analysis can aid in diagnosis, predict prognosis, and disclose subsequent clonal evolution. Three different cell culture methods: direct harvest, nonsynchronized culture, and synchronized culture are usually prepared if the nucleated cell counts in marrow blood are sufficient. Synchronized culture is the first choice of method in myeloid malignancies, whereas the direct method can be omitted if the cell count is low. The aseptic culture technique is strictly followed until harvesting procedure. For synchronized culture, uridine and fluorodeoxyuridine are added as blocking reagents and released by thymidine on the following day. Harvesting steps of the cultures involved colcemid exposure, hypotonic treatment, and Carnoy's fixation. The cells are then ready for slide making and banding for chromosomal analysis.

Key words Myeloid malignancies, Chromosome preparation, Cytogenetic culture, Synchronization culture, Metaphase harvesting

1 Introduction

Myeloid malignancies include acute myeloid leukemia (AML), myeloproliferative neoplasm (MPN), and myelodysplastic syndrome (MDS). The new classification of hematopoietic and lymphoid neoplasms was first introduced in 2001 by the World Health Organization (WHO), the Society for Hematopathology and the European Association for Haematopathology [1, 2]. In addition to the assessment on morphology and cytochemistry of the neoplastic cells as adopted by the French-American-British (FAB) system for the classification of acute myeloid leukemia (AML) since 1976 [3], the new classification of myeloid neoplasm has incorporated genetic information to establish specific disease entities and predict the prognosis more accurately. Many cases of AML are found to have recurring genetic abnormalities that affect cellular pathways of myeloid cells. In 2008, WHO revised the classification of myeloid neoplasm to provide an updated version based on recent data [4]. Additional chromosomal rearrangements are further updated the category of AML with recurrent genetic

Thomas S.K. Wan (ed.), *Cancer Cytogenetics: Methods and Protocols*, Methods in Molecular Biology, vol. 1541,
DOI 10.1007/978-1-4939-6703-2_2, © Springer Science+Business Media LLC 2017

Table 1
WHO classification of acute myeloid leukemia with recurrent genetic abnormalities [5]

AML with t(8;21)(q22;q22.1); *RUNX1-RUNX1T1*
AML with inv(16)(p13.1q22) or t(16;16)(p13.1;q22); *CBFB-MYH11*
AML with *PML-RARA*
AML with t(9;11)(p21.3;q23.3); *MLLT3-KMT2A*
AML with t(6;9)(p23;q34.1); *DEK-NUP214*
AML with inv(3)(q21.3q26.2) or t(3;3)(q21.3;q26.2); *GATA2, MECOM*
AML (megakaryoblastic) with t(1;22)(p13.3;q13.3); *RBM15-MKL1*
AML with *BCR-ABL1* (provisional entity)
AML with mutated *NPM1*
AML with biallelic mutations of *CEBPA*
AML with mutated *RUNX1* (provisional entity)

abnormalities in 2016 revision (Table 1) [5]. Cytogenetic analysis of bone marrow cells is important during initial evaluation for diagnosis and prediction of prognosis. Patients with AML harboring t(15;17)(q22;q21), t(8;21)(q22;q22), and inv(16)(p13.1q22)/t(16;16)(p13.1;q22) are associated with relatively favorable outcomes, whereas those with inv(3)(q21q26.2)/t(3;3)(q21;q26.2), MLL rearrangement (except t(9;11)(p22;q23)), deletion of 5q, monosomies of chromosome 5 and/or 7, or complex karyotypes are associated with poorer prognoses [6].

Bone marrow aspirate in heparin or in culture medium should be sent to the laboratory as soon as possible without delay at room temperature. White cell count is adjusted to 1×10^6 cells/mL of culture medium. At least two different culture methods, nonsynchronized and synchronized, are set up if white cell count is adequate. If insufficient cells are present in the specimen, synchronized culture is preferred for myeloid malignancy.

The principle of cell cycle synchronization is to block the cells at the synthesis (S) phase causing an accumulation of many cells at this particular stage and release the cells on the next day so that many cells enter mitosis at approximately the same time. Better banding quality and longer chromosomes can thus be achieved. Fluorodeoxyuridine (FdU) and uridine prevent the synthesis of thymidine by blocking the action of thymidylate synthetase, an important enzyme in the production of thymidine. Cells are then blocked in S-phase in the cell cycle. These blocking reagents are usually added 16–20 h before harvesting. On the next morning, thymidine is added to release the block and the cells can resume their cell cycles. The block is removed 4–5 h before harvesting to let the cells go through the remaining cell cycle and enter into mitosis.

Harvesting begins with the addition of mitotic spindle inhibitor that depolymerizes the microtubules, which make up the spindle fiber. The chromosomes are freed from the metaphase plate without the spindle fiber, thus allowing them to float freely within the cytoplasm. As a result, the cells are arrested at metaphase. Colcemid is an analog of colchicine which is less toxic and is the most commonly used mitotic inhibitor nowadays. After the mitotic arrest, cells are centrifuged and resuspended in hypotonic solution. This hypotonic treatment causes swelling and lysis of the red blood cells, which facilitates better metaphase spreading. The final step involves fixing the cells using freshly prepared Carnoy's fixative. The cells become dehydrated while the cell membrane is hardened in the fixation process. The cells are washed with Carnoy's fixative until a clear solution is obtained. Fixed cells can be kept in −20 °C for slide making and banding over years [7–9].

2 Materials

2.1 Equipments

1. Class 2 biological safety cabinet (*see* **Note 1**).
2. Humidified 37 °C, 5% CO_2 incubator (*see* **Note 2**).
3. Bench-top automated cell counter (*see* **Note 3**).
4. Centrifuge.
5. Water bath.
6. Sterile 25-cm^2 flask with ventilation cap (*see* **Note 2**).
7. Sterile 15-mL centrifuge tubes.
8. Sterile transfer pipettes.

2.2 Reagents

All containers and distilled water used in reagents 1–5 should be sterile.

1. Growth medium: 1000 mL of RPMI 1640 medium (*see* **Note 4**), 180 mL of fetal calf serum, 12 mL of penicillin & streptomycin, 12 mL of preservative-free heparin (1000 IU/mL), 12 mL of L-glutamine. Store aliquots at −20 °C for 2 months.
2. Chang medium BMC. Store aliquots at −20 °C (*see* **Note 5**).
3. Working fluorodeoxyuridine (FdU): Dissolve 10 mg of FdU (M.W. 246.2) in 40 mL of distilled water as super-stock (1 mM). Pass through 0.45 μm filter to sterilize and store 1 mL aliquots at −20 °C for 2 years. Add 9 mL of distilled water to 1 mL of super-stock as stock solution (100 μM). Pass through 0.45 μm filter to sterilize and store 1 mL aliquots at −20 °C for 2 years. Add 9 mL of distilled water to 1 mL of

stock solution as 10 μM working solution. Store at 4 °C for 1 month.

4. Working uridine: Dissolve 97.7 mg of uridine (M.W. 244.2) in 100 mL of distilled water as stock solution (4 mM). Pass through 0.45 μm filter to sterilize and store 1 mL aliquots at −20 °C for up to 2 years. Add 9 mL of distilled water to 1 mL aliquot as 0.4 mM uridine working solution. Store at 4 °C for 1 month.
5. Working thymidine: Dissolve 24.22 mg of thymidine (M.W. 242.2) in 10 mL of distilled water as stock solution (10 mM). Pass through 0.45 μm filter to sterilize and store 1 mL aliquots at −20 °C for up to 2 years. Add 9 mL of distilled water to 1 mL aliquot as 1 mM thymidine working solution. Store at 4 °C for 1 month.
6. 1× Phosphate buffered saline (PBS): Dissolve 8 g of NaCl, 0.2 g of KCl, 0.92 g of Na_2HPO_4, and 0.2 g of KH_2PO_4 in 1 L of distilled water. Adjust pH to 7.2.
7. Colcemid (KaryoMax, Gibco):10 μg/mL solution (*see* **Note 6**).
8. 0.054 M (0.4%) Potassium chloride (KCl): Dissolve 4 g of KCl (M.W. 74.55) in 1 L of distilled water (*see* **Note 7**).
9. Carnoy's fixative: Freshly prepare 3:1 (v/v) absolute methanol/glacial acetic acid (*see* **Note 8**).

3 Methods

Carry out all procedures in a Class 2 safety cabinet using the aseptic culture technique until cell harvest. Pre-warm all medium at 37 °C.

3.1 Measurement of Nucleated Cell Count and Cell Washing

1. 1–2 mL of bone marrow aspirate is collected in a preservative-free heparin bottle or in 8 mL of growth medium (*see* **Note 9**).
2. Note the volume of bone marrow.
3. Mix 50 μL of bone marrow with 450 μL of saline or culture medium. Measure nucleated cell count of the bone marrow using bench-top cell analyzer.
4. Calculate the nucleated cell in bone marrow as follows:
   white cell count in analyzer (10^6/mL) × 10 (dilution factor) × volume of bone marrow (mL).
5. Add approximate 1×10^7 total nucleated cells to each 10 mL of culture (*see* **Note 10**). Set up direct harvest, synchronized culture, and nonsynchronized culture if adequate amount of nucleated cells is available (*see* **Note 11**).

6. Take out appropriate volume of bone marrow into a sterile 15-mL centrifuge tube.
7. Wash the bone marrow with growth medium. Make up the volume to 10 mL and centrifuge at 200 × *g* for 10 min.
8. After centrifugation, remove supernatant and resuspend the cell pellet in 1 mL.
9. Proceed each tube for direct harvest (*see* Subheading 3.2), nonsynchronized culture (*see* Subheading 3.3), and synchronized culture (*see* Subheading 3.4).

3.2 Direct Harvest

1. Add 9 mL of growth medium and 50 μL of colcemid.
2. Incubate in 37 °C water bath for 45 min.
3. Proceed with cell harvest (*see* **steps 5–14** in Subheading 3.5).

3.3 Nonsynchronized Culture

1. Add 5 mL of Chang medium and 4 mL of growth medium.
2. Transfer all the contents to the culture flask.
3. Incubate in 37 °C, 5% CO_2 incubator for 1–3 days.
4. Proceed with cell harvest (*see* Subheading 3.5).

3.4 Synchronized Culture

1. Add 5 mL of Chang medium and 4 mL of growth medium.
2. Transfer all the contents to the culture flask.
3. Add 100 μL of working FdU and 100 μL of working uridine to the culture after at least 2 h incubation preferably to let the cells acclimatize the culture environment. Otherwise, these reagents can be added on the following day.
4. Incubate in 37 °C 5% CO_2 incubator overnight.
5. Add 100 μL of working thymidine in the next morning. Incubate for further 5–7 h prior harvesting.
6. Proceed with cell harvest (*see* Subheading 3.5).

3.5 Cell Harvest

1. Add 30 μL of colcemid to a 15-mL centrifuge tube (*see* **Note 12**).
2. Transfer culture to the centrifuge tube.
3. Incubate in 37 °C water bath for 30 min.
4. Pre-warm 0.4% KCl to 37 °C.
5. After incubation, centrifuge the culture at 200 × *g* for 10 min.
6. Discard supernatant and resuspend the pellet.
7. Add pre-warmed 0.4% KCl and top up to 10 mL.
8. Incubate in 37 °C water bath for 16 min.
9. After incubation, add 1 mL of Carnoy's fixative with inverted mixing (see **Note 13**).

10. Centrifuge at 200 × *g* for 10 min.
11. Discard supernatant.
12. Add 8–10 mL of Carnoy's fixative with inverted mixing and incubate for 10 min at room temperature.
13. Repeat **steps 10-11** at least twice until the suspension appears clear.
14. Store at −20 °C for subsequent slide making and banding.

4 Notes

1. Class 2 biological safety cabinet is characterized by a vertical laminar flow of air, which is filtered through a high efficient hepa filter. It can protect both the worker and specimen from microbial contamination.
2. An open culture system is used in this protocol which allows gaseous exchange between the air inside the flask and the environment within the incubator. It helps to maintain the pH of the culture media between 7.2 and 7.4 by the reaction of sodium bicarbonate in the medium and CO_2 environment of the incubator. A trough of water is needed to place on the lowest shelf of the incubator to avoid evaporation of the medium. Vented flasks with 0.2 μm membrane filter are used to allow gaseous interchange and protect from microbial contamination.
3. Dilute the marrow blood with PBS or culture medium before aspirating into the cell counter to avoid clotting of the analyzer. Alternatively, the nucleated cell count can also be achieved manually by using hemocytometer.
4. RPMI 1640 medium was originally developed to culture human leukemic cells in suspension and as a monolayer. It requires supplement with 10% fetal bovine serum (FBS) and uses a sodium bicarbonate buffer system (2.0 g/L). A 5% CO_2 incubator is used to maintain optimum pH for cell growth.
5. Chang medium BMC is intended for use in primary culture of clinical human bone marrow cells for karyotyping. It consists of RPMI medium 1640, FBS, hepes buffer, L-glutamine, giant cell tumor conditioned medium, and gentamicin sulfate (Irvine Scientific).
6. Gibco KaryoMAX colcemid solution is a 10 μg/mL *N*-desacetyl-*N*-methylocolchicine solution made up in Hanks' balanced salt solution (HBSS). It prevents spindle formation during mitosis, arresting cells in metaphase so that the chromosomes can be separated for cytogenetic studies and in vitro diagnostic procedures. The mechanism of action is similar to that of colchicine, but with lower mammalian toxicity.

7. Alternative hypotonic solutions are 0.075 M KCl, water, 0.4% sodium citrate, or dilute medium.
8. Carnoy's fixative must be freshly prepared since methanol reacts with acetic acid to form methyl acetate on prolonged standing, which may lead to improper drying and spreading of the chromosomes. They should be kept in air-tight containers to prevent water being absorbed.
9. Fresh bone marrow aspirate, preferably the first portion, should be sent to the laboratory as soon as possible at room temperature. Bone marrow aspirate in EDTA bottle is unsatisfactory specimen as EDTA is toxic to the cells that may not yield viable culture.
10. Too high nucleated cell count in the culture may lead to depletion of nutrients in the medium. Conversely, low cell count in the culture does not grow well and will result in inadequate metaphase available for chromosomal analysis.
11. Synchronized culture is the best choice for myeloid malignancies where direct method usually fails if the cell count is insufficient. In acute promyelocytic leukemia, the abnormality t(15;17)(q22;q21) is usually not present in the direct method.
12. The longer exposure and higher concentration of colcemid produce greater contraction of the chromosome.
13. This step is called pre-fix. If this step is missing, Carnoy's fixative can also be added at **step 12** in Subheading 3.5. However, a few drops of fixative need to be added first with thorough agitation of the cell pellet before adding the rest of fixative to avoid cell clumping. This may require a skillful technique.

References

1. Jaffe ES, Harris NL, Stein H, Vardiman JW (eds) (2001) World Health Organization classification of tumours. Pathology and genetics of tumours of hematopoietic and lymphoid tissues. IARC, Lyon
2. Vardiman JW, Harris NL, Brunning RD (2002) The World Health Organization (WHO) classification of the myeloid neoplasms. Blood 100(7):2292–2302
3. Bennett JM, Catovsky D, Daniel MT et al (1976) Proposals for the classification of the acute leukaemia: French-American-British. Cooperative Group. Br J Haematol 33:451–458
4. Swerdlow SH, Campo E, Harris NL et al (eds) (2008) WHO classification of tumours of hematopoietic and lymphoid tissues. IARC, Lyon
5. Arber DA, Orazi A, Hasserjian R et al (2016) The 2016 revision to the World Health Organization classification of myeloid neoplasms and acute leukemia. Blood 127(20):2391–2405
6. Grimwade D, Hills RK, Moorman AV et al (2010) Refinement of cytogenetic classification in acute myeloid leukaemia: determination of prognostic significance of rare recurring chromosomal abnormalities among 5876 younger adult patients treated in the United Kingdom Medical Research Council trials. Blood 116(3):354–365
7. Dunn B, Mouchrani P, Keagle M (eds) (2005) The cytogenetic symposia, 2nd edn. Association of Genetic Technologists, Olathe, KS
8. Dunn B, McMorrow LE (2008) Cytogenetic study guide. Foundation for Genetic Technology, Lenexa, KS
9. Hopwood VL, Gu J, Zhao M (eds) (2011) The cytogenetic technology program: A comprehensive review in clinical cytogenetics. MD Anderson Cancer Center, Houston, TX

Chapter 3

Chromosome Preparation for Acute Lymphoblastic Leukemia

Mary Shago

Abstract

The chromosome abnormalities observed in acute lymphoblastic leukemia have been demonstrated to contribute to patient management and treatment stratification. This chapter provides a basic protocol for the procurement, culture, harvest, and slide preparation of bone marrow aspirate and unstimulated peripheral blood specimens.

Key words Acute lymphoblastic leukemia, Cytogenetics, Fluorescence in situ hybridization (FISH), Cell culture, Slide preparation

1 Introduction

Acute lymphoblastic leukemia (ALL), a malignancy of precursor lymphoblasts, may be observed at any age, but is predominantly a childhood disease [1]. A B-cell lineage origin is identified in approximately 80–85 % of cases, while 15 % derive from T-cell precursors. The genetic basis of ALL is diverse; however, multiple recurrent categories of cytogenetic abnormalities have been defined [2]. Along with age, white blood cell count, and immunophenotype, cytogenetics provides a key prognostic indicator in patients presenting with ALL. The difficulty of obtaining sufficient good quality metaphase cells for analysis from the bone marrow aspirate and peripheral blood specimens of ALL patients is well known. Although genomic and molecular techniques such as microarray, reverse transcriptase-PCR (RT-PCR), and sequencing can also be valuable tools for the investigation of these samples, cytogenetic analysis provides a rapid overview of the genetics of ALL patients, and remains an integral component of the diagnostic workup.

This chapter provides a basic method for the preparation of ALL samples for cytogenetic G-banding and fluorescence in situ hybridization (FISH) analyses. Both direct preparation and 24-h

Thomas S.K. Wan (ed.), *Cancer Cytogenetics: Methods and Protocols*, Methods in Molecular Biology, vol. 1541, DOI 10.1007/978-1-4939-6703-2_3, © Springer Science+Business Media LLC 2017

culture procedures are included. Although a greater number of metaphase cells may be obtained from the cultures, the direct preparation provides a rapid source of material for FISH analysis, and the mitotic index is generally high enough to yield metaphase cells for G-banding and FISH analyses. The cellular concentration in ALL cultures is a critical factor in obtaining optimal material for analysis, and a simple method for cell count and culture setup using a hemocytometer is described. Obtaining good quality metaphase spreads for ALL cells is very challenging because of the low mitotic index and generally poor chromosome morphology. There are many different methods for slide preparation; use of the Thermotron Cytogenetic Drying Chamber for this purpose assists with the control of a number of variables that influence slide making [3]. A slide preparation protocol for sequential G-banding-to-FISH analysis is included, as FISH analysis is often used to confirm an abnormality suspected by G-banding, or to demonstrate a cryptic abnormality. Although bone marrow aspirate is always the preferred specimen for the analysis of ALL, unstimulated peripheral blood specimens may be used in place of bone marrow aspirate provided that the patient has circulating lymphoblasts in the peripheral blood.

2 Materials

2.1 Anticoagulant Used in Bone Marrow Aspiration

Sodium heparin, preservative-free, 100 USP units/mL.

2.2 Receiving Specimens in Transport Medium or Transferring Specimens to Transport Medium

1. Ready to use (RTU) medium: 500 mL of RPMI 1640, 60 mL of fetal bovine serum, 6 mL of 10,000 IU penicillin/10,000 μg/mL streptomycin, 6 mL of 100× MEM nonessential amino acid solution, and 6 mL of 200 mM L-glutamine.
2. Bone marrow transport medium: Add 0.4 mL of 1000 USP units/mL sodium heparin to 100 mL of RTU RPMI 1640 (final concentration 4 U/mL). Aliquot 5 mL into 10-mL sterile transport vials with white screw caps. Label each vial with expiry date (1 month from date of preparation). Store at 4 °C.

2.3 Setting Up Direct Preparations of Bone Marrow Aspirate Specimens

1. Tubes, 10-mL with one flattened side.
2. Tubes, 14-mL round-bottom polypropylene.
3. P1000 Micropipette and tips.
4. Timer.
5. Incubator 37 °C, 5 % CO_2.
6. Colcemid KaryoMax, 10 μg/mL ready to use (Invitrogen).
7. 1× Trypsin-EDTA (0.05 %)/0.53 mM EDTA.

8. 0.062 M KCl: Add 0.47 g of KCl to 100 mL of distilled water. Mix by swirling until dissolved.
9. MarrowMax Bone Marrow Medium (Gibco).

2.4 Setting Up 24-h Cultures of Bone Marrow Aspirate Specimens

1. Biosafety cabinet.
2. Hemocytometer (Neubauer counting chamber) and coverslips.
3. P200 and P10 Micropipettes and tips.
4. Phase contrast microscope.
5. Incubator 37 °C, 5% CO_2.
6. 2% acetic acid: Add 2 mL of glacial acetic acid into 98 mL of distilled water. Aliquot into 0.95 mL portions in polypropylene round-bottom tubes and store at 4 °C for up to 3 months.
7. Tubes – 10 mL with one flattened side.
8. MarrowMax Bone Marrow Medium (Gibco).
9. RTU RPMI 1640 (*see* Subheading 2.2).

2.5 Harvesting Direct Preparations or 24-h Cultures of Bone Marrow Aspirate Specimens

1. Biosafety cabinet.
2. Centrifuge.
3. Vacuum/Erlenmeyer flask suction.
4. Incubator 37 °C, 5% CO_2.
5. Electronic pipette filler and 10 mL sterile pipettes.
6. Carnoy's fixative: Combine three parts of methanol to one part of glacial acetic acid (v/v).
   Store at −20 °C for the direct preparation harvest and at room temperature for the 24-h culture harvest.
7. Colcemid KaryoMax, 10 μg/mL ready to use (Invitrogen).
8. 0.062 M KCl, pre-warmed to 37 °C (*see* Subheading 2.3).

2.6 Preparing Slides for G-banding Analysis or for FISH Analysis

1. Thermotron (CDS-5 Cytogenetics Drying Chamber).
2. Centrifuge.
3. Biosafety cabinet.
4. Phase contrast microscope.
5. Vacuum/Erlenmeyer flask suction.
6. Carnoy's fixative (*see* Subheading 2.5).
7. Slide racks.
8. High quality frosted microscope slides.
9. 9-in. and 6-in. glass Pasteur pipettes.
10. Lint-free tissues.
11. Rubber Pasteur pipette bulbs.

12. Diamond tipped pencil.
13. P10 micropipette and tips.

2.7 Aging of Slides and G-banding

1. Slide racks.
2. Oven (60 °C).
3. Oven (90 °C).
4. Desiccator cabinet with drierite desiccant crystals.
5. Electronic hot plate/stirrer.
6. Coplin jars.
7. Air jet.
8. 1 M NaCl stock solution: Add 58.4 g of NaCl to 1 L of distilled water.
9. 0.15 M NaCl: Add 900 mL of 1 M NaCl stock solution to 5.1 L of distilled water.
10. Pancreatin stock: Combine 2.5 g of Pancreatin and 100 mL of 0.15 M NaCl in an Erlenmeyer flask. Add small magnetic stir bar, and stir for 30 min on electronic stirrer. Transfer to two 50-mL blue-capped conical tubes. Centrifuge for 8 min at 470×*g* to pellet undissolved pancreatin. Aliquot supernatant into screw cap cryotubes and store at −20 °C.
11. 1× Hanks' balanced salt solution.
12. Pancreatin working solution: Dilute 2 mL of pancreatin stock solution into 50 mL of 1× Hanks' balanced salt solution in Coplin jar.
13. Gurr buffer tablets, pH 6.8: Dissolve 1 tablet in 1 L of distilled water.
14. Protocol Wright Giemsa/Giemsa Stain: Combine 6 mL of Protocol Wright Giemsa stain, 2.5 mL of Giemsa stain, 20 mL of distilled water, and 30 mL of Gurr buffer (pH 6.8) in a Coplin jar. Filter the Protocol Wright Giemsa and Giemsa stains using Grade 1, 125 mm filter paper as these components are added.

2.8 Preparation of Slides for Sequential G-band-to-FISH Analysis

1. Coplin jars.
2. Citrisolv (Fisher).
3. Carnoy's Fixative (*see* Subheading 2.5).
4. 100% ethanol, 80% ethanol, 70% ethanol.
5. 2× Saline-sodium citrate (SSC), pH 7.0.
6. 1× Phosphate-buffered saline (PBS), pH 7.4.
7. 1× PBS/$MgCl_2$: Combine 475 mL of 1× PBS with 25 mL of 1 M $MgCl_2$. Store at 4 °C for up to 1 week.
8. 1% Formaldehyde/1×PBS/$MgCl_2$: Add 1.35 mL of 37% formaldehyde to 50 mL of 1× PBS/$MgCl_2$. Store at 4 °C for up to 1 week.

3 Methods

3.1 Instructions for the Hematology/Oncology Team

1. To prevent clotting, coat the syringe that will be used to draw the bone marrow specimen with 0.2–0.5 mL (20–50 U) of 100 units/mL preservative-free sodium heparin.
2. The sample drawn for the cytogenetics laboratory should be the first or second draw. If samples for other tests must be drawn prior to the cytogenetics sample, relocate the needle before obtaining the sample to obtain an adequately cellular sample.
3. Obtain 2–3 mL of bone marrow aspirate.
4. Invert the syringe gently a few times to distribute the heparin into the sample.
5. If bone marrow aspirate cannot be obtained and the patient has circulating lymphoblasts, draw 5–10 mL of peripheral blood in a sodium heparin tube.
6. Keep the specimen at room temperature. Transport to the cytogenetics laboratory.

3.2 Transferring Bone Marrow Aspirate Specimens to Transport Medium

1. If it is not possible to process the specimen at the time of receipt, add up to 2 mL (maximum) of bone marrow aspirate to each bone marrow transport vial.
2. Mix the vial gently to ensure that the aspirate is diluted into the transport media and washed off the wall of the tube.
3. Store the specimen at room temperature and process the next day.

3.3 Receiving Specimens in Transport Medium

1. Centrifuge the tube at 185 × *g* for 10 min.
2. Aspirate all but ~2 mL of supernatant (without disturbing the pellet).
3. Resuspend the pellet by manual shaking and proceed to Subheading 3.4.

3.4 Setting Up Direct Preparations of Bone Marrow Aspirate Specimens

1. Label two 14-mL round-bottom tubes D1 and D2; label a 10 mL flat-side tube C1.
2. Add 20 μL of colcemid, 0.625 mL of thawed 1× trypsin–EDTA (0.05%), and 10 mL of pre-warmed 0.062 M KCl to tubes D1 and D2. Invert to mix.
3. Add 5 mL of MarrowMax Bone Marrow Medium to tube C1.
4. Gently invert the specimen syringe or tube to ensure even distribution of heparin with the bone marrow aspirate.
5. Follow the instructions below for samples of ~2 mL or more. For samples of 1.5 mL or less, *see* **Note 1**.
6. Add 20 drops (total 1 mL) of bone marrow aspirate to the C1 tube. Leave C1 tube at room temperature until ready to set up 24-h cultures (*see* Subheading 3.5).

7. Add eight drops (0.4 mL) to the D1 tube and add ten drops (0.5 mL) to the D2 tube.
8. If the reason for referral is neutropenia/pancytopenia or the patient has just finished chemotherapy, and >3 mL are available, add two to three additional drops of bone marrow aspirate into the D1 and D2 tubes.
9. Invert the tubes to mix and place in the 37 °C incubator for 25 min.
10. Proceed to Subheading 3.6.

3.5 Setting Up 24-h Bone Marrow Aspirate Cultures

The concentration of white blood cells in bone marrow aspirate specimens is variable. Superior results are obtained when culture cell concentrations are optimized (*see* **Note 2**).

1. Calculate the white blood cell (mononuclear cells) number using a hemocytometer. Invert tube C1 gently to mix. Remove 50 μL from C1 and add to 0.95 mL of 2% glacial acetic acid. Shake gently to mix. Wait approximately 1 min for the color to change from pink to brown. Place a clean coverslip on the hemocytometer slide. Remove 10 μL of the mixture with a micropipette and add into the hemocytometer side opening. Capillary action will spread sample over the surface. Use a phase contrast microscope at 100× magnification to assess cell count. Visually inspect slide to ensure that all corners have equivalent cell density. Count all the round and refractile cells in one of the large four corner squares (each large square is divided into 16 small squares). If the count is less than 10, or if the cells are distributed unevenly, count all the cells on the 4 corner squares and divide by 4 to obtain the average result (*see* **Note 3**).
2. Prepare cultures from the C1 tube of bone marrow aspirate/medium according to the guidelines in Table 1.
3. Incubate cultures overnight at 37 °C with tubes lying on the side, flat bottom down. After a minimum of 24 h of culture, proceed to Subheading 3.7. Harvesting of all bone marrow aspirates received in a day can be done 24 h after the last bone marrow aspirate received.

3.6 Harvesting Bone Marrow Aspirate Direct Preparations

1. All harvesting is done in the biosafety cabinet until the fixative stage. Fixative is added and aspirated in the fume hood.
2. After the 25 min incubation at 37 °C, centrifuge the D1 and D2 tubes at 185*g* for 8 min.
3. Aspirate the supernatant, leaving 1.0–1.5 mL of the suspension.
4. Resuspend the pellet manually by shaking vigorously, ensuring that the pellet is completely resuspended.

Table 1
Setting up 24-h bone marrow aspirate cultures according to hemocytometer cell count

Hemocytometer cell count	Action	Dilution factor
<5 cells	Use tube C1 and proceed to Subheading 3.5, **step 3**	–
5–15 cells	Set up two tubes. Invert C1 tube gently to mix cells. Use a disposable pipette to remove one half of the volume in C1 and add to another flat-sided culture tube labeled C2. Add enough MarrowMax Bone Marrow Medium to C1 and RTU-RPMI to C2 so that the final volume is 5 mL. Proceed to Subheading 3.5, **step 3**	1/2 (0.5–1.5 × 10^6 cells per mL)
15–30 cells	Set up two tubes. Remove one half of the volume in C1 and add to another flat-sided culture tube labeled C2. Add enough MarrowMax Bone Marrow Medium to C1 and RTU-RPMI to C2 so that the final volume is 10 mL. Proceed to Subheading 3.5, **step 3**	1/4 (0.75–1.25 × 10^6 cells per mL)
30–50 cells	Set up four tubes. Estimate the total volume in C1 and add one-quarter to each of three flat-sided culture tubes labeled C2, C3, C4. Add enough MarrowMax Bone Marrow Medium to C1 and RTU-RPMI to tubes C2, C3, and C4 so that the final volume is 10 mL. Proceed to Subheading 3.5, **step 3**	1/8 (0.75–1.25 × 10^6 cells per mL)
~100 cells	Invert C1 to mix and label "Original." Take a new tube and label C_{dilute}. Remove 2 mL from C1 original and place into C_{dilute}. Add 2 mL MarrowMax Bone Marrow Medium to C_{dilute}. Label 4 tubes C1-C4. Add 0.25 mL from C_{dilute} to C1, 0.50 mL to C2, 1 mL to C3, and 2 mL to C4. Add enough MarrowMax Bone Marrow Medium to C1 and RTU-RPMI to tubes C2, C3, and C4 so that the final volume is 10 mL. The original C1 and C_{dilute} can be stored at 4 °C in case additional cultures are required. Proceed to Subheading 3.5, **step 3**	1/20, 1/13, 1/10, 1/8 (1, 1.5, 2, and 2.25 × 10^6 cells per mL)
~200 cells	Invert C1 to mix and label "Original." Take a new tube and label C_{dilute}. Remove 2 mL from C1 original and place into C_{dilute}. Add 6 mL MarrowMax Bone Marrow Medium to C_{dilute}. Label five tubes C1–C5. Add 1 mL from C_{dilute} to C1, 1.5 mL to C2, 2.0 mL to C3, 2.25 to C4, and 0.5 mL to C5. Add enough MarrowMax Bone Marrow Medium to C1 and RTU-RPMI to tubes C2, C3, C4, and C5 so that the final volume is 10 mL. The original C1 and C_{dilute} can be stored at 4 °C in case additional cultures are required. Proceed to Subheading 3.5, **step 3**	1/40, 1/26, 1/20, 1/16, and 1/80 (1, 1.5, 2, 2.25 × 10^6, and 0.5 × 10^6 cells per mL)

5. Add 1 mL of cold (−20 °C) Carnoy's fixative slowly to each tube, drop by drop, with shaking between each drop, until the suspension turns brown. Prepare fixative fresh daily and store at −20 °C between uses.
6. Add 10 mL of Carnoy's fixative to each tube and invert gently to mix.

7. Place the tubes in the freezer (−20 °C) for a minimum of 1 h. Samples may be left overnight at this stage.
8. Centrifuge at 185 × *g* for 8 min.
9. For the second fixation, repeat **steps 3** (aspirate), **4** (resuspend), **6** (add fixative), and **8** (centrifuge).
10. For the third fixation, repeat **steps 3** (aspirate), **4** (resuspend), and **6** (add fixative).
11. Store tubes in the freezer (−20 °C) until slides are to be made. Slide making can proceed immediately if need be.

3.7 Harvesting 24-h Bone Marrow Aspirate Cultures

1. All harvesting is done in the biosafety cabinet until the fixative stage. Fixative is added and aspirated in the fume hood.
2. Remove 24-h culture tubes from the incubator and add 60 μL of colcemid to each tube containing 10 mL of media. If the volume is 5 mL, add 30 μL of colcemid. Mix by gently inverting tubes.
3. Place in the incubator for 30 min at 37 °C.
4. Centrifuge for 10 min at 265 × *g*.
5. Aspirate supernatant, leaving 1.0–1.5 mL of suspension in the tube.
6. Resuspend the pellet manually by shaking vigorously, ensuring that the pellet is completely resuspended.
7. Add 8 mL of pre-warmed (37 °C) 0.062 M KCl, and incubate for 16 min in the 37 °C incubator.
8. Remove tubes from the incubator and add 0.5 mL of fixative at room temperature (prefix) slowly to each tube. Gently invert to mix.
9. Centrifuge for 8 min at 185 × *g*.
10. Aspirate the supernatant, leaving 1.0–1.5 mL of suspension in the tube. Resuspend pellet.
11. Slowly add six to eight drops of room temperature Carnoy's fixative using a Pasteur pipette while gently shaking the tube by hand.
12. Add 8 mL of room temperature Carnoy's fixative.
13. Place the tubes in the freezer (−20 °C) for a minimum of 1 h.
14. Centrifuge tubes for 8 min at 185 × *g*.
15. For the second fixation, repeat **steps 10** (aspirate and resuspend), **12** (add fixative), and **14** (centrifuge).
16. For the third fixation, repeat **steps 10** (aspirate and resuspend) and **12** (add fixative).
17. Store tubes in the freezer (−20 °C) until slides are to be made.

3.8 Preparing Slides for G-banding Using the Thermotron

1. Set the Thermotron slide drying chamber to 30 °C, 45 % relative humidity, and allow to equilibrate for at least 15 min.
2. Centrifuge the tubes of fixed cells at 185 ×*g* for 8 min.
3. Carefully aspirate all but 0.5–1 mL, leaving the pellet undisturbed. The amount aspirated will depend on the size of the pellet. Resuspend fixed cell pellets by shaking the tube side to side.
4. Place fixed cell suspension tubes in a rack outside the Thermotron, and work on only one patient's direct preparations/cultures at a time within the Thermotron.
5. Place a tube of fresh room temperature fixative into the Thermotron.
6. Place clean 9-in. glass Pasteur pipettes with rubber bulbs into each direct preparation or culture tube and a 6-in. glass Pasteur pipette with rubber bulb into the tube of fresh fixative.
7. Set clean dry microscope slides flat in the Thermotron chamber. Label the slides with patient identifiers and direct preparation/culture information.
8. Add a drop of fixative to the front of the slide and wipe with a lint-free tissue.
9. Use the glass Pasteur pipette to ensure that the cells are in suspension by drawing the cell suspension up and down several times. Remove a small amount. Holding the pipette at a 30° angle and approximately 1 cm from the slide, add one drop of cell suspension slowly, placing the drop toward the labeled end of the slide. Replace Pasteur pipette in the suspension tube.
10. Allow the suspension to spread out. As the cell suspension ring starts to retract, immediately add one drop of fixative on the top of the cell suspension.
11. Once the first spot is dry, add another drop of cell suspension further down the slide.
12. Allow the suspension to spread out. As the cell suspension ring starts to retract, immediately add one drop of fixative on the top of the cell suspension.
13. Do not move the slide until completely dry.
14. Slides are evaluated under a phase microscope. It may be necessary to scan the slide to observe a metaphase cell. Chromosomes should be dark and well spread (*see* **Note 4**).
15. Make three to four slides per direct preparation/culture to begin. The total number of slides made for the case will depend upon the mitotic index and the quality of the metaphase cells obtained.
16. Age the slides according to the instructions in Subheading 3.10.

3.9 Preparing Slides for FISH Analysis Using the Thermotron

1. Centrifuge the tubes of fixed cells at 185 × *g* for 8 min. Aspirate all but 0.5–1 mL of the suspension.
2. Place fixed cell suspension tubes in a rack outside the Thermotron, and work on only one patient's direct preparations/cultures at a time within the Thermotron.
3. Place a tube of fresh room temperature fixative into the Thermotron. Insert a 6-in. glass Pasteur pipette with rubber bulb into the tube.
4. Draw a circle (about 10–12 mm in diameter) with a diamond-tipped pencil on the back of a precleaned slide (*see* **Note 5**).
5. Add a drop of fixative to the front of the slide and wipe with a lint-free tissue.
6. Resuspend the fixed cell pellet by shaking the tube side to side or by using the micropipette.
7. Add 3 μL of fixed cell suspension to the center of the circle, followed by one drop of fixative. Allow the slide to dry.
8. Evaluate the slide under the phase contrast microscope. Metaphase chromosomes should appear flat and dark, without visible cytoplasm surrounding the chromosomes. Ensure that there are an adequate number of nuclei for interphase FISH. If the slide is too concentrated, add fixative to the fixed cell suspension to dilute. If the slide is too dilute, return the slide to the Thermotron and repeat the process of adding 3 μL of fixed cell suspension followed by one drop of fixative. Allow to dry.
9. Slides with debris or streaks of cytoplasm will be improved by placing the slide on a 90° angle on top of tissues in the Thermotron and rinsing with several mL of fixative. Allow to dry and evaluate under the phase contrast microscope.
10. Label slides and proceed to Subheading 3.10.

3.10 Aging of Slides

1. If slides are to be used for G-banding, place slides in the oven overnight at 60 °C (range of 55–65 °C). Place slides in the desiccator until banding is performed.
2. FISH slides are aged for 1–3 days at room temperature (minimum of overnight). If same-day slides are required, *see* **Note 6**. For long-term storage of FISH slides, place in a slide box and store at −20 °C to keep the slides fresh.

3.11 G-Banding Using Pancreatin and Protocol Wright Giemsa/Giemsa Stain

1. Prepare the following coplin jars in sequence for staining: Jar 1: pancreatin, Jar 2: 0.15 M NaCl, Jar 3: 0.15 M NaCl, Jar 4: Protocol Wright Giemsa/Giemsa, Jar 5: distilled water, Jar 6: distilled water.
2. Place slide(s) into Jar 1 (pancreatin) for 20–30 s.
3. Dip slide(s) into Jar 2 (0.15 M NaCl) and remove.

4. Dip slide(s) into Jar 3 (0.15 M NaCl) and remove.
5. Place slide(s) into Jar 4 (Protocol Wright Giemsa/Giemsa) for 25–30 s.
6. Dip slide(s) into Jar 5 (distilled water) and remove.
7. Dip slide(s) into Jar 6 (distilled water) and remove.
8. Air dry, or use an air jet to dry the slides.
9. Check under a light microscope to assess pancreatin digestion and the darkness of the stain. If the stain is too light, lengthen the time in the Protocol Wright-Giemsa/Giemsa stain (*see* **Note 7**).
10. Proceed with microscope analysis.

3.12 Preparation of Slides for Sequential G-band-to-FISH Analysis

Sequential FISH analysis on a previously G-banded and analyzed slide is a very useful technique to confirm a chromosome rearrangement suspected by G-banding, or for the characterization of a cryptic chromosome rearrangement (*see* **Note 8**).

1. Add fresh Citrisolv to a Coplin jar in the fumehood.
2. To remove oil from the slide, place the slide in the Citrisolv and leave for 15 min.
3. Leave slide to dry in the fumehood. If necessary, repeat until the slide is clean.
4. Destain slide by placing into fixative in a Coplin jar for 30 s. Allow slide to dry.
5. Rehydrate the slide in a descending ethanol series (100, 80, and 70 %) for 2 min each. Use the air jet to gently dry the slide.
6. Place slide in 2× SSC at 37 °C for 15–20 min.
7. Post-fix the slide in 1 % formaldehyde/1× PBS/$MgCl_2$ for 15 min at room temperature to maintain chromosome morphology.
8. Wash the slide in 1× PBS for 5 min at room temperature.
9. Dehydrate slide in 70, 80, and 100 % ethanol for 2 min each.
10. Use the air jet to dry the slide and proceed to FISH analysis.

4 Notes

1. If the amount of sample is very small (<1.5 mL), prepare the C1 tube according to the instructions in Subheading 3.4, and perform the hemocytometer count (*see* Subheading 3.5) prior to setting up the direct preparation tubes. If the count is >5 cells, set up the D1 tube only and proceed with setup of the 24-h cultures. If the count is less than five cells, do not set up direct preparations. Add the remainder of the specimen to the C1 tube, redo the cell count, and set up the 24-h cultures accordingly.

2. A cell count should be determined for each bone marrow specimen. Too few cells in culture will result in suboptimal cell conditioning and poor growth, while a very high cell concentration will exhaust the culture nutrients and will impact cell growth. An overall cell density of ~1×10^6 cells/mL is recommended to optimize the quality of metaphase cell preparation. For a leukemia patient with a high white blood cell count, it is advisable to set up cultures with various cell concentrations, as it is difficult to predict which cellular concentration will yield the best mitotic index.
3. The number of cells contained in the sample is calculated using the following formula: Number of cells per mL equals cell number counted in one large square $\times 10 \times 20$ (sample dilution factor) $\times 10^3$ (hemocytometer factor that converts mm^3 to mL) [4].
4. If the metaphase cells are very tight, add the drop of fixative sooner after the drop of cell suspension. The timing of the drop of fixative depends on the tightness of the metaphase spreads. The tighter the metaphase spread, the earlier the drop of fixative is to be added. In addition, the height from which the suspension is dropped can be increased to try to improve spreading of tight metaphase cells.
5. The fixed cell suspension may be resuspended and transferred to an Eppendorf tube for centrifugation in a microfuge if further concentration of the cells is required. For FISH analysis, the goal is to have plenty of interphase and metaphase cells to score on a small, predefined area of the slide. The laboratory may mark the slides, or may use slides with pre-drawn circles for FISH. This will minimize the amount of probe required to cover the target area. If the slide is too dilute, return the slide to the Thermotron and repeat the process of adding 3 μL of fixed cell suspension followed by one drop of fixative. Allow to dry. This may be repeated a number of times if necessary.
6. Slides for G-banding may be rapidly aged for 90 min at 90 °C (range of 85–95 °C); however, it is more difficult to obtain consistent sequential FISH results from rapidly aged slides. If FISH setup is required the same day as slide-making, age slides in the oven at 60 °C (range of 55–65 °C) for 10–20 min.
7. The time in pancreatin will depend on the specimen, and on how slides were made. Test one slide and assess before proceeding with several slides from the same specimen. Under-digested chromosomes have indistinct bands with little contrast. They are usually fuzzy in appearance. Over-digested chromosomes have sharp bands and often appear frazzled at the ends, with extreme contrast between landmark bands and very pale chromosome ends. Extremely over-digested chromosomes are very pale after staining and may appear ghost-like

and swollen. Appropriately stained chromosomes are neither too dark nor too pale to analyze at the microscope. There should be a fair amount of contrast with a wide range of gray values. Judging slides takes practice, time, and experience. Adjust pancreatin times by at least 5 s increments.

8. Aging slides at a lower temperature prior to G-banding (60 °C overnight) is necessary for reliable sequential G-banding-to-FISH analysis. The technologist may mark the area of the slide where the cells of interest were found to minimize the area where FISH probe is to be applied. The procedure is superior on slides with under-digested chromosomes. Over-digested metaphase cells may not hybridize well with FISH probes. The slide must be clean with all traces of oil removed for the subsequent denaturation/hybridization to be successful.

Acknowledgments

I would like to thank all the members of the Hospital for Sick Children Cytogenetics Laboratory for their assistance and advice on the preparation of this chapter, especially Natacha Mosler, Daniel Antinucci, Xiaoyan Wu, Wendy Cockett, Sophie Zhao, Assya Pavlova, and Jennifer Brown.

References

1. Swerdlow SH, Campo E, Harris NL et al (eds) (2008) WHO classification of tumours of haematopoietic and lymphoid tissues. IARC, Lyon
2. Harrison CJ (2009) Cytogenetics of paediatric and adolescent acute lymphoblastic leukaemia. Br J Haematol 144(2):147–156
3. Spurbeck JL, Zinsmeister AR, Meyer KJ et al (1996) Dynamics of chromosome spreading. Am J Med Genet 61(4):387–393
4. Barsh MJ, Knutsen T, Spurbeck JL (eds) (1991) The AGT cytogenetics laboratory manual, 3rd edn. Lippencot-Raven, Philadelphia

Chapter 4

Chromosome Preparation for Chronic Lymphoid Malignancies

Dorota Koczkodaj and Agata A. Filip

Abstract

Conventional cytogenetics is invariably one of the most important methods used in diagnostics of chronic lymphoproliferations. It complements fluorescence in situ hybridization (FISH) and molecular analysis. Presence of particular chromosomal alterations in chronic lymphocytic leukemia enables patients' stratification into appropriate cytogenetic risk groups and influences treatment decisions. In other non-Hodgkin lymphomas cytogenetic analyses are employed also in minimal residual disease assessment.

As lymphocytes in chronic lymphoid malignancies are characterized by low proliferation rate in vitro, it is critical to induce their division in the culture properly. Here, we describe methods of lymphocyte isolation from patient's samples, conditions of cell culture, and the most commonly used mitogens for B- and T-lymphocytes in hemato-oncologic analyses.

Key words Non-Hodgkin lymphomas, Cell cultures, Mitogens for B- and T-lymphocytes, Harvesting techniques

1 Introduction

Chronic lymphocytic leukemia (CLL) and other non-Hodgkin lymphomas affect primarily older patients. They are defined as heterogeneous group of malignancies of lymphatic system consisting of many different conditions, and they may be classified by their aggressiveness or the origin of the leukemic lymphocytes. Recent World Health Organization (WHO) classification of tumors of hematopoietic and lymphoid tissues groups lymphomas not only by cell type, but also defining phenotypic, molecular, or cytogenetic characteristics [1].

Chromosome aberrations are the independent prognostic factors, which allow stratifying CLL patients with respect to clinical course, time to first treatment (TTT), and overall survival (OS). Standard methods utilized for the detection of genomic chromosome alterations involve conventional cytogenetics, i.e., chromosome banding analysis (CBA) and fluorescence in situ hybridization

Thomas S.K. Wan (ed.), *Cancer Cytogenetics: Methods and Protocols*, Methods in Molecular Biology, vol. 1541,
DOI 10.1007/978-1-4939-6703-2_4, © Springer Science+Business Media LLC 2017

(FISH). CBA identify chromosomal aneuploidies, deletions, additions, as well as translocations and complex karyotypes (≥3 alterations). Routine classical cytogenetics techniques are often ineffective in CLL patients, because of low proliferative activity of CLL lymphocytes in vitro, even in cultures supplemented with specific B-cell mitogens [2, 3]. Metaphase spreads are frequently of poor quality, or the dividing cells are found to be normal T-lymphocytes [4]. Hence, this is necessary to apply mitogen cocktails for B-lymphocytes that would increase the mitotic index both in CLL and in other B-cell lymphoma cases. One of the most effective duets developed so far is Interleukin 2 (IL-2)/CpG-oligonucleotides DSP30 (CPG-ODN DSP30) combo. The effect of CpG-ODN DSP30 is based on their similarity to bacterial DNA and their immunostimulatory properties. Together with IL-2 they were shown to induce proliferation of B-CLL lymphocytes and, noteworthy, this phenomenon was not so evident in normal B-lymphocytes [5]. In turn, cytogenetics in T-cell lymphoma will require mitogens specific for T-lymphocytes.

Many laboratories prepare their own procedures of cell culture and composition of mitogen cocktails. In this chapter, we present standards of cell culture and chromosome analyses employed in diagnostics of NHL patients.

2 Materials

2.1 Culture Medium

The composition of culture medium depends on the type of malignant cells and the purpose of the culture. For CBA it is important to remember appropriate mitogens.

1. Transport medium: Mix 100 mL of Eagle's minimal essential medium (EMEM), 1 mL of antibiotics (100 U/mL penicillin and 50 μg/mL streptomycin), and 2500 IU heparin (*see* **Note 1**). The volume of transport medium for standard sample of bone marrow and lymph node/tumor section is 5 mL.
2. Culture medium for CLL cells: Mix 84 mL of RPMI 1640 containing 2 mM L-Glutamine and 10 mM HEPES, 15 mL of heat inactivated fetal calf serum (FCS) or fetal bovine serum (FBS), and 1 mL of antibiotics (100 U/mL penicillin and 50 μg/mL streptomycin). An appropriate volume of mitogens should be added when setting up cultures for CLL cells (see Subheading 2.2.1). Routinely used combination of mitogens for CLL cells includes: (a) mixture of 2 μM/L CpG-ODN DSP30 and 0.04 μg/mL IL-2 (*see* Subheading 2.2.1) [6, 7], and (b) enriched mitogen cocktail involves Pokeweed mitogen (PWM), 12-0-tetradecanoylphorbol (TPA), Calcium Ionophore, and CPG-ODN DSP30 (*see* Subheading 2.2.1) [8]. Standard mitogens used for constitutional karyotyping,

like Phytohemagglutinin (PHA), are not recommended, as they induce division of T-lymphocytes. For ready to use medium storage, *see* **Note 2**.

3. Culture medium for lymphoma cells: Mix 84 mL of Eagle's minimal essential medium (EMEM), 15 mL of heat inactivated fetal calf serum (FCS) or fetal bovine serum (FBS), and 1 mL of antibiotics (100 U/mL penicillin and 50 μg/mL streptomycin). An appropriate volume of mitogens should be added when setting up cultures for lymphoma cells (*see* Subheading 2.2.1). For ready to use medium storage, *see* **Note 2**.

2.2 Cell Culture Mitogens

2.2.1 CLL Lymphocyte Mitogens Preparation

1. IL-2: Dissolve 50 μg of IL-2 in 1 mL of sterile water (50 ng/μL) as a stock solution. Use 8 μL IL-2 stock solution for 10 mL of cell culture medium (final concentration 0.04 μg/mL).
2. CpG-ODN DSP30 (with DNA sequence: TCGTCGCTGTCTCCGCTTCTTCTTGCC): Dissolve 20 μM lyophilized CpG-ODN DSP30 in 25 mL of sterile distilled water as *stock 1*. Take out 1 μL of stock 1 and add 99 μL of water as *stock 2*. Then, take out 1 μL of stock 2 and add 99 μL of water as *stock 3*. Finally, use 1 μL of stock 3 for 10 mL of culture medium (final concentration of 2 μmol/L).
3. Calcium Ionophore (4-bromo-calcium ionophore): Dissolve 1 mg of calcium ionophore in 1 mL of ethanol as a stock solution. Use 1 μL of stock solution for 10 mL of culture medium (final concentration 7.5×10^{-7} M).
4. PWM: Dissolve 5 mg of PWM in 5 mL of PBS as stock solution. Use 25 μL of this solution for 10 mL of culture medium (final concentration 2.5 μg/mL).
5. TPA: Dissolve 10 μg of TPA (12-0-tetradecanoylphorbol) in 1 mL of sterile water as a stock solution. Use 10 μL of this solution for 10 mL of culture medium (final concentration 10 ng/mL).

2.2.2 Lymphoma Cell Mitogens Preparation

Depending on the initial diagnosis, for lymphoma cell cultures the appropriate mitogens for B-lymphocytes or for T-lymphocytes are used.

1. For B-lymphocytes
   TPA (12-O-tetradecanoylphorbol 13-acetate): Use 10 μL of stock solution for 10 mL of culture medium (final concentration 10 ng/mL).
2. For T-lymphocytes
   PHA (Phytohemagglutinin): Use 100 μL of stock solution for 10 mL of culture medium (final concentration of 1–2%, v/v).

2.3 Harvesting

1. 0.075 M KCl hypotonic solution: Dissolve 2.8 g of KCl in 500 mL of distilled water. Keep warmed at 37 °C for use.
2. Carnoy's fixative (methanol/glacial acetic acid, 3:1 v/v): Mix 300 mL of methanol with 100 mL of glacial acetic acid. Store at −20 °C.

3 Methods

3.1 Sample Collection and Storage

Metaphases of malignant cells may be obtained from different types of affected tissues including: peripheral blood, bone marrow, lymph node biopsy sample collected during fine needle aspiration, lymph node/tumor section, and pleural/peritoneal effusion. Samples should be collected before chemotherapy (or after the break during the course of treatment). The time and conditions of shipping the sample to the laboratory are crucial, which may affect cell viability and their proliferative activity. Samples should not be frozen or stored at 4 °C more than 24 h.

Peripheral blood (4–10 mL), bone marrow (1–2 mL), or pleural/peritoneal effusion is collected to Lithium heparinized tubes. Bone marrow can also be transferred to a sterile tube containing 5 mL of transport medium with heparin. Biopsy samples and lymph node sections (0.5 cm × 0.5 cm) have to be placed in transport medium with heparin (5 mL), in sterile conditions.

3.2 Cell Preparation for Cultures

Cell preparation and cell cultures have to be handled in sterile conditions, using laminar flow cabinet and separate room for cell culture.

3.2.1 Peripheral Blood

Lymphocytes concentrated by gravity blood sedimentation or lymphocytes isolated by density gradient centrifugation may be used for culture.

1. Gravity sedimentation.
   Leukocytes can be separated by gravity blood sedimentation. After standing for 40–80 min at room temperature or 37 °C (the tube has to be held vertically), leukocytes remain in the plasma above the red cell pellet. For the volume of 10 mL of culture medium in culture flask, 0.3–0.5 mL of leukocyte-rich plasma should be added.
2. Isolation of leukocytes by centrifugation (buffy layer culture).
   (a) In the centrifuge tube carefully apply two volumes of whole blood diluted 1:1 with PBS to one volume of separation medium (i.e., Ficoll hypaque or Lymphoprep) to retain the boundary between phases.
   (b) Spin at room temperature, 800 × *g* for 25 min.

(c) The mononuclear cells (mostly leukocytes and platelets) will settle as the pale layer below the plasma supernatant, on the top of erythrocytes.

(d) Carefully collect this layer with sterile pipette or wide bore syringe.

(e) Wash three times with RPMI 1640 medium supplemented with antibiotics (100 U/mL penicillin and 50 μg/mL streptomycin).

(f) Count the cells using hemocytometer (e.g., Bürker or Thom hemocytometer) (*see* **Note 3**). Cell concentration in the culture medium should range $1\text{–}2 \times 10^6$ cells/mL.

3.2.2 Bone Marrow

The sample of 2 mL may be divided into two to three culture flasks in 10 mL of culture medium each.

3.2.3 Lymph Node Biopsy Sample

Depending on the density, the sample in 5 mL of transport medium may be divided into two to three culture flasks in 5 mL of culture medium each.

3.2.4 Lymph Node/Tumor Section

1. Section of 0.5 cm × 0.5 cm should be fragmented mechanistically into small particles (sterile scissors may be used).
2. The sample may then be divided into two to three culture flasks in 10 mL of culture medium each.

3.2.5 Pleural/Peritoneal Effusion

1. Centrifuge the sample at room temperature, 350 × *g* for 7 min.
2. Resuspend in 2 mL of culture medium and depending on the size of the pellet divide into two to three culture flasks in 5 mL of culture medium each.

3.3 Duration of Culture

The duration of culture depends on the type of cells and the purpose of the culture. In general, use 1 h for lymphomas and 24 h for CLL cultures for FISH analysis. For conventional karyotyping, lymphoma cells are cultured for 24–72 h, and CLL cells for 3–5 days. All cultures should be incubated in 37 °C humidified incubators with 5 % CO_2.

3.4 Cell Harvesting

To obtain a sufficient number of metaphases for analysis, it is recommended to use mitotic spindle inhibitor, like colchicine or its analog colcemid, which blocks the dividing cells between metaphase and anaphase. It is added before cell harvesting for 1–1.5 h. In general, the time of incubation with colcemid is proportional to the mitotic index, but prolonged incubation results in chromosome shortening.

3.4.1 Incubation with Mitotic Spindle Inhibitor

1. After appropriate time (*see* Subheading 3.3), add 100 μL of colcemid for 10 mL of culture (final concentration 0.1 μg/mL), mix gently, and incubate at 37 °C for 1–1.5 h (*see* **Note 4**).

2. Transfer the culture to centrifuge tube and spin at room temperature, 300 × *g* for 10 min.
3. Decant the supernatant and leaving 1 mL of medium above the cell pellet.
4. Mix gently to resuspend the cells.

3.4.2 Hypotonic Treatment and Fixation

Hypotonic pretreatment swells the cells and helps to degrade erythrocytes.

1. Using vortex add slowly (drop by drop) 10 mL of warm (37 °C) 0.075 M KCl solution to the cell suspension.
2. Incubate at 37 °C for 20 min for CLL cells and 30 min for lymphoma cells.
3. Spin the cells at room temperature, 300 × *g* for 10 min.
4. Discard the supernatant.
5. Using vortex slowly (drop by drop) add 10 mL of cold (−20 °C) Carnoy's fixative (methanol/glacial acetic acid, 3:1, v/v).
6. Spin the cells at room temperature, 300 × *g* for 10 min.
7. Discard the supernatant.
8. Add 10 mL of cold (−20 °C) Carnoy's fixative.
9. Spin the cells at room temperature, 300 × *g* for 10 min. Repeat **steps** 7 and **8** for two times.
10. After the last centrifugation, discard the supernatant and add small amount of fixative (1–2 mL, depending on the density of cells) and mix gently. Cell suspension should be opaque. It is now ready for dripping onto the slides.
11. Unused cell suspension in fixative may eventually be stored at −20 °C in a capped tube for further analysis.

3.5 Slide Preparation

Cell suspension should be dropped (one to two drops) using pipette on degreased microscopic slides, which may be purchased from the manufacturers or specifically pretreated (*see* **Note 5**).

Slide should be checked with the microscope with respect to density of cell layer, add more fixative if the cells are too dense (Fig. 1). Let the slides air-dry.

3.6 Chromosome Staining

There are two most common banding techniques utilized in chromosome analysis in hemato-oncology, that is G- and R-banding (*see* Chap. 6)

4 Notes

1. Lithium or sodium heparin is the anti-coagulant of choice. Commercial heparin tubes to sample blood contain 25 IU/

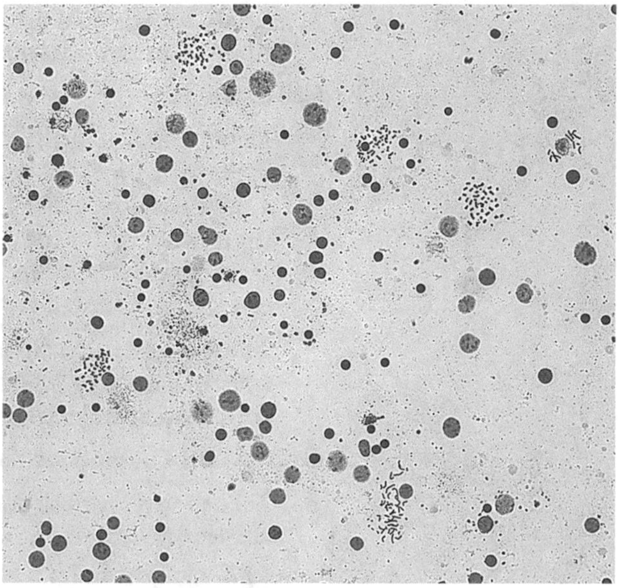

Fig. 1 The expected density of cell layer (magnification 125×)

mL unfractionated heparin. 1 mg of unfractionated heparin is equal to 100 IU. Powdered heparin may be dissolved in PBS or EMEM.

2. Medium supplemented with FBS/FCS may be stored for longer periods of time at −20 °C and warmed up to 37 °C before use. Mitogens should be added when setting up cultures.
3. Counting the cells using the hemocytometer:
   Clean hemocytometer and coverslip with alcohol before use. Moisten the coverslip with water and affix to the hemocytometer. The presence of Newton's refraction rings under the coverslip indicates proper adhesion.

   (a) Preparing cell suspension:

   - Gently mix the cell suspension to ensure the cells are evenly distributed.
   - Take out 0.5 mL of cell suspension using a 5-mL sterile pipette and place in an Eppendorf tube.
   - Take 100 μL of cells into a new Eppendorf tube and add 400 μL of 0.4% trypan blue (final concentration 0.08%). Mix gently.
   - Using a pipette, take 100 μL of trypan blue-treated cell suspension and apply to the hemocytometer. Very gently fill both chambers and allow the cell suspension to be completely drawn out by capillary action.

- Using a brightfield microscope, focus on the grid lines of the hemocytometer with a 10× objective.

(b) Cell counting:

- Count the live, unstained cells (live cells do not take up trypan blue) in one set of 16 squares (Fig. 2). Count only the cells placed within a square or on the right-hand or bottom boundary line. Following the same guidelines, dead cells stained with trypan blue can also be counted for a viability estimate if required.
- Move the hemocytometer to the next set of 16 corner squares and carry on counting until all four sets of 16 corner squares are counted.

(c) Calculation of number of viable cells per mL:

- Take the average cell count from each of the sets of 16 corner squares.
- Multiply by 10,000.
- Multiply by five to correct for the 1:5 dilution from the trypan blue addition.

  The final value is the number of viable cells/mL in the original cell suspension.

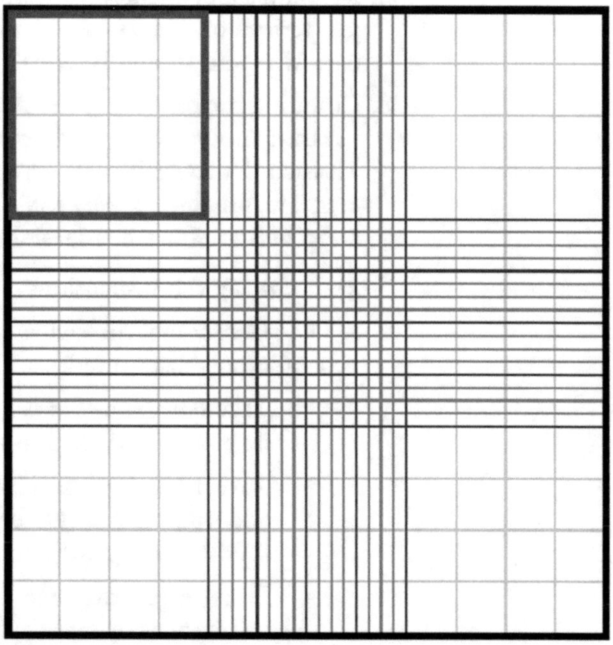

Fig. 2 Bürker hemocytometer grid diagram indicating one of the sets of 16 squares that should be used for counting (in *red*)

4. It is also possible to use ten times lower final concentration of colcemid (i.e., 0.01 μg/mL) for 24 h before harvesting.
5. Pretreatment of slides may involve soaking in detergent solution, alcohol, chromic acid, or ether to remove traces of grease, use of frosted slides (stored in the fridge), or use of wet slides (soaked in water).

References

1. Campo E, Swerdlow SH, Harris NL et al (2011) The 2008 WHO classification of lymphoid neoplasms and beyond: evolving concepts and practical applications. Blood 117:5019–5032. doi:10.1182/blood-2011-01-293050
2. Morgan R, Chen Z, Richkind K et al (1999) PHA/IL2: an efficient mitogen cocktail for cytogenetic studies of non-Hodgkin lymphoma and chronic lymphocytic leukemia. Cancer Genet Cytogenet 109:134–137
3. Gahrton G, Robert KH, Friberg K et al (1980) Nonrandom chromosomal aberrations in chronic lymphocytic leukemia revealed by polyclonal B-cell-mitogen stimulation. Blood 56:640–647
4. Decker T, Schneller F, Hipp S et al (2002) Cell cycle progression of chronic lymphocytic leukemia cells is controlled by cyclin D2, cyclinD3, cyclin-dependent kinase (cdk) 4 and the cdk inhibitor p27. Leukemia 16:327–334
5. Decker T, Schneller F, Kronschnabl M et al (2000) Immunostimulatory CpG-oligonucleotides induce functional high affinity IL-2 receptors on B-CLL cells: costimulation with IL-2 results in a highly immunogenic phenotype. Exp Hematol 28:558–568
6. Dicker F, Schnittger S, Haferlach T et al (2006) Immunostimulatory oligonucleotide-induced metaphase cytogenetics detect chromosomal aberrations in 80% of CLL patients; a study of 132 CLL cases with correlation to FISH, IgV_H status, and CD38 expression. Blood 108:3152–3160
7. Shi M, Cipollini MJ, Crowley-Bish PA et al (2013) Improved detection rate of cytogenetic abnormalities in chronic lymphocytic leukemia and other mature B-cell neoplasms with use CpG-oligonucleotide DSP30 and interleukin 2 stimulation. Am J Clin Pathol 139:662–669
8. Koczkodaj D, Popek S, Zmorzyński SZ et al (2016) Detection of chromosomal changes in chronic lymphocytic leukemia using classical cytogenetic methods and FISH: application of rich mitogen mixture for lymphocyte cultures. J Investig Med 64:894–898. doi:10.1136/jim-2015-000050

Chapter 5

Cytogenetic Harvesting of Cancer Cells and Cell Lines

Roderick A.F. MacLeod, Maren E. Kaufmann, and Hans G. Drexler

Abstract

We describe an evidence-based approach toward optimizing chromosome preparation from cancer cells and cell lines. The procedures described here emphasize the utility of both cell culture—to maximize the yields of the dividing cells needed to harvest mitotic metaphase chromosome preparations and how an empirical evaluation of hypotonic treatments enables optimal conditions to be efficiently determined.

Key words Cancer chromosomes, Cell culture, Hypotonic treatment, Fixation, Slide making

1 Introduction

1.1 Background

Despite their uncontrolled proliferation and numerous dividing cells, cancer cells nevertheless often yield chromosome preparations inferior to those from benign tissue, a discrepancy seldom encountered by molecular biological approaches for which cell cycle stage is largely immaterial. As well as cell cycle dependence, the legion variety of cell types encountered in cancer—each clone being effectively unique—defeats a "one size fits all" approach. Thus, cytogenetic harvesting of cancer cells should be tailored to the individual needs of each intractable cell or cell type.

Thanks to the advent of fluorescence in situ hybridization (FISH), cytogenetics now bridges the gap between classical and pure molecular biological methodologies. It is now apparent that in addition to point mutations, a major force in carcinogenesis is the production of molecular gene alterations by chromosome rearrangements, which if recurrent, may be used diagnostically. Accordingly, a standard work on the cytogenetics of human cancer [1] has been published to cover the field, in which the fourth edition to date requires 27 authors when compared to merely 2 in the second edition. As well as in hematopoietic cancers, recurrent chromosome changes have now been described in solid tumors enabling target gene identification. Hence, rarer and poorly characterized tumors lacking known cytogenetic involvement have

Thomas S.K. Wan (ed.), *Cancer Cytogenetics: Methods and Protocols*, Methods in Molecular Biology, vol. 1541,
DOI 10.1007/978-1-4939-6703-2_5, © Springer Science+Business Media LLC 2017

acquired heightened research interest to those seeking novel cancer mechanisms. Intractable tumors may be particularly challenging to harvest, or bear the most subtle cytogenetic changes where chromosome quality is at a premium. Cancer cytogenetics helps interpretation of genomic array data by providing a window onto individual cells and intercellular heterogeneity [2].

A basic cytogenetic requirement is the provision of dividing cells which must be arrested at mitosis when individual chromosomes and their structure become microscopically visible enabling cancer chromosome rearrangements to be discerned. We are now able to tackle these complexities thanks to FISH-based methodologies which, in turn, demand chromosome preparations of the best quality possible. Clinical cytogenetic protocols rarely allow the empirical optimization of cell harvest conditions since repeat diagnostic samples are seldom available. These exigencies may in some cases be obviated by recourse to cell culture which enables cell numbers to be expanded. Cancer cell lines offer infinite replication and repetition by providing unlimited material, allowing analyses of a scope and depth that usually denied to those working with primary cancer cells.

Our experience has taught us that cell harvest conditions, especially choice of hypotonic treatments, are the most critical to success with intractable cell types. Hence, a little effort invested in optimizing these conditions to individual cultures is well worth the effort.

1.2 Harvesting Aims

The complex chromosomal rearrangements of cancer cells often present a challenge to cytogenetic analyses and require multiple rounds of FISH to achieve meaningful results. Such approaches are greatly facilitated by cryopreservation, of metaphase cell suspensions at −20 °C, microscope slides bearing such metaphases at −80 °C, and living cells themselves in liquid nitrogen at −196 °C. Microscope slides bearing metaphase-enriched cell suspensions are the bread and butter of cytogenetics and their assessment underlies any scheme for evidence-based hypotonic optimization. Hence, mitotic metaphase chromosomes must be analyzed rationally. Consequently, three key criteria that are likely to impact on subsequent analyses are metaphase quantity, chromosome spreading, and chromosome morphology.

1. Metaphase quantity (*see* Fig. 1a, b): To enrich metaphase numbers growing cultures are treated with colcemid: its key activity—microtubule depolymerisation—inhibits formation of mitotic spindles leading to metaphase arrest. Colcemid is toxic limiting the degree of effective exposure. Other agents have been proposed, e.g. vinblastine or colchicine, but they have proved to be more expensive or even more toxic.

   To quantify mitotic sufficiency (on a scale of A to C), as a rule of thumb, low power (100×) fields should carry on average

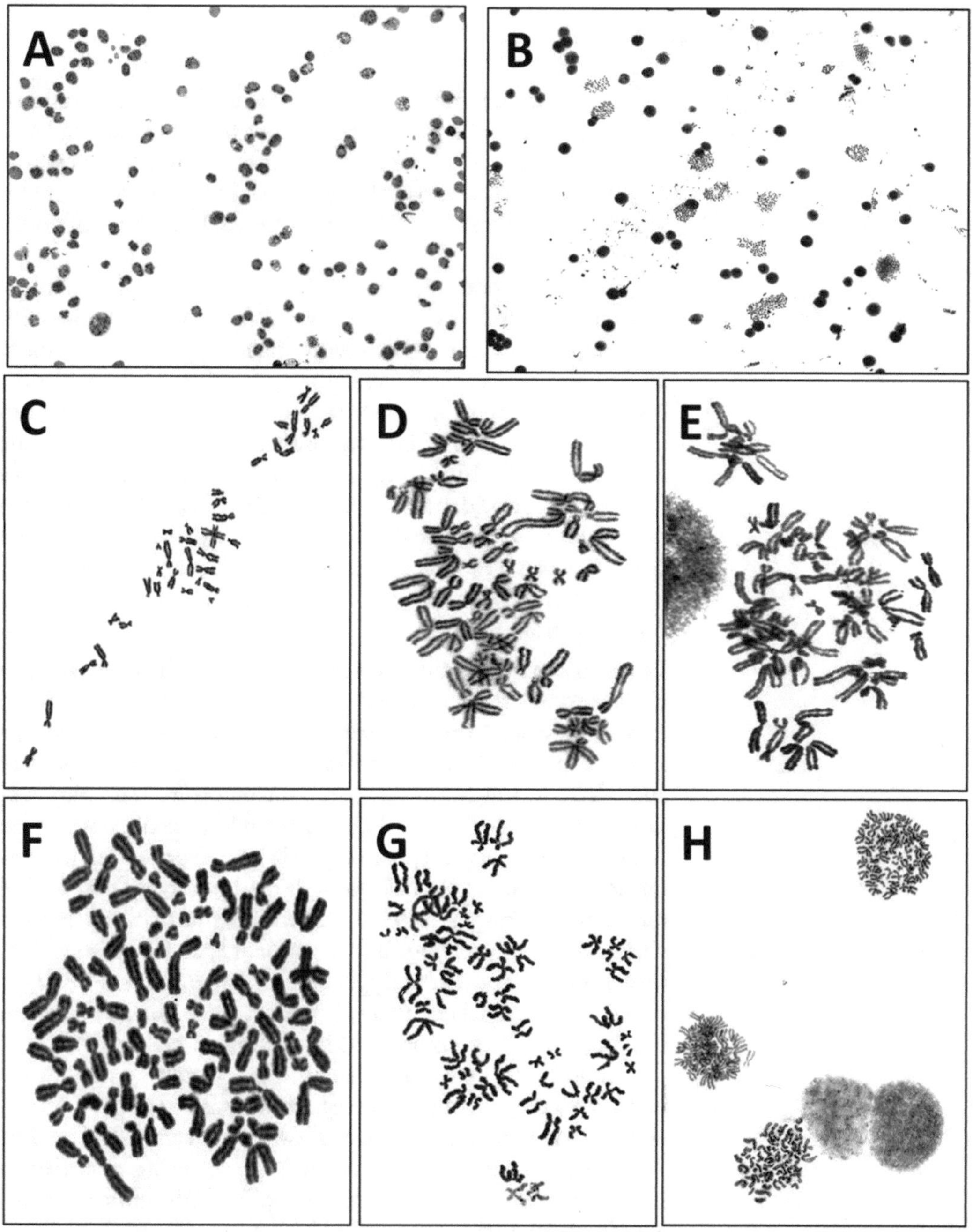

Fig. 1 Impact of harvesting conditions on harvesting mitotic metaphase chromosomes for cytogenetic analysis. (**a, b**) Images show how severe hypotonic treatments can deplete harvests of mitotic cells which easily might be misinterpreted as "low mitotic index." While cells shown in (**a**) were subjected to "standard" hypotonic treatment (0.075 M KCl for 7 min) which effectively burst mitoses, those shown in (**b**) received a milder treatment (1:1 = 0.075 M KCl + 0.9 % sodium citrate, 1 min). **(c–e)** The metaphase images show different levels of spreading without great impact on chromosome quality. Image (**c**) is clearly broken due to overlong hypotonic exposure with concomitant chromosome loss. That in (**e**) shows excessive crossovers hampering analysis, while that in (**d**) allows chromosomes to be easily seen without undue risk of chromosome loss. **(f–h)** Images illustrate chromosome quality. While in (**f**) chromosomes are adequately spread and chromatids lie in parallel. The *solid* in appearance of chromosomes in (**f**) is likely to yield good G-banding and FISH, while those in (**g**) and (**h**) are substandard. The arms of those in image (**g**) lie akimbo, a configuration inimical to subsequent G-banding or FISH. In (**h**) spreading and morphology are clearly substandard, the chromosomes too small and overlaid for analysis. Counterintuitively perhaps, the poor chromosomes in (**h**) were produced after an overly harsh hypotonic treatment

at least one usable metaphase to be deemed "A"; one per horizontal row scores a "B"; while fewer than that gets a "C." "AB" or better is necessary for G-banding, while "B" is necessary for chromosome painting and "A" for the most challenging FISH-based methods, if only to justify the additional outlay involved.

In our experience, counterintuitively perhaps, the most common ground for mitotic insufficiency is not lackadaisical proliferation, rather an overly harsh hypotonic treatment which increases the cell breakage and yields a "chromosome soup." Hence, the appropriate responses to lack of metaphases should include the following measures: (a) increasing the amount of "soft" buffer (e.g., sodium citrate) at the expense of "harsh" KCl, avoidance of warm incubation at 37 °C, or even performing this step on ice; (b) reducing incubation times down to even a few seconds; and (c) reducing the amount of hypotonic used in relation to residual medium remaining after centrifugation.

2. Chromosome spreading (*see* Fig. 1c, e): To facilitate analysis chromosomes must ideally lie grouped together and evidence mitotic integrity: broken cells which have lost chromosomes serve to confuse analysis and may yield false ascertainment of aneuploidies. On the other hand, chromosomal superimposition—"crossovers"—should be avoided lest detail be sacrificed thereby. To improve spreading cells are exposed to what is termed "hypotonic shock", though the underlying biophysical mechanisms linking it to chromosome morphology remain elusive [3]. After hypotonic treatment, nuclei release their chromosomal contents. Hypotonic treatments must be finely tuned to individual cell types, however, since excessive nuclear breakage may be accompanied by chromosome losses.

   Importantly, we have found that matching hypotonic treatments to individual cell requirements is the single controllable factor which contributes most to chromosome quality. This requires testing replicate cell cultures using a variety of hypotonic treatments to determine optimal conditions, repeating if necessary until successful [4].

   In addition to hypotonic tuning, chromosome spreading may be controlled by local humidity and viscosity encountered by fixed cells when they hit the target microscope slide. Hence, slides should be cleaned by washing in diluted HCl, followed by ethanol and polishing using a lint-free cloth. Precleaned slides are then kept at −20 °C until immediately before use, their thin frost layers turning rapidly to moisture which encourages spreading. Paradoxically, overly spread metaphases and those remaining tight may both, again, be caused by overly harsh hypotonic treatments. In extreme cases, so much inherently sticky DNA is released that metaphases are effectively cocooned by it. The same considerations and remedial measures are applied again as described in the preceding section.

3. Chromosome quality (*see* Fig. 1f–h): The third basic criterion described here is best defined pictorially. Although the term "quality" is subjective, "good chromosome quality" is seldom in doubt. Ideally, chromosomes should appear dense under phase contrast or after solid staining, but never retractile with troublesome halos. Arms should lie straight in parallel, never akimbo, as this impairs band formation and is associated with "fluffiness" inimical to banding resolution.

   There is little doubt that cancer chromosome quality fails to match normal cells, whether lymphocytes, keratinocytes, or amniocytes. This shortcoming is often blamed on the altered chromatin states involved in gene dysregulation present in cancer. Alternatively, the immature cell types giving rise to various cancers may be unsuited to standard hypotonic treatments. Poor chromosome quality may be due to the use of suboptimal media or fetal bovine serum (FBS) supplements in certain cases (*see* **Note 1**).

1.3 Cells and Culture

Cells may be harvested directly from tumor biopsies or after culture. In the case of continuous cell lines, cultures are long-term and the number of population cell doublings is seldom—if indeed ever—known with any precision. Clonal heterogeneity which is a key characteristic of cancer cell populations may be lost during passage, but a recent study showing long-term subclonal stability suggests that this fear may be overstated [5]. In the case of primary cancer cells, short-term cultures (usually <72 h) may be used to expand the mitotic cell fraction. If cancer samples also contain normal stroma tissue, the risk of its inadvertent analysis at the expense of the neoplastic moiety demands special consideration, e.g., via cytogenetic data, though this is obviously uninformative when poor quality hampers detection.

1. Primary cancer cells: These may grow in suspension like most hematopoietic cancers, or only when attached to plastic or glass substrates like epithelial tumors. Suspension cells are easier to handle and maintain because they may be processed directly while adherent cells must be detached, either mechanically, e.g., using a scraper, enzymatically using trypsin, or by some other proteolytic enzyme or combination thereof. Some cells grow semi-adherently and may be detached simply by vigorous shaking. Mitotic metaphases used for karyotyping are the most loosely attached cell types in adherent cultures and may also be dislodged mechanically at high yields. A few more demanding hematopoietic cell types are best cultivated on semisolid agar which must be removed by washing prior to harvest.

Nevertheless, some primary cancers are more difficult than others to harvest successfully, e.g., breast, neuroblastoma, and prostate cancers; while among hematopoietic tumors, Hodgkin lymphoma cells have proved conspicuously intractable due to their relative paucity and difficulty of separation from reactive T-cells. Accordingly, much of what we know about the cytogenetics of several such intractable cancers is based on continuous cell lines. Hence, those failing to accomplish successful harvesting should consult the primary literature for tips or tricks needed for certain cell types.

2. Cancer cell lines: A guesstimated approximate 10^4 human cancer cell lines have been established to date. As only a tiny minority have been analyzed in any detail, untold cell lines await extended cytogenetic investigation to reveal their hidden charms. Data thus acquired are cumulative when rendered accessible via publication and may be used as portals for hunting new cancer genes, developing new targeted therapies, and performing in vitro functional assays in cells bearing the selfsame changes, a unique advantage of cell lines over primary cancers.

   However, a word of caution is necessary concerning cell provenance. A significant proportion of cell lines in circulation has been misidentified, either by cross-contamination at the hands of would-be "originators" [6], or downstream by careless recipients [7]. Tyros should be wary of cell lines obtained from other than their originators or reputable cell repositories, since misidentification remains a chronic problem. A tool has been developed [8] for checking cell line identity via STR-DNA profiling (www.dsmz.de). Moreover, under the auspices of the International Cell Line Authentication Committee (ICLAC) a database of known misidentified cell lines to serve as a guide for the wary is regularly updated (http://iclac.org/databases/cross-contaminations/).

   In addition to characterizing new cell examples, reasons for performing cytogenetic analysis in cancer cell lines include: (a) ascertainment and resolution of subtle rearrangements escaping detection in primary cancer cells; (b) authentication and stability studies; and (c) genotoxicity studies.

   A common misconception concerning cancer cell lines is that since they are "immortal" this seeming robustness renders them impervious to harvesting difficulties. However, such is not the case. Hence, it is of the utmost importance that cell lines be carefully maintained and fed regularly. In the case of leukemia/lymphoma cell lines, cells should not be over-diluted to prevent colony collapse due to growth factor starvation, or bottlenecking selection leading to loss of heterogeneity and fixation of potentially atypical subclones. Bottlenecking selection along with cross-contamination may contribute significantly to reports of "genetic instability"—a charge sometimes laid unjustly at the door of cell lines.

1.4 Cell Culture

For the advice on cancer cell culture, including the choice of laminar flow safety cabinets and incubators, readers are urged to consult one of the many available specialist works now available [9, 10]. The most critical component of cell culture systems is probably the fetal bovine serum (FBS), which is normally added at 10–20 % unless otherwise specified. Serum samples should be batch tested for their ability to support growth of several fastidious sentinel cell lines (*see* **Note 1**). The remaining 80–90 % is made up of culture medium. We generally use Dulbecco's Minimal Essential Medium (DMEM) for adherently growing cells and Roswell Park Memorial Institute (RPMI) 1640 Medium for leukemia or lymphoma cells. McCoy's 5A medium is a good all-round medium for those unable to keep dedicated media. Certain additional supplements may be required for long-term cultures together with antibiotics (e.g., penicillin/streptomycin) for primary cells where replacement would be difficult after contamination.

2 Materials

Unless otherwise indicated, reagents may be stored at 4 °C up to 4 weeks.

1. Complete culture medium: RPMI 1640, 20 % FBS, and penicillin/streptomycin.
2. 100× colcemid (*N*-Deacetyl-*N*-methylcolchicine) solution: 4 μg/mL colcemid stock solution. Store refrigerated for up to 1 year.
3. 100× FdU (5-fluoro-2′-deoxyuridine)/uridine (1-β-D-ribofuranosyluracil) stock solution: Mix one part of 25 μg/mL FdU with three parts of 1 mg/mL uridine. Store refrigerated for up to 1 year.
4. 100× thymidine [1-(2-deoxy-β-D-ribofuranosyl)-5-methyluracil] stock solution: Dissolve 50 mg of thymidine in 100 mL of autoclaved TE buffer (10 mM Tris–HCl, pH 7.5 and 1 mM EDTA). Filter-sterilize through 0.22 μm filter.
5. 0.5 g/L trypsin/0.2 g/L EDTA: For removal and dispersal of adherent cells, store at −20 °C up to 6 months.
6. Hypotonic solution: Mix 5.59 g/L KCl solution with 9.0 g/L sodium citrate solution in different ratios as required; KCl solution : sodium citrate solution (v/v) = 20:1, 10:1, 1:1, 1:10 and 1:20, allowing time to reach desired temperature shortly before use.

7. Carnoy's fixative: Mix absolute methanol and glacial acetic acid at 3:1. Use freshly but can be stored at 4 °C or on ice up to 4 h.
8. Slides (frosted ends for labeling): Wash mechanically overnight in warm ion-free detergent; rinse twice in deionized water; oven-dry, and leave overnight in 70% ethanol. Slides should then be polished using a lint-free cloth (or non-shredding tissue) and wrapped in aluminum foil. Store at −20 °C until use (*see* **Note 2**).
9. Phosphate buffered saline (PBS): Adjust to pH 6.8 for Giemsa solution or pH 7.2 for cell washing.
10. Giemsa stain: Add 5 mL of Giemsa stain solution in 100 mL of PBS (pH 6.8). Filter before use.
11. Light microscope with phase-contrast illuminator and equipped with 10× (phase contrast), 40× (phase contrast), and 50× (brightfield–dry) objectives (*see* **Note 3**).
12. 100-mL glass Coplin jars.

3 Methods

Perform in a class II safety cabinet due to aerosol and cross infection risks issues.

3.1 Sample Types

Clinical samples may be for diagnostics or research. For research purposes, separate informed patient consent must be obtained in advance and ethical approval documented in accordance with local regulations.

No matter whether samples are diagnostic or experimental, remote clinical pathology laboratories should be provided in advance with sufficient sterile universal tubes for transport. Tubes containing culture medium and double-strength antibiotics should be provided by the recipient cytogenetics lab and bear its address label. A brief note on storage conditions, sample handling, and contact details should be attached to accommodate staff changes. For nearby clinical facilities, autonomous choices of container may suffice.

A little time spent on explaining reasons for requesting tumor material is well invested and may be critical in persuading clinicians/pathologists that nondiagnostic requests are worthy of their consideration. A judicious offer of collaboration may be warranted. When cell lines are being analyzed, ethical issues are less of a problem, particularly when long established.

However, cell line provenance should be characterized and documented along with evidence of authentication and its date. This is not merely good laboratory practice but mandated by scientific journals and funding agencies, increasingly.

Tumor type impacts optimal culture conditions. In general, epithelial and leukemia/lymphoma cells are cultivated at higher densities than mesenchymal tumors. In the following protocol, procedures comprise two successive parts. Firstly, cytogenetic culture protocols tailored to four different sample types: liquid tumors (*see* Subheading 3.2), solid tumors (*see* Subheading 3.3), adherent cell lines (*see* Subheading 3.4), and suspension cell lines (*see* Subheading 3.5). Secondly, the shared harvesting protocol for all these sample types (*see* Subheading 3.6).

3.2 Cytogenetic Culture for Cancer Cells in Suspension

Apart from hematopoietic malignancies, cancer cells in suspension also include tumor effusions and ascites. Unless growth factor requirements for these fastidious cell types are known in advance, direct harvest of cancer cells (<24 h) is preferred instead of long-term cell culture.

1. Dilute blood/bone marrow/effusion/ascites 1:10 in complete culture medium. Dilution ratios need to be greater where viscosity is an issue. Alternatively, incubate overnight with FdU to promote chromosome stretching (*see* **Note 4**).
2. Add colcemid (final concentration 40 ng/mL) to 75-cm^2 flasks culture. Incubate at 37 °C for 1–3 h, or exceptionally overnight.
3. Proceed to Subheading 3.6.

3.3 Cytogenetic Culture for Solid Tumor Cells

To maximize growth potential, specimens are usually cut up into small pieces which are either explanted into culture flasks, or disaggregated enzymatically. Samples are thus first cross-cut with sterile scalpels on a large Petri dish (or lid) and carefully transferred dry to culture flasks before adding culture medium. Alternatively, tissue fragments may be further disaggregated in enzyme cocktail prior to seeding. While disaggregation is assisted by prolonging enzyme exposure times, gains may be offset by losses in viability. These losses may be minimized by recourse to a "cold cocktail" protocol, whereby tissue fragments are marinated in enzyme cocktail at 4 °C for several hours (allowing deep penetration while mitigating toxicity) prior to the incubation step at 37 °C which thus induces rapid cell release [11].

3.3.1 Direct Explant in Culture Flask

1. Wash sample in PBS to remove extraneous matter. Discard wash.
2. Mince tissue into 2–4 mm fragments in a sterile Petri dish (or lid) by cross-cutting.
3. Carefully transfer tumor fragments to culture flasks using sterile Pasteur pipet to allow explants adhere to bottom for 1 h before adding complete culture medium.
4. Proceed to **step 8** in Subheading 3.3.2.

3.3.2 Disaggregate in Enzyme

1. Wash sample in PBS to remove extraneous matter. Discard wash.
2. Mince tumor into 2–4 mm fragments in a sterile Petri dish (or lid) by cross-cutting.
3. Transfer fragments into 10-mL centrifuge tubes containing filtered (pore size 20 μM) trypsin/collagenase in culture medium plus double strength antibiotic at 4 °C (*see* **Note 5**).
4. Refrigerate 1–3 h to allow deep tissue penetration according to fragment size, type, and sensitivity. Overnight refrigeration is sometimes necessary.
5. Incubate at 37 °C for 15–30 min or until medium is opaque. Incubation >45 min should be avoided.
6. Add 20% FBS to inactivate enzymes.
7. Centrifuge at 400×*g* for 5 min.
8. Resuspend in complete culture medium.
9. Incubate at 37 °C in 5% CO_2 humidified incubator until half confluent, replenishing medium when necessary, and at any rate prior to harvest.
10. When 3/4 confluent or medium persistently yellow, cultures are ready for harvest. Alternatively, incubate overnight with FUDR to promote chromosome stretching (*see* **Note 4**).
11. Add colcemid (final concentration 40 ng/mL) and incubate for 1–3 h.
12. Proceed to Subheading 3.6.

3.4 Cytogenetic Culture for Adherent Cell Lines

Although mitotic cells may be dislodged by shaking adherent cultures, enzymatic dislodgement is preferable to yield larger pellets for washing. Mitotic cells are removed mechanically first and enzymatically detached afterwards.

1. Add colcemid (final concentration 40 ng/mL) to flask for 1–3 h.
2. Shake 175-cm^2 flask vigorously to detach mitoses. Decant medium into a 50-mL centrifuge tube. Place the tube on a rack. Alternatively, it can be incubated overnight with FUDR to promote chromosome stretching (*see* **Note 4**).
3. Rinse the flask with 3–5 mL of PBS and add to the tube holding mitoses. Add 5–10 mL trypsin–EDTA which barely covering flask bottom and gently swirl before placing inside an incubator at 37 °C for 5–10 min until sheets of cells begin to detach.
4. Shake the flask vigorously until sheets of cells are fully detached and separated. NB: incomplete disaggregation, as produced by premature shaking, should be avoided to minimize clump

formation inimical to successful passage. Pour the contents of the 50-mL tube containing mitoses back into the flask allowing FBS therein to inactivate the trypsin. Decant into 4 × 10-mL tubes for centrifugation.

5. Proceed to Subheading 3.6.

3.5 Cytogenetic Culture for Suspension Cell Lines

While suspension cultures are easier to harvest, their chromosome banding qualities seldom match those of adherently growing cells. Moreover, suspension cultures require more careful attention than adherent cultures. Hence, backup cultures should be maintained to facilitate repetition.

1. Add colcemid (final concentration 40 ng/mL) to recently fed (<24 h) 75-cm^2 cultures and incubate for 1–3 h.
2. Decant culture (~40 mL) into 4 × 10-mL tubes for centrifugation.
3. Proceed to Subheading 3.6.

3.6 Cell Harvesting for All Sample Types

1. Centrifuge at 400 × *g* for 5 min, and discard supernatant.
2. Resuspend cell pellets gently by tapping with forefinger. Add 5–10 mL from a predetermined range of hypotonic solutions (*see* **Note 6**).
3. Incubate tubes for allotted times: initially from 1 to 5 min (*see* Table 1).
4. Centrifuge and discard supernatant. Resuspend pellet gently and carefully add ice-cold Carnoy's fixative, at first dropwise (critical!), and then faster until the tube is nearly full.
5. Hold on ice for 1–2 h to allow fixation to take place.
6. Equilibrate to room temperature to minimize clumping. Centrifuge at 400 × *g* for 5 min.
7. Wash cell pellet with Carnoy's fixative.
8. Store tubes containing fixed cells overnight at 4 °C in fresh Carnoy's fixative.

3.7 Slide Preparation

1. Next day, equilibrate tubes to ambient temperature. Centrifuge at 400 × *g* for 5 min.
2. Wash cell pellet twice with Carnoy's fixative.
3. Resuspend cells in just enough fixative, typically 1–2 mL, to produce a slightly milky suspension.
4. Remove four precleaned slides (one per harvest tube) from storage at −20 °C and place atop a plastic freezer block held at a slight incline off horizontal (~10°) tilted away from the operator by insertion of a pipet underneath the proximal edge.
5. Breathe heavily on slides so that they steam up.

Table 1
Harvesting record sheet for U-2932 (DSM ACC 633)

				Hypotonic treatment					Results			Slides and suspensions				
Date	Harvest no.	Colcemid time	Tube	KCl	Na Citrate	Other	Temp	Min	Q	Spr	Morph	Total	Untr	60 °C GTG	−80 °C FISH	−20 °C Susp
18.09.2012	1a	3 h	10 mL	100	–	–	RT	5	B	AA	B-	–	–	–	–	Reserve only
	1b			–	100	-		5	A	A	C	–	–	–	–	–
	1c			100	–	–	37 °C	5	C	C	C	–	–	–	–	–
	1d			–	100	–		5	B	B	C	–	–	–	–	–
G-banding: *unsuitable*[a]				Repeat: *yes*					Action: discard; *try KCl:NaCit 20:1 and 1:1*							
04.10.2012	2a	3 h	10 mL	90	10	–	RT	5	A	AA	B+	–				
	2b			50	50	–		5	A	A	AB		*1*	*8*	*7*	Yes 2 mL
	2c			90	10	–		1	A	A	AB					
	2d			50	50	–		1	A	AB	AB	–				
G-banding: *yes, was OK*				Repeat: *no*					Action: *mix tubes 2b and 2c discard rest*							

Abbreviations for results assessment: *Q* quantity of metaphases is defined as follows "A," ≥1 metaphase per low power (~100×) microscope field; "*B*" ≥1 metaphase per low power field, "*C*" ≤1 metaphase per row power field. *Spr* spreading is defined as: "A," optimal with all or most chromosomes separately visible; "AA" (possibly usable for FISH), as "A," but mostly broken; "B" (usable), with most metaphases showing crossed-over chromosomes; and "C" (unusable), with no chromosomes separately visible. *Morph* Chromosome morphology, "A" (good), with parallel, solid, clearly separated chromatids; "B" (average); and "C" (poor) with amorphous or refractile chromatids when viewed under phase-contrast. Intermediate quantities and qualities are defined by "AB," "BC," etc

Other abbreviations: *GTG* G-banding, *temp* temperature, *RT* room temperature, *susp* cell suspension, *untr* untreated

[a] In the case of U-2932, although the first harvest was discarded, it provided information to direct the choice of hypotonic buffers in second harvest toward a more satisfactory conclusion

6. Immediately, by holding the pipet just above the slides, carefully place two drops of cell suspension onto each slide—the first about one third, the second about two-thirds along to yield a figure-of-eight pattern. Do not flood.
7. Immediately lift both pairs of slides, one in each hand. Breathe on them once more (optional) to maximize spreading if deemed necessary from subsequent evaluation.
8. Further to improve spreading if deemed necessary, gently ignite residual fixative by flaming with a camping stove or Bunsen burner. On no account allow slide to become warm, as this may compromise subsequent G-banding and FISH. (Note: This step demands a degree of finesse to avoid burning fingers!)
9. Label slides using a sharp hard pencil and air-dry by leaving to stand vertically for 10 min.
10. Examine slides by phase-contrast microscopy (*see* **Note 3**) and assess each hypotonic treatment individually (*see* **Note 6**).
11. Prepare slides from best scoring treatments, mixing tubes if necessary. Slides are generally used for three main purposes: (a) solid Giemsa staining to facilitate determination of modal chromosome number and identify supernumerary chromosomes which may be performed directly (*see* Subheading 3.8)-store at room temperature; (b) G-banding (*see* Chap. 6); (c) FISH (*see* Chaps. 11, 13, 14, 16)-store at −80 °C.
12. Store remaining cell suspensions at −20 °C in sealed 2-mL microfuge tubes filled to the brim with fixative. Under such conditions, suspensions remain stable for several years; we have performed FISH successfully using 5-years-old suspensions. Cryopreserved cell suspensions must be centrifuged and resuspended in fresh fixative prior to slide making.

3.8 Ploidy Studies

Once established during tumorigenesis, modal chromosome numbers of cancer cells remain surprisingly stable and provide first pass evidence of identity and tumorigenicity [12]. Extended counting enables subclones to be identified, whether polyploid iterations of the stem clone, or deviant clones signifying heterogeneity [5].

4 Notes

1. FBS: In our experience, given the variable quality of FBS commercially supplied on offer, this vital ingredient should be batch tested using sentinel cell line(s) prior to purchase. The order should then be sufficiently large so as to cover foreseeable needs. At the DSMZ we have assembled a panel of fastidious sentinel cell lines for assessing FBS quality, namely:

HEK-293 (DSM ACC 305) embryonal kidney cells; 380 (DSM ACC 29) B-cell precursor acute lymphoblastic leukemia (BCP-ALL); BV-173 (DSM ACC 20) BCP-ALL; KU-812 (DSM ACC 378) chronic myeloid leukemia; and PEER (DSM ACC 6) T-cell ALL. The growth of parallel cultures supplemented respectively with candidate and tried-and-tested FBS is monitored and the batch yielding the best proliferation ordered.

2. Slide making: The key to successful slide making lies, unsurprisingly perhaps, on the slides themselves. Even from the most reputable manufacturers, "precleaned" slides all-too-often disappoint. Where the slides yield inconsistent spreading or chromosome qualities acid washing is warranted. A sign of unclean slides are autofluorescent streaks or lines causing background signal with FISH.
   (a) Soak slides overnight in 1 M HCl at 55 °C in a nonmetallic vessel.
   (b) Allow to equilibrate to room temperature. Wash in double-distilled water. Repeat.
   (c) Sonicate for 30 min. Repeat twice in double-distilled water.
   (d) Soak 1 h in 50% ethanol.
   (e) Soak 1 h in 70% ethanol.
   (f) Store in 95% ethanol until use.
3. Microscopic evaluation: Well-honed microscopy skills are the key to successful slide evaluation upon which evidence-based hypotonic optimization rests in turn. The microscope should be equipped with both brightfield and phase-contrast condenser systems. Assuming 10–12× ocular magnification, objectives should include those with 10–20× and 40–50× magnifications and with phase-contrast compatibility. These two magnification ranges are needed for assessing mitotic sufficiency ("quantity") and "spreading" plus "quality" respectively. In addition a high power (50×) epiplan or equivalent objective is needed for evaluating stained or banded chromosomes. The microscope should be configured to a computer as images may be recorded to provide a check on consistency over time.
4. FdU harvesting: In general, the most optimal morphologies result from hypotonic treatments comprising less than half sodium citrate. Hypotonic buffers containing more sodium citrate tend to result in suboptimal chromosomal morphologies that fail to produce acceptable G-banding or FISH. Some types of cancer cells and derived cell lines often yield stumpy chromosomes that resist improvement by altering hypotonic mixtures. In these types of cells, FdU pretreatment may be

warranted. Accordingly, incubate cultures overnight with FdU (final concentration 250 ng/mL) and uridine (final concentration 10 μg/mL). The next morning, resuspend in fresh medium with added thymidine (final concentration 5 μg/mL) to reverse the blockade and harvest 7–9 h later.

5. Enzymatic tissue disaggregation: Although trypsin/collagenase is our default cocktail, individual laboratories tend to have their own preferred enzyme combinations. Among those commonly used is the following: 1:1 0.15% collagenase 1a plus 0.15% DNase 1.

6. Evidence-based choice of hypotonic treatment: In our experience, finding the right hypotonic treatment is the single most important step in successful harvesting of cancer cells for cytogenetics [4]. Cancer cells, perhaps reflecting their diversity, are pickier than untransformed cells. It is, therefore, necessary to record carefully the conditions adopted for preceding failed harvests before embarking on a new course. To assist in such an evidence-based process, we use a datasheet that records three key features of successful harvests (*see* Table 1): (a) Quantity: mitotic sufficiency (*see* Fig. 1a, b); (b) Spreading: minimizing the chromosomal overlap while retaining nuclear integrity (*see* Fig. 1c–e); (c) Quality: optimizing the level of discernible detail (*see* Fig. 1f–h).

   In the case illustrated in Table 1, reasonable preparations were only obtained at the second attempt using the standard protocol. Although all four hypotonic combinations yielded adequate numbers of metaphases at the second attempt, only tubes 2b and 2c yielded satisfactory spreading and morphology and were finally mixed for subsequent slide preparation. A total of 16 slides were prepared: 8 for G-banding, 1 for Giemsa staining alone (to check for the presence of smaller chromosomal elements that G-banding sometimes render invisible, such as so-called double minute chromosomes that may harbor oncogenes), and 7 for FISH. In addition, the remaining cell suspension in fixative was stored at −20 °C for future use. Slides with sparse yields of metaphases are unsuitable for FISH where probe costs are often critical. For slowly dividing cell lines (doubling times >48 h), colcemid times can be increased to 6 h first, then to 17 h (overnight), reducing colcemid concentrations simultaneously by half to minimize toxicity. However, paucity of metaphases is usually the result of depletion by overly harsh hypotonic treatments. Paradoxically, we find that reducing hypotonic exposures to 1 min and, if necessary, performing this step in microfuge tubes to facilitate speedy centrifugation to reduce total hypotonic incubation times may improve spreading and yield by enabling survival of fragile cells which might otherwise be lost. Tight metaphases with an excess of overlapping chromosomes might be useful for FISH but are unsuitable for G-banding. In such cases, spreading can sometimes be improved by the following measures: (a) adopting harsher hypotonic treatments, whether by increasing the proportion of KCl to 100%, increasing the hypotonic time up to 15 min, or by performing the latter at 37 °C instead of ambient temperature; (b) gentle flaming often assists spreading and, contrary to received wisdom, has little or no deleterious effect on G-banding or FISH; (c) dropping mitotic suspensions from a height brings scant improvement in spreading. "Offensively" heavy breathing performed both immediately before and after dropping benefits spreading by increasing local humidity levels; (d) excessive spreading, on the other hand, is often cured by reducing the proportion of KCl, shortening hypotonic treatment times, retaining more of the original medium from the first centrifugation prior to addition of hypotonic buffer, or simply increasing the density of fixed cell suspensions to limit "elbow room."

References

1. Heim S, Mitelman F (eds) (2015) Cancer cytogenetics, 4th edn. Wiley, Hoboken, NJ
2. Dai H, Ehrentraut S, Nagel S et al (2015) Genomic landscape of primary mediastinal B-Cell lymphoma cell lines. PLoS One 10: e0139663
3. Tijo JH, Levan A (1956) The chromosome number of man. Hereditas 42:1–6
4. MacLeod RAF, Kaufmann M, Drexler HG (2007) Cytogenetic harvesting of commonly used tumor cell lines. Nat Protoc 2:372–382
5. Quentmeier H, Amini RM, Berglund M et al (2013) U-2932: two clones in one cell line, a tool for the study of clonal evolution. Leukemia 27:1155–1164
6. MacLeod RAF, Dirks WG, Matsuo Y et al (1999) Widespread intraspecies cross-contamination of human tumor cell lines arising at source. Int J Cancer 83:555–563
7. Drexler HG, Dirks WG, MacLeod RAF (1999) False human hematopoietic cell lines: cross-contaminations and misinterpretations. Leukemia 13:1601–1607
8. Dirks WG, Drexler HG (2013) STR DNA typing of human cell lines: detection of intra- and interspecies cross-contamination. Methods Mol Biol 946:27–38
9. Cree IA (ed) (2011) Cancer cell culture: methods and protocols. Methods Mol Biol 731: 1–245
10. Freshney RI (2011) Culture of animal cells: a manual of basic technique and specialized applications, 6th edn. Wiley, Hoboken, NJ
11. MacLeod RAF (1993) Rapid monolayer primary cell culture from tissue biopsy: the cold cocktail method, Cell & tissue culture laboratory procedures. Wiley, Chichester, pp 3E: 2.1–3E:2.8
12. MacLeod RAF, Nagel S, Scherr M et al (2008) Human leukemia and lymphoma cell lines as models and resources. Curr Med Chem 15:339–359

Chapter 6

Chromosome Bandings

Huifang Huang and Jiadi Chen

Abstract

Chromosome banding is an essential technique used in chromosome karyotyping to identify normal and abnormal chromosomes for clinical and research purposes. Giemsa (G)-, reverse (R)-, and centromere (C)-banding are the most commonly dye-based chromosome-banding techniques. G-banding involves the staining of trypsin-treated chromosomes and R-banding involves denaturing in hot acidic saline followed by Giemsa staining. C-banding is specifically used for identifying heterochromatin by denaturing chromosomes in a saturated alkaline solution followed by Giemsa staining. Different banding techniques may be selected for the identification of chromosomes.

Key words Chromosome banding, Karyotyping, G-banding, R-banding, C-banding

1 Introduction

In 1960, Nowell and Hungerford [1–3] identified that the Philadelphia chromosome was consistently associated with chronic myeloid leukemia, ushering in a new era in the field of cancer genetic diagnosis. As we know, identification of chromosomal abnormalities is crucial not only for the diagnosis and prognosis in different types of cancer but also for the monitoring of minimal residual disease and/or relapse [4]. Karyotyping is now mandatory for the newly diagnosed hematological malignancies especially leukemia [5]. Karyotyping is also widely accepted as the gold standard for genetic analysis as it is the most comprehensive method for chromosomal characterization nowadays, even for the developing countries. Chromosomes are analyzed in metaphase through recognition of banding patterns. A band is defined as the part of a chromosome that is clearly distinguishable from adjacent segments by appearing dark or light after banding techniques. A band that stains darkly with G-band method (Fig. 1) may stain lightly with R-band method (Fig. 2). Thus, a continuous series of dark and light bands are present on chromosomes [6]. Banding techniques can be divided into two main types: (1) those generating bands

Thomas S.K. Wan (ed.), *Cancer Cytogenetics: Methods and Protocols*, Methods in Molecular Biology, vol. 1541,
DOI 10.1007/978-1-4939-6703-2_6, © Springer Science+Business Media LLC 2017

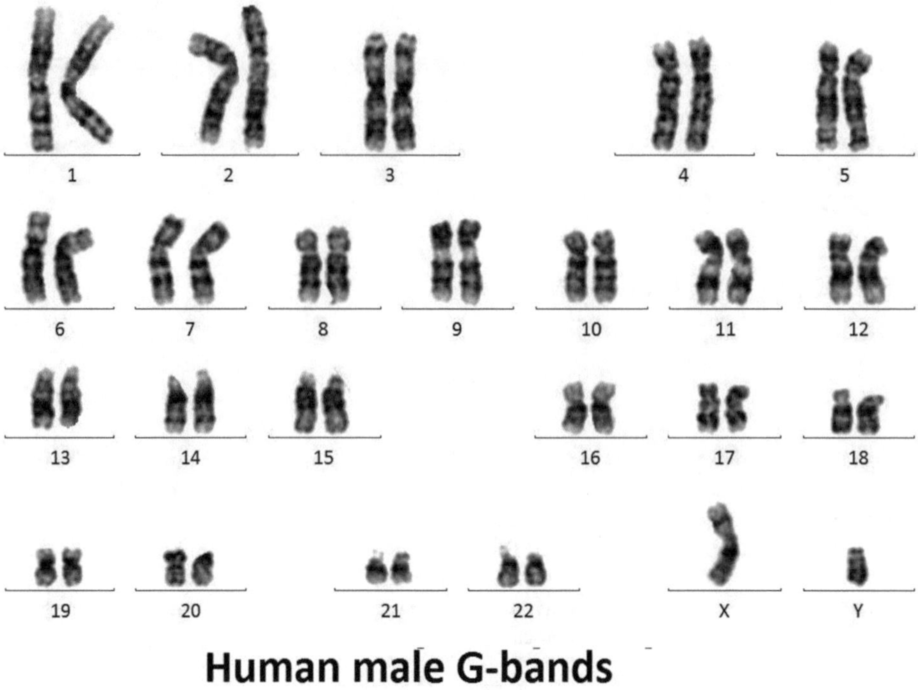

Fig. 1 G-banded human karyogram showing 22 pairs of autosomes, X and Y sex chromosomes

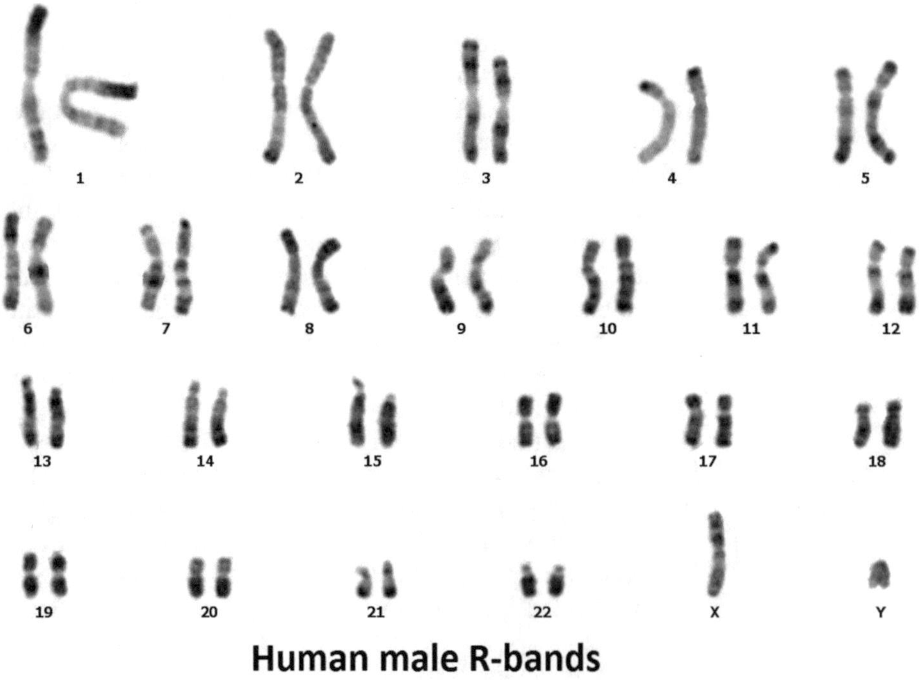

Fig. 2 R-banded human karyogram showing 22 pairs of autosomes, X and Y sex chromosomes

distributing along the whole chromosome, such as G- and R-banding, and (2) those staining specific chromosome structures with a limited number of bands, such as C-banding (Fig. 3).

G- and R-banding are the most commonly used karyotyping techniques for the identification of chromosome number, translocations, deletions, inversions, or amplifications of chromosome segments [7]. G-banding involves the staining of trypsinized chromosomes with Giemsa. The AT-rich regions will appear dark whereas the GC-rich regions appear light [8]. R-banding involves denaturing chromosomes in hot acidic saline followed by Giemsa staining. This method preferentially denatures AT-rich DNA and consequently stains nondenatured GC-rich regions. Therefore, G-bands and R-bands are largely complementary. G-banding is the most widely used technique nowadays while R-banding is preferred in some European countries. Although chromosome morphology is poorly visualized in R-banding, it can identify abnormalities at the ends of chromosomes that are often present in leukemia [4].

G-banded chromosomes are usually used as standard reference for chromosome banding [9]. Bands are consecutively numbered from the centromere on both of the short (p) and the long (q) arms [10, 11]. The total number of bands or "resolution" in the human karyotype depends on the condensation of chromosomes and the stage of mitosis. A resolution of 350–500 bands corresponds to chromosomes in the late metaphase and high resolution (about 850 bands) corresponds to chromosomes in the mid-prophase. A

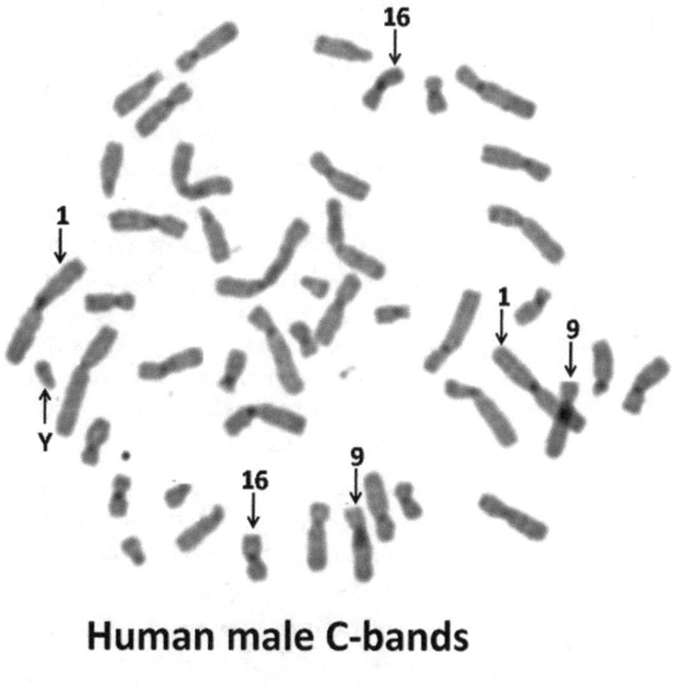

Fig. 3 C-banded human metaphase showing the constitutive heterochromatic regions of chromosomes 1, 9, 16 and Y are *darkly stained*

2000-band resolution chromosome band may contain approximately 1.5 Mb of DNA, whereas a 350-band resolution chromosome may contain 7–10 Mb of DNA [12]. A skilled cytogeneticist should be able to spot a deletion of 5–10 Mb of DNA.

C-banding is usually used to identify heterochromatin. The main C-bands are present on the long arm of the Y chromosome and close to the centromeres of chromosomes 1, 9, and 16. The sizes of these C-bands may differ between individuals. C-banding can detect pericentric inversions of chromosomes 1, 9, and 16 and identify Y chromosome [13, 14].

The following protocol of chromosome banding is used in our laboratory. Readers may modify this protocol according to their experimental conditions.

2 Materials

All solutions should be prepared using ultrapure water and analytical grade reagents and may be stored at room temperature (unless otherwise indicated). All waste materials should be disposed according to the local or institutional regulations.

1. 2.5% Trypsin: Add 2.5 g of trypsin to 100 mL of physiological saline. Mix it slightly (*see* **Note 1**). Store the solution at 4 °C overnight. On the following day, aliquot the solution into 0.5-mL tubes and store them at –20 °C.
2. Phosphate buffer (pH 6.8): Add approximately 100 mL of water to a 1-L graduated cylinder or a glass beaker (*see* **Note 2**). Add 19.08 g of Na_2HPO_4 and 1.82 g of KH_2PO_4 to the cylinder and fill the cylinder with water (about 900 mL). Mix thoroughly (*see* **Note 3**) and make up to 1 L with distilled water. Adjust the pH to 6.8 with HCl or NaOH.
3. Earle's solution: Add approximately 100 mL of water to a 1-L graduated cylinder or glass beaker. Add 6.8 g of NaCl, 0.4 g of KCl, 0.164 g of $NaH_2PO_4{\cdot}2H_2O$, 0.2 g of $MgSO_4{\cdot}7H_2O$, 1.0 g of glucose, 0.225 g of Na_2HPO_4, 0.01 g of phenol red, and 0.2 g of $CaCl_2$ to the cylinder. Fill the cylinder with distilled water (about 900 mL). Mix thoroughly and make up to 1 L with distilled water. Adjust the pH to 6.8 with HCl or NaOH (*see* **Note 4**).
4. 5% $Ba(OH)_2$ alkaline solution: Add 25 g of $Ba(OH)_2$ into a bottle with 500 mL of distilled water. Mix thoroughly to ensure that $Ba(OH)_2$ is completely dissolved (*see* **Note 5**).
5. 2× Saline sodium citrate (SSC): Add 17.5 g of NaCl and 88.2 g of sodium citrate to a cylinder with 100 mL of distilled water. Add distilled water to a volume of about 900 mL. Mix thoroughly and make up to 1 L with distilled water. Adjust pH to 7.0 with HCl or NaOH.

6. Carnoy's fixative: Methanol and glacial acetic acid (3:1, v/v). The solution should be freshly prepared and used within a few hours (*see* **Note 6**).
7. Microscope slide (*see* **Note 7**).
8. Giemsa stain.
9. Coplin jars.

3 Methods

3.1 Metaphase Spreading

The preferable air temperature and humidity for achieving optimal chromosome spreading are 25 °C and 50–55% respectively.

1. Slides are first soaked in concentrated sulfuric acid, followed by washing with distilled water and soaked in 75% alcohol overnight.
2. Change the Carnoy's fixative before spreading. Centrifuge the cell suspension at 300 × g for 5 min. Discard the supernatant and add a few drops of fresh Carnoy's fixative solution to obtain a slightly cloudy suspension (*see* **Note 8**).
3. Generally, four slides are spread with cells for each patient. A variety of methods are available to spread cell suspension on slides. Here is a method used in our lab. Slides are first dipped in 20% alcohol. Then two drops of cell suspension are sequentially dropped from the height of about 30–50 cm onto the slide at positions of one third and two thirds of the slide length respectively (*see* **Note 9**). The slide is briefly waved above a flame to speed up the drying process. The slide is labeled with the patient's identity number and method of preparation with code D for direct preparation and code C for short-term culture (*see* **Note 10**).
4. Check the cell density and chromosomes spreading on the first slide prepared using a microscope under the 10× objective.
5. Adjust the density of the cell suspension accordingly if necessary.

3.2 Banding

3.2.1 G-banding

Slides for G-banding need to be aged for a few days. We can speed up the process by incubating the slides in an oven at 75 °C for 2 h (*see* **Note 11**).

1. Prepare solutions in the following order in a series of Coplin jars.
   (a) 50 mL of phosphate buffer, pH 6.8 with 0.5 mL of 2.5% trypsin (*see* **Note 12**).
   (b) 50 mL of physiological saline.
   (c) 50 mL of distilled water with 5 mL of Giemsa stain.
2. Place the jars in water bath at 37 °C for 15 min.

3. Dip the slide into the trypsin solution and gently shake the slide in the solution for 10–15 s (*see* **Note 13**).
4. Rinse the slide with physiological saline in Coplin jar for a few seconds.
5. Stain the slide with Giemsa stain in the Coplin jar for 1 min (staining time may vary depending on the concentration and strength of the Giemsa stain).
6. Rinse the slide briefly in tap water.
7. Blow the slide with an electric fan.
8. Scan the metaphases whether the chromosomes have clear G-banding. If G-banding is not clear enough, adjust the time for trypsin digestion and Giemsa staining for the following slides.

3.2.2 R-banding

1. Place Earle's solution (*see* **Note 14**) in the water bath at 87.5 °C (*see* **Note 15**) for at least 30 min.
2. Slides are placed in the Earle's solution for 100 min (*see* **Note 16**).
3. Take out the slides. Briefly rinse them in tap water.
4. Air dry the slides.
5. Stain the slides with 50 mL of 10% Giemsa stain solution in a Coplin jar for 1 h.
6. Take out the slides. Briefly rinse them in tap water.
7. Air dry the slides. Then, assess the metaphases under a microscope.

3.2.3 C-banding

1. Incubate the slide in an oven at 75 °C for 2 h.
2. Prepare 50 mL of 5% $Ba(OH)_2$ (saturated) alkaline solution and 50 mL of 2× SSC solution in two Coplin jars.
3. Place the jars in water bath at 60 °C for 0.5 h.
4. Place the slide in alkaline solution for 10 s to several min (see **Note 17**).
5. Take out the slide. Briefly rinse it in tap water.
6. Incubate the slide with 50 mL of 2× SSC solution in Coplin jar for 1 h.
7. Take out the slide. Briefly rinse it in tap water.
8. Stain the slide with 50 mL of 10% Giemsa stain solution in Coplin jar for 5–10 min.
9. Air dry the slide and assess the metaphases.

4 Notes

1. Vigorous mixing will give rise to bubbles.
2. Adding small amount of water first help to dissolve easily.

3. A magnetic stirrer may help mixing more easily and thoroughly.
4. Earle's solution should be stored at −20 °C. Avoid freeze and thaw repeatedly.
5. The chromosomes should be saturated by the $Ba(OH)_2$ alkaline solution.
6. Carnoy's fixative should be freshly prepared to achieve a good metaphase spread.
7. Precleaned slides are essential to obtain a good spread. The slides should be cleaned again prior to use.
8. The characters or numbers written on the opposite side of the tubes can still be read. Cell density can be adjusted by adding fresh Carnoy's fixative (for dilution) or centrifugation (for concentration).
9. The height of dropping should be at least 30–50 cm to obtain a good spread.
10. The other two ways of spreading cell suspensions onto slides are as follows: (a) Cold slides are used. Release two drops of cell suspension from the height of approximately 30–50 cm onto a slide at positions of one third and two thirds of the slide length respectively. The slide is briefly waved above a flame to speed up the drying process. Label the slide accordingly. (b) Label dry slides and place them flat on a slide tray. Add one drop of cell suspension to each slide. Then, immediately blow gently or "huff" on the slides.
11. Alternative ways to age slides are: (a) Incubate slides in an oven at 60 °C overnight; (b) Incubate slides in an oven at 90 °C for 1 h; (c) Incubate slides in an oven at 100 °C for 20 min.
12. The concentration of trypsin working solution is 0.25 %.
13. Time for pretreatment with trypsin should be adjusted for each case according to the spreading technique used, age of slide, degree of contraction of chromosomes, and chromosome morphology. Too long or too short pretreatment time will result in poor banding resolution. Sometimes pretreatment time may be as long as 1 min.
14. The pH of the Earle's solution must be 6.8; otherwise, the quality of R-banding will be poor.
15. For R-banding, the temperature of water bath must be accurately adjusted to 87.5 °C.
16. Each laboratory should explore the temperature according to its own conditions to obtain ideal R-banding.
17. The time for denaturing in alkaline solution depends on the age of slide. A temperature gradient must be established based on experience.

References

1. Gonon-Demoulian R, Goldman JM, Nicolini FE (2014) History of chronic myeloid leukemia: a paradigm in the treatment of cancer. Bull Cancer 101(1):56–67
2. Wan TS (2014) Cancer cytogenetics: methodology revisited. Ann Lab Med 34(6): 413–425
3. Sudoyo AW, Hardi F (2011) Cytogenetics in solid tumors: lessons from the Philadelphia Chromosome. Acta Med Indones 43(1): 68–73
4. Bernheim A (2010) Cytogenomics of cancer from chromosome to sequence. Mol Oncol 4(4):309–322
5. Swansbury J (2003) Introduction. In: Swansbury J (ed) Cancer cytogenetics: methods & protocols. Humana, Clifton, NJ
6. Ushiki T, Hoshi O, Iwai K et al (2002) The structure of human metaphase chromosomes: its histological perspective and new horizons by atomic force microscopy. Arch Histol Cytol 65(5):377–390
7. Craig JM, Bickmore WA (1993) Chromosome bands-flavours to savour. BioEssays 15: 349–354
8. Saitoh Y, LaemmLi UK (1994) Metaphase chromosome structure: bands arise from a differential folding path of the highly AT-rich scaffold. Cell 76(4):609–622
9. Francke U (1994) Digitized and differentially shaded human chromosome ideograms for genomic applications. Cytogenet Cell Genet 65(3):206–218
10. McGowan-Jordan J, Simons A, Schmid M (eds) (2016) ISCN 2016: An International System for Human Cytogenomic Nomenclature. S. Karger, Basel. [Reprint of Cytogenet and Genome Res 149(1–2)]
11. Simons A, Shaffer LG, Hastings RJ (2013) Cytogenetic nomenclature: changes in the ISCN 2013 compared to the 2009 edition. Cytogenet Genome Res 141(1):1–6
12. Yunis JJ (1981) Mid-prophase human chromosomes: the attainment of 2000 bands. Hum Genet 56:293–298
13. Imai HT (1991) Mutability of constitutive heterochromatin (C-bands) during eukaryotic chromosomal evolution and their cytological meaning. Jpn J Genet 66(5):635–661
14. Wijayanto H, Hirai Y, Kamanaka Y et al (2005) Patterns of C-heterochromatin and telomeric DNA in two representative groups of small apes, the genera Hylobates and Symphalangus. Chromosome Res 13(7):717–724

Chapter 7

Chromosome Recognition

Thomas S.K. Wan, Eleanor K.C. Hui, and Margaret H.L. Ng

Abstract

Chromosomal analysis of human cells serves to characterize aberrations of chromosome number and structure. Individual chromosome can be identified precisely by recognition of its morphological characteristics and staining patterns according to specific landmarks, regions, and bands as described in the ideogram. Since the quality of metaphases obtained from malignant cells is generally poor for karyotyping, a practical and accurate chromosome recognition training guide is mandatory for a trainee or newly employed cytogenetic technologist in a cancer cytogenetics laboratory. The most distinguishable bands for each chromosome are described in detail in this chapter with an aim to facilitate quick and accurate karyotyping in cancers. This is an indispensable chromosome recognition guide used in a cancer cytogenetics laboratory.

Key words Chromosomal analysis, Chromosome pattern, Chromosome recognition, G-banded karyotyping

1 Introduction

The technique of autoradiography had been used in an attempt to improve on the identification of individual chromosomes in the early 60s. However, neither chromosome morphology nor autoradiography provided unequivocal identification. At that time, these non-banded chromosomes can only be arranged into seven readily distinguishable groups (A–G groups) in descending order based on the characteristics of size and centromere location [1]. The major breakthrough in chromosomal identification came only after the demonstration by Casperson et al. [2] that each chromosome has its own unique anatomy by virtue of its banding pattern in 1970. The Fourth International Congress on Human Genetics held in Paris in 1971 was a critical developmental milestone in chromosome recognition [3]. In this landmark achievement, an internationally agreed system for describing the banding pattern of chromosomes was established, by which each homologous chromosome pair can be identified precisely by specific landmarks, regions, and bands as described in the ideogram.

Thomas S.K. Wan (ed.), *Cancer Cytogenetics: Methods and Protocols*, Methods in Molecular Biology, vol. 1541,
DOI 10.1007/978-1-4939-6703-2_7, © Springer Science+Business Media LLC 2017

The chromosomes are arranged in a karyotype based on the respective centromere position, band pattern, and length of the chromosome arms. Chromosome numbers are designated corresponding to decreasing size, except for chromosome 21 that is smaller than 22. The location of the centromere is a key feature described in the chromosome morphology: (1) metacentric chromosome refers to a centromeric location near the middle of the chromosome with a ratio of short arm to long arm of 1:1 to 1:1.3; (2) submetacentric chromosome refers to a centromeric location closer to one end of the chromosome than the other with a ratio of short arm to long arm of 1:1.3–1:7; (3) acrocentric chromosome refers to a centromeric location near the end of the chromosome with a ratio of short arm to long arm >1:7, also a secondary constriction, or stalk, may separate satellites from the proximal short arm [4]. Regions and bands are numbered consecutively from the centromere outward along each chromosome arm. The symbols p and q are used to designate the short and long arms of each chromosome respectively [5].

Since the morphology of metaphases obtained from malignant cells is generally ambiguous and complex, it poses an added challenge to cancer cytogeneticists in chromosome recognition, particularly when the metaphase quality is inferior. The chromosome morphology, length, and banding resolution of cancer cells show a high diversity. It is important to analyze a wide spectrum of metaphase cells of varying chromosomal qualities to avoid missing detection of the abnormal clone or subclones as normal metaphase cells with better chromosomal resolution may coexist. It often takes a new cytogenetic technologist several weeks to months to become competent and confident in recognizing normal and specific abnormal patterns of chromosomes. The most distinguishable bands for each normal human chromosome are described and highlighted on the partial chromosome and the corresponding ideogram in this chapter. This is an indispensable practical training guide for trainees or newly employed cytogenetic technologists.

2 Chromosome Identification

2.1 Group A

Group A consists of chromosomes 1-3 and they are usually identified by their size and centromeric index of chromosome (Fig. 1).

2.1.1 Chromosome 1

Chromosome 1 is the largest chromosome and is metacentric.

1. p-arm: The most distinctive feature is the large and light-staining region on the distal half of the p-arm. In the proximal half of the p-arm, there are two distinct dark bands.
2. q-arm: There are three evenly spaced dark bands with the most proximal one showing the highest staining density. The dark heterochromatic region is just below the centromere.

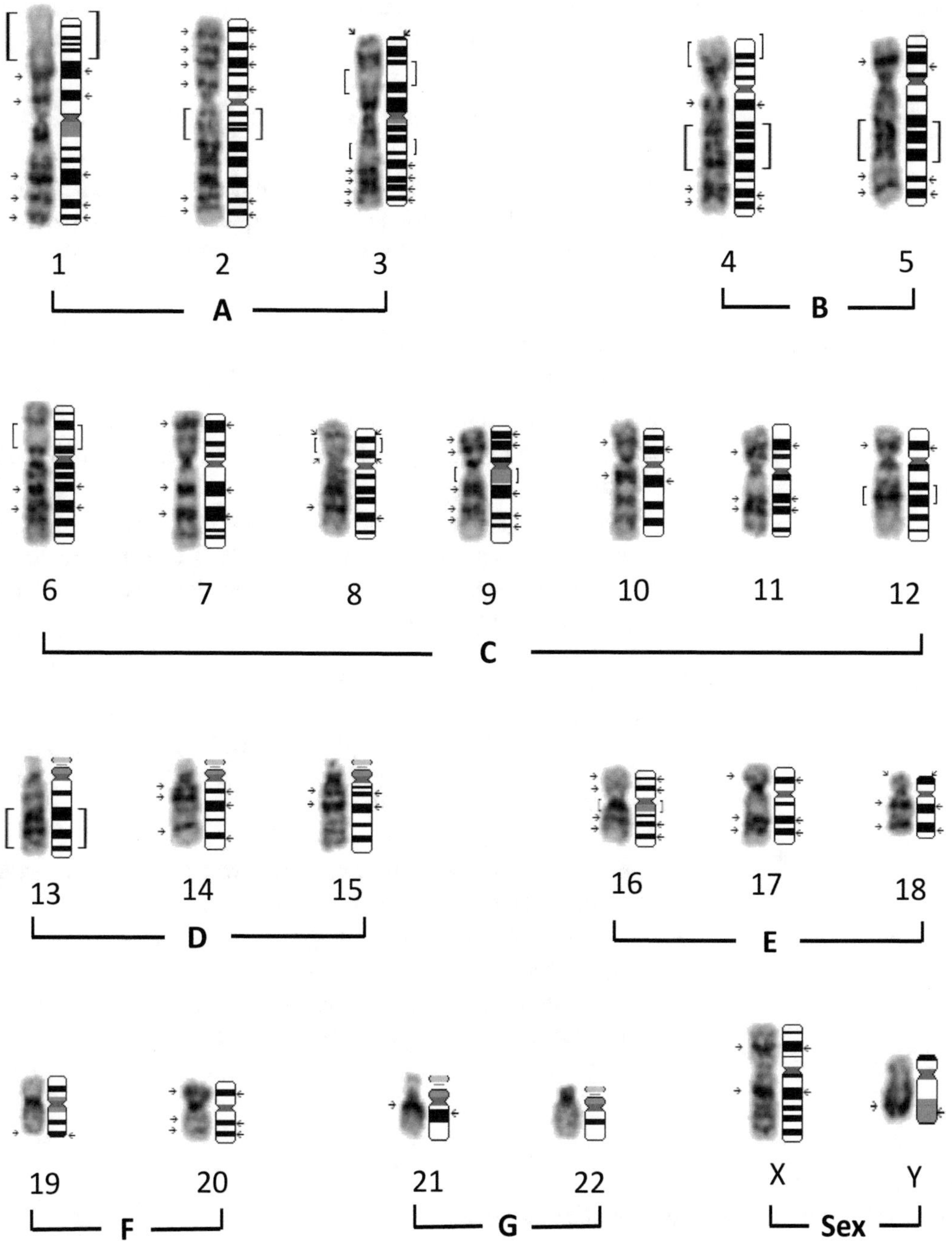

Fig. 1 Landmarks of G-banded human chromosomes

2.1.2 Chromosome 2

Chromosome 2 is the largest submetacentric chromosome. It has few obvious bands; it often looks uniformly dark unless the morphology is good.

1. p-arm: It contains four distinct dark bands that span the whole arm.
2. q-arm: It starts with a light-staining region with three low density dark bands. The distal end of the q-arm is characterized by the presence of two evenly spaced dark bands of equal density.

2.1.3 Chromosome 3

Chromosome 3 is the second largest metacentric chromosome and it may be difficult to differentiate p-arm and q-arm.

1. p-arm: A distinct dark band cap sits at the telomeric end of the p-arm whereas one cluster of light bands is centrally located.
2. q-arm: One cluster of light bands is located proximal to the center. There are three to four dark bands (depend on band level) in the distal third of the q-arm and these dark bands are larger than those on the p-arm.

2.2 Group B

Group B consists of chromosomes 4 and 5, which are not easily distinguishable from each other (Fig. 1). Both of them are submetacentric; the ratio of p-arm:q-arm length is approximately 1:3. The strategic approach in distinguishing chromosome 4 from chromosome 5 is shown in Table 1.

2.2.1 Chromosome 4

1. p-arm: A broad "pure" light band followed by two dark bands of medium density is present.
2. q-arm: A darker "shoulder" band just below the centromere could be identified. Centrally located are four closely spaced dark bands of medium density, which may blend together. Also, the distal end contains two dark bands of similar density.

Table 1
Strategy in distinguishing between chromosomes 4 and 5

	Chromosome 4	Chromosome 5
A characteristic light cap	Yes	No
No. of dark band in p-arm	Two (lighter)	One (darker)
A dark band "shoulder" in q-arm	Yes	No
Two dark bands at the distal q-arm	Similar stain density	Lower one darker

2.2.2 Chromosome 5

1. p-arm: It is characterized by the presence of a distinct central dark band.
2. q-arm: There are three central closely spaced dark bands of medium density, which may blend together. The distal end of the q-arm also harbors two dark bands of different densities, in which the lower one is darker than the upper one.

2.3 Group C

Group C consists of submetacentric chromosomes 6–12 (Fig. 1).

2.3.1 Chromosome 6

Chromosome 6 is one of the three largest chromosomes in this group

1. p-arm: Presence of a distinctive cluster of broad light bands is evident.
2. q-arm: Presence of several dark bands including two central dark bands of high densities could be noted.

2.3.2 Chromosome 7

Chromosome 7 is comparable in size to chromosome 6 but may look similar to chromosome 9.

1. p-arm: A high density dark band near the telomeric end is prominent.
2. q-arm: Two prominent high density dark bands, one located 1/3 and the other 2/3 of the way down the arm, are present.

2.3.3 Chromosome 8

Chromosome 8 is similar in size to chromosome 10.

1. p-arm: A small cluster of light bands with two low density dark bands on either side of the cluster of light bands usually giving them a square appearance is characteristic.
2. q-arm: There are two major dark bands on the q-arm with different intensities and the distal one is noticeably darker.

2.3.4 Chromosome 9

Chromosome 9 is similar in size to chromosome 11. In 5–10% of the population, there is an inherited pericentric inversion of chromosome 9 with the heterochromatic region being relocated from below to above the centromere [6]. This is not known to have any significant clinical implications.

1. p-arm: Two dark bands located in the upper 1/2–2/3 of the arm are noted.
2. q-arm: A triangular heterochromatic band that is light to pale gray in staining is found just below the centromere. It also has three distinct dark bands; one is below the heterochromatic region followed by a broad light band; the other two are distal to the broad light band. Telomeric end shows a broad "pure" light band.

2.3.5 Chromosome 10

Chromosome 10 is similar in size to chromosome 8.

1. p-arm: It is characterized with a distinct central dark band.
2. q-arm: There are three evenly spaced dark bands and the proximal one is darkest.

2.3.6 Chromosome 11

Chromosome 11 is similar in size to chromosome 9.

1. p-arm: It is characterized with one distinct dark band in the middle.
2. q-arm: Two distinct dark bands are centrally located, which may blend together to form one large broad dark band.

2.3.7 Chromosome 12

Chromosome 12 has a ratio of p-arm:q-arm length of 1:3, being the smallest p-arm in group C.

1. p-arm: A broad dark band is present.
2. q-arm: A dark band right below the centromere followed by a large broad light-staining region is characteristic.

2.4 Group D

Group D consists of chromosomes 13–15. The satellite region on these chromosomes is small and polymorphic. Only q-arms are used to distinguish between these chromosomes (Fig. 1).

2.4.1 Chromosome 13

q-arm has three distinctive dark bands in the lower half; however, sometimes they may be fused into one large broad dark band.

2.4.2 Chromosome 14

q-arm has a pair of dark bands, one near the centromere and one near the telomere, giving it a more rectangular or square shape.

2.4.3 Chromosome 15

The upper half of the q-arm is darker. There are two distinctive dark bands in the upper half of the q-arm.

2.5 Group E

Group E consists of submetacentric chromosomes 16–18, where discrimination is usually not difficult (Fig. 1).

2.5.1 Chromosome 16

The appearance of chromosome 16 looks close to metacentric and similar to chromosome 19. It has a conspicuous and very dark heterochromatic band just below the centromere.

1. p-arm: It bears two low density dark bands.
2. q-arm: It carries three evenly spaced dark bands.

2.5.2 Chromosome 17

Chromosome 17 is lighter in color than chromosome 16 or 18.

1. p-arm: It harbors a central dark band of medium density.
2. q-arm: It carries two high density dark bands in the distal area followed by a paler band on the telomeric end.

2.5.3 Chromosome 18

1. p-arm: It exhibits a characteristic dark band cap.
2. q-arm: There are one or two dark bands in the proximal and distal end of the arm usually giving them a square appearance.

2.6 Group F

Group F consists of the smallest metacentric chromosomes 19 and 20, and they are similar in size and shape (Fig. 1).

2.6.1 Chromosome 19

Chromosome 19 is very light in color with a dark pericentric region. Both p-arm and q-arm are characterized with a central dark band of very low density. The difference between them is that the telomere of the p-arm fades into the background whereas the telomere of the q-arm has a distinctive edge to it.

2.6.2 Chromosome 20

1. p-arm: There is a distinct broad dark band of medium to high density in the middle to distal end.
2. q-arm: It carries two dark bands.

2.7 Group G

Group G consists of the smallest acrocentric chromosomes 21 and 22 (Fig. 1).

2.7.1 Chromosome 21

Chromosome 21 is the smallest chromosome and even smaller than chromosome 22. It has a broad and high density dark band in the proximal end of q-arm.

2.7.2 Chromosome 22

Chromosome 22 is a very light in color acrocentric chromosome with a dark pericentric area. q-arm bears a central dark band of low density.

2.8 Sex Chromosomes

Chromosome X is comparable to chromosomes 6 and 7 in terms of size and centromere position (Fig. 1).

2.8.1 Chromosome X

1. p-arm: There is a dark band in the middle of the pale p-arm.
2. q-arm: It harbors a broad and high density dark band at approximately equal distance from the centromere as the prominent dark band in the p-arm. They are of similar stain density. No distinct pale band at the end of the q-arm is evident.

2.8.2 Chromosome Y

Chromosome Y is submetacentric. Its overall size varies from being smaller than chromosome 21 to about the size of chromosome 13 (Fig. 1). The heterochromatic region is uniformly dark and distinctly located at the telomeric end of the q-arm.

References

1. Hamerton JL, Klinger HP, Mutton DE et al (1963) The London Conference on the Normal Human Karyotype, 28th–30th August, 1963. Cytogenetics 2:264–268
2. Casperson T, Zech L, Johansson C (1970) Differential binding of alkylating fluorochromosomes in human chromosomes. Exp Cell Res 60:315–319
3. Paris Conference (1971): Standardization in human cytogenetics. Cytogenetics 11:317–362
4. Kuffel DG, Carison AW, Stupca PJ et al (2007) Training guide for chromosome recognition. J Assoc Genet Technol 33(2):62–68
5. McGowan-Jordan, Simons A, Schmid M (eds) (2016) ISCN (2016): An International System for Human Cytogenomic Nomenclature. S. Karger, Basel. [Reprint of Cytogenet Genome Res 149(1–2)]
6. Wan TS, Ma SK, Chan LC (2000) Acquired pericentric inversion of chromosome 9 in essential thrombocythemia. Hum Genet 106:669–670

Chapter 8

Applications of Fluorescence In Situ Hybridization Technology in Malignancies

Montakarn Tansatit

Abstract

The molecular characterization of nonrandom recurrent cytogenetic abnormalities has identified numerous disease-related genes involved in hematologic and lymphoid malignancies. Cytogenetic analysis has become essential for disease diagnosis, classification, prognostic stratification, and treatment guidance. Fluorescence in situ hybridization (FISH) has greatly enhanced the field and enabled a more precise determination of the presence and frequency of genetic abnormalities. The advantages of FISH compared to standard cytogenetic analysis are that FISH can be used to identify genetic changes that are too small to be detected under a microscope, does not require cell culture, and can be applied directly on fresh or paraffin-embedded tissues for rapid evaluation of interphase nuclei. The application of FISH with a variety of chromosome-specific DNA probes helps to further define molecular subclasses and cytogenetic risk categories for patients with particular hematologic malignancies. FISH analysis is useful in identifying genetic abnormalities undetectable by conventional chromosomal analysis and monitoring residual disease during treatment and follow-up. Therefore, FISH has become an indispensable tool in the management of hematologic malignancies.

Key words Fluorescence in situ hybridization, FISH, Chromosomal abnormality, Hematologic malignancy

1 Introduction

Cytogenetic analysis has played a pivotal role in the diagnostic process for hematologic malignancies. Cytogenetic diagnostics is an invaluable addition to routine laboratory testing and clinical evaluation. A cytogenetic analysis provides important prognostic and predictive information and guides therapeutic decisions by setting the basis for individual treatment options that target cancer-specific genetic abnormalities or their products, as well as helps to assess therapeutic effectiveness by monitoring genetic remission or progression [1].

The chromosomal analysis of bone marrow cells using various cytogenetic techniques has become an integral part of the careful examination of virtually any group of patients with a particular hematologic disorder. A complete cytogenetic analysis of bone

Thomas S.K. Wan (ed.), *Cancer Cytogenetics: Methods and Protocols*, Methods in Molecular Biology, vol. 1541,
DOI 10.1007/978-1-4939-6703-2_8, © Springer Science+Business Media LLC 2017

marrow cells is essential during the initial evaluation for establishing a baseline karyotype. Some specific cytogenetic abnormalities are closely and uniquely associated with morphologically and clinically distinct subsets of leukemia or lymphoma, as well as with their prognosis. The identification of a nonrandom recurrent chromosomal abnormality is a powerful approach for diagnosing and defining molecular subclasses and cytogenetic risk categories for patients with these disorders, selecting the appropriate therapy and monitoring the efficacy of therapeutic regimens [2, 3].

The information derived from cytogenetic studies has resulted in a new classification of tumors of the hematopoietic and lymphoid tissues, developed by the World Health Organization (WHO) and based on genetic subtyping of diseases. WHO's recent classification of myeloid and lymphoid neoplasms utilizes morphology, immunophenotype, genetics, and clinical features to define disease entities of clinical significance [4]. Conventional cytogenetic analysis, which enables the detection of both balanced and unbalanced chromosomal rearrangements, is still recognized as the gold standard of genetic diagnostics in hematologic malignancies [5]. In some cases, the analysis is inconclusive due to low cell yield, low mitotic index, and poor quality of metaphases in the samples.

2 Fluorescence In Situ Hybridization (FISH)

FISH is a molecular diagnostic technique that utilizes labeled DNA probes to detect or confirm gene or chromosome abnormalities. FISH is often utilized for both research and diagnosis of hematological malignancies and solid tumors. Conceptually, FISH is a very straightforward technique whereby a DNA probe is hybridized to its complementary sequence on chromosomal preparations previously fixed on microscope slides. The sample DNA (metaphase chromosomes or interphase nuclei) is first denatured, and a denatured fluorochrome-labeled probe of the region of interest is added to the denatured sample and hybridized with the sample DNA at the target site as it re-anneals back into a double-stranded DNA (Fig. 1). The hybridization probe is a short fragment of DNA that is labeled with a fluorochrome. The probe signal can be visualized with a fluorescence microscope, and the sample can be scored for the presence or absence of the signal. The major advantage of FISH is that the technique can be performed on dividing (metaphase) cells where individual chromosomes can be distinguished or on non-dividing (interphase) cells. This feature of FISH allows obtaining results more expeditiously than other techniques such as karyotyping. FISH probes are commonly prepared from bacterial artificial chromosome (BAC) clones. A typical FISH probe can be 10–100 kilobase pairs (kb) of DNA in length. FISH can be used to map loci on specific chromosomes, detect both structural

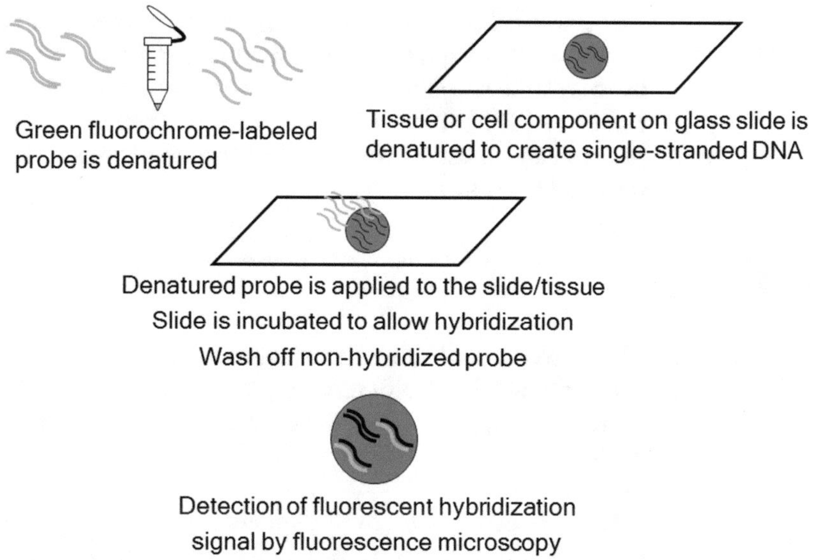
Green fluorochrome-labeled probe is denatured
Tissue or cell component on glass slide is denatured to create single-stranded DNA
Denatured probe is applied to the slide/tissue
Slide is incubated to allow hybridization
Wash off non-hybridized probe
Detection of fluorescent hybridization signal by fluorescence microscopy

Fig. 1 A schematic representation of the FISH technique. A DNA probe is labeled with a fluorochrome. The probe and target DNA on the slide are denatured, and the probe is allowed to hybridize with the target. The fluorescence signal is detected with a fluorescence microscope

chromosomal rearrangements and numerical chromosomal abnormalities, and reveal cryptic abnormalities such as deletions as small as 200–500 kb [6]. Applications of FISH technology encompass a wide range of molecular cytogenetic investigations including the detection of numerical and structural chromosomal abnormalities, identification of marker chromosomes, and detection of gene deletions and gene amplifications. These aberrations have clinical implications for numerous genetic diseases, such as leukemias, lymphomas, solid tumors, autism, and other developmental disorders.

Using FISH, defined numerical and structural chromosomal aberrations can be detected even in fixed interphase cells. Interphase FISH enables researchers to cytogenetically analyze tumors in cases where cytogenetic analysis is hampered by the low mitotic activity of leukemic cells or poor chromosome morphology [7]. Interphase FISH has proven to be valuable not only to detect chromosomal changes pathognomonic for acute myeloid leukemia but also to provide novel insight into cytogenetic abnormalities of chronic lymphocytic leukemia [8] and multiple myeloma. In these diseases, previously underestimated chromosomal abnormalities (in particular, deletions of *TP53* gene and 11q23) were shown to be of major prognostic significance.

The potential of almost all FISH applications has been greatly enhanced by the development of the multicolor FISH assay for the simultaneous detection of numerical and structural chromosomal abnormalities. This approach is particularly useful when structural chromosomal aberrations involving different chromosomal regions are to be elucidated or when several numerical aberrations need to be detected in parallel. One of the most important considerations in FISH analysis is the choice of probes. A wide range of probes can be used, from whole genome probes to small cloned probes (1–10 kb).

3 Types of FISH Probes

There are broadly three categories of FISH probes as follows, each of which has a different range of applications: whole chromosome painting probes, repetitive sequence probes, and locus-specific probes.

3.1 Whole Chromosome Painting (WCP) Probes

WCP probes refer to the hybridization of fluorochrome-labeled chromosome-specific probes, which are actually collections of smaller probes, each of which binds to a different sequence along the length of a target chromosome. In particular, recent advances in chromosome painting to color karyotyping can now be applied as hybridization-based karyotype analysis. WCP probes are available for every human chromosome, allowing the simultaneous painting of the entire genetic complement in 24 colors. WCP probes promptly led to the development of the following two independent FISH imaging systems: fluorochrome-specific optical filters, termed multicolor FISH (mFISH) [9], and interferometer-based spectral imaging, introduced as spectral karyotyping or SKY [10]. In SKY, the image acquisition is based on a combination of epifluorescence microscopy, charge-coupled device (CCD) imaging, and Fourier spectroscopy that enables the measurement of the entire emission spectrum with a single exposure at all image points. In mFISH, separate images are captured for each of the five fluorochromes using narrow band-pass microscope filters; these images are then combined using dedicated software. In both techniques, unique pseudocolors are assigned to the chromosomes based on their specific fluorochrome signatures [11]. Both systems have been invaluable in diagnostic and research applications and differ only in the way they capture and analyze multicolor images; therefore, the same set of probes can be used. WCP probe sets allow the visualization of individual chromosomes in metaphase cells and the identification of both numerical and structural chromosomal aberrations in human pathological specimens with high sensitivity and specificity. The chromosome painting approaches are helpful in elucidating the pattern of chromosomal rearrangements in tumor cytogenetics. In tumor metaphases with highly rearranged chromosomes, karyotype interpretation often requires great efforts because the shuffling of chromatin produces a banding pattern that obscures the original band sequence [12]. The limitation of conventional banding approaches results in a high number of so-called derivative and marker chromosomes in the analysis of tumor metaphase chromosomes. WCP probes have been successfully used for confirmation, refinement, and/or characterization of translocations; searching for cryptic rearrangements; and characterization of marker chromosomes in clinical genetics and tumor cytogenetics (Fig. 2). In contrast, the chromosome painting technique is not helpful for the analysis of interphase cells because the signal domains are very large and diffuse.

Based on the same principle as mFISH, multicolor banding (mBAND) has been developed. The mBAND technique can be used to elucidate the pattern of chromosomal rearrangements and characterize chromosome breakpoints observed in many types of tumors (Fig. 3). The mBAND DNA probes contain a mixture of region-specific partial chromosome paint probes (PCPs) that are generated by microdissection of a particular chromosome and are labeled with three to five different fluorochromes. The neighboring PCPs partially overlap each other. Consequently, the overlapping of the neighboring PCPs decreases the fluorescence intensity toward the margins of the signals leading to a consistent variation of fluorescence intensity ratios along the longitudinal axis of the chromosomes. These unique color combinations can be identified with the mFISH/mBAND module of the FISH imaging software. The software interprets the combination of fluorochromes to distinguish each chromosome and produce a pseudo-color image specific for each chromosome or region.

3.2 Repetitive Sequence Probes

Repetitive sequence probes hybridize to specific chromosomal regions or structures, which contain short sequences and are present in many thousands of copies. Examples of this type of probes are telomeric probes targeting tandem repeat (TTAGGG) sequences present on all human chromosome ends or alphoid/centromeric probes that target the alpha (α) and beta (β) satellite sequences, which flank the centromeres of human chromosomes. Alphoid or centromeric repeat probes are generated from the repeated sequences found in the middle of each chromosome. In most instances, these sequences are distinct, such that an alpha satellite probe derived from one chromosome will not hybridize to another chromosome. Centromeric probes, which target all human centromeres, are also available. Satellite DNA probes hybridize to multiple copies of the repeat unit present at the centromeres, resulting in two very bright fluorescence signals in both metaphase and interphase diploid cells. These probes are useful as chromosome enumeration probes to determine whether an individual has the correct number of chromosomes, hence making centromeric enumeration probes (CEP) particularly valuable for the detection of monosomy, trisomy, and other aneuploidies in both leukemias and solid tumors [13].

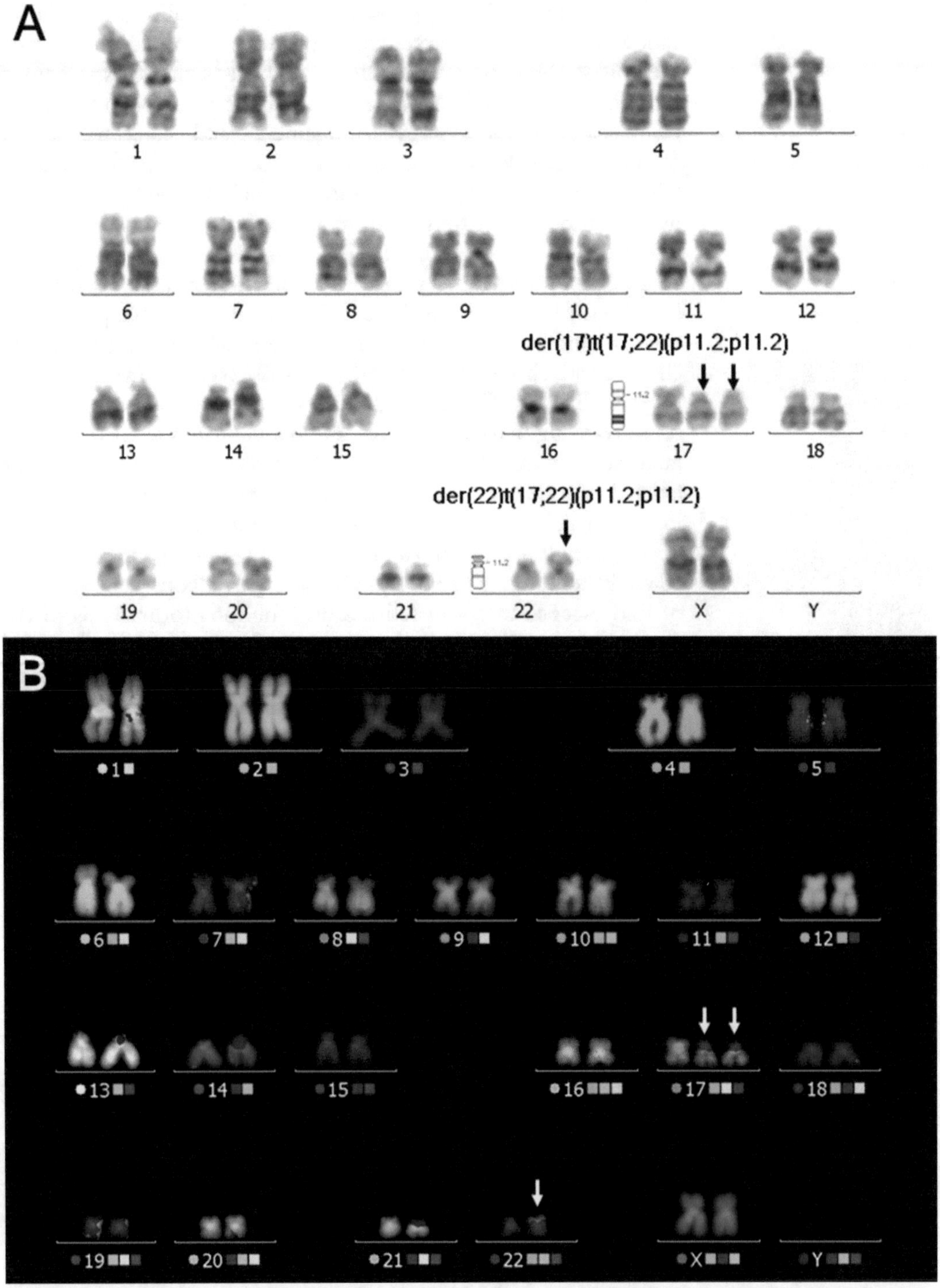

Fig. 2 (**a**) GTG-banding analysis showed an aberrant karyotype 47,XX,+der(17)t(17;22)(p11.2;p11.2),t(17;22). The *arrows* indicate the derivative chromosomes. (**b**) Multicolor FISH (mFISH) analysis confirmed that both derivative chromosomes 17 were composed of chromosomal fragment from chromosome 22 attached to the short arm of chromosome 17 and that derivative chromosome 22 contained small chromosomal fragment from chromosome 17

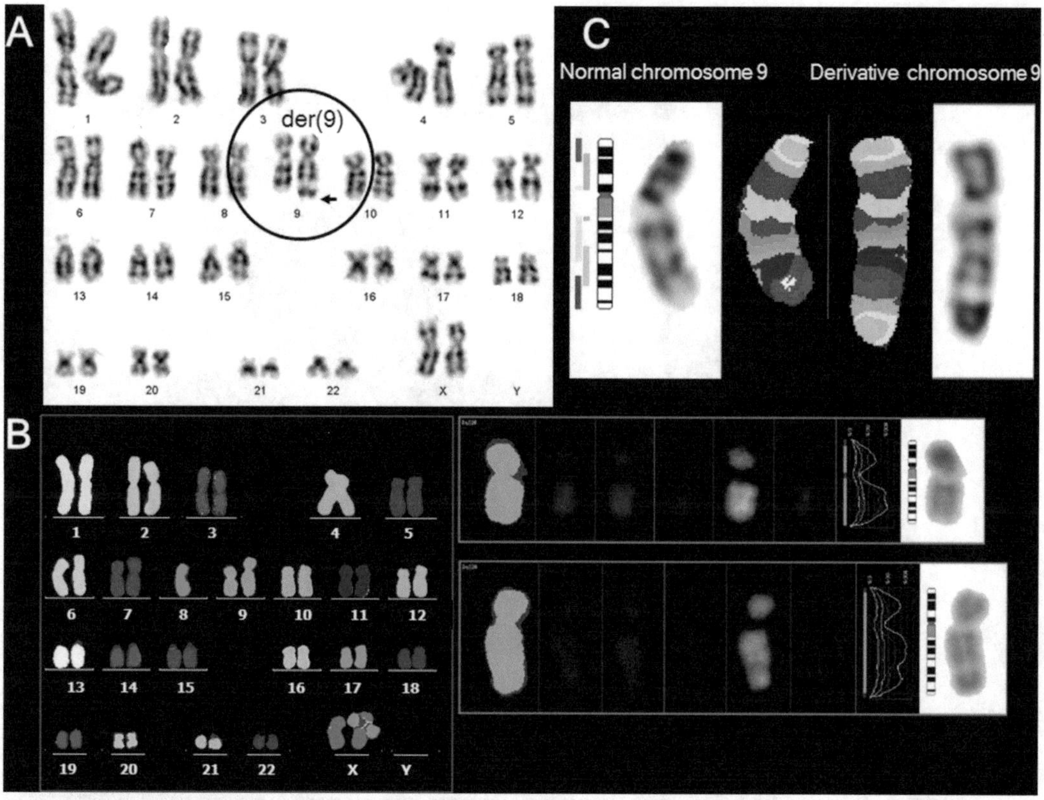

Fig. 3 (**a**) Karyotype of G-banded chromosomes showed the normal chromosome 9 and a derivative chromosome 9. (**b**) mFISH confirmed that the extra chromosomal fragment of the derivative chromosome 9 was all of chromosome 9 origin. (**c**) mBAND showed the duplicated of 9p13-pter chromosomal fragment on 9qter

3.3 Locus-Specific Probes

The third category of probes, locus-specific probes, consists primarily of genomic clones, which vary in size depending on the nature of the cloning vector, from plasmids (1–10 kb) to the larger P1-plasmid artificial chromosome (PAC), yeast artificial chromosome (YAC), and bacterial artificial chromosome (BAC) vectors (80 kb to 1 Mb) [14]. Locus-specific probes target specific genes of interest in oncology and constitutional syndromes. Gene-specific probes are ideal for the rapid identification of a range of chromosomal aberrations across the genome. These probes can be used to determine whether a gene is amplified, deleted, or present in a normal copy number (Fig. 4). Probes in this category are also particularly useful for detecting structural rearrangements, such as specific chromosomal translocations or inversions in both metaphase and interphase cells using a combination of locus-specific probes with the mFISH strategy. A variety of locus-specific FISH probes have been generated for different diagnostic applications. There are mainly two types of dual-color locus-specific probes for the detection of chromosomal translocations depending on the

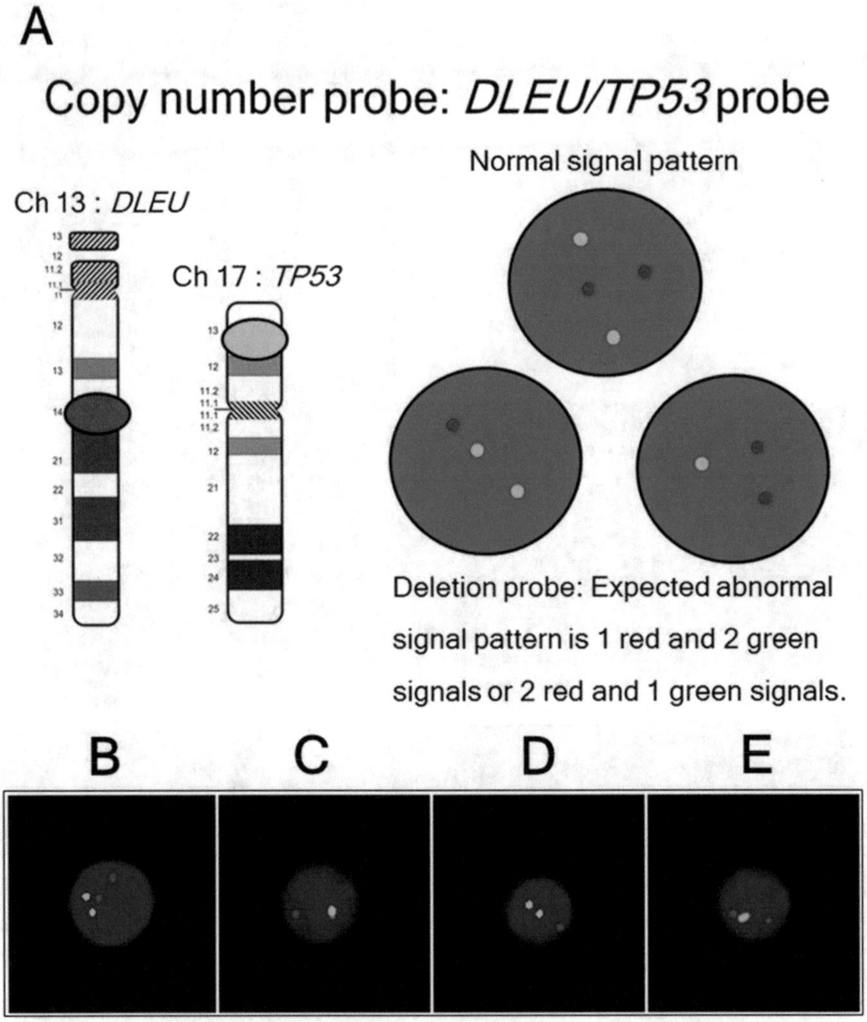

Fig. 4 (**a**) A schematic illustration of the *DLEU1/TP53* FISH probe designed to identify the human *DLEU1* and *TP53* genes located on chromosome bands 13q14.2 and 17p13.1, respectively, to detect rearrangements or abnormal copy number of the *DLEU1* gene and the *TP53* gene, which are commonly observed in B-cell chronic lymphocytic leukemia (CLL) and other malignancies. (**b**) Normal signal pattern: two copies of both genes are present in a nucleus. (**c**) Deletion of one of the *DLEU1* and *TP53* loci. (**d**) Deletion of one of the *DLEU1* locus. (**e**) Deletion of one of the *TP53* locus

translocation partner as follows: fusion probes and break-apart probes. Fusion probes are suitable to detect known specific translocation partners and the alternative break-apart probes are preferable in cases of multiple translocation partners.

3.3.1 Dual-Color, Single-Fusion Probes

Recurrent and specific chromosome translocations can be identified in cells by means of genomic probes that are derived from the two genetic breakpoints. For example, the fusion-signal FISH technique was initially devised for the identification of the t(9;22), known as the Philadelphia translocation, in peripheral blood and bone marrow cells of chronic myeloid leukemia (CML) patients to detect minimal residual disease after bone marrow transplantation [15]. A locus-specific probe for the breakpoint cluster region (*BCR*) gene at 22q11.2 labeled with a green fluorochrome and a locus-specific probe for the Abelson murine leukemia viral oncogene homolog 1 (*ABL1*) gene at 9q34 labeled with a red fluorochrome will appear as a bright yellow spot (single-fusion signal, the combination of green and red fluorochromes) on derivative chromosome 22 in leukemic cells viewed by fluorescence microscopy, indicating the presence of the *BCR-ABL1* fusion gene as a result of t(9;22)(q34;q11.2). Interphase FISH can be used to detect any chromosome abnormality for which an appropriate probe is available. The disadvantage of the single-fusion FISH technique is an inherently high false-positive rate that occurs as a result of coincidental colocalization of two signals, which actually consists of two separate signals in a 3-dimensional nucleus, but they are viewed as a single colocalized signal due to the 2-dimensional analysis of the nucleus [3].

As discussed above, the single-fusion probe for *BCR-ABL1* contains the 5′ portion of the *BCR* gene exhibiting green fluorescence and the 3′ portion of the *ABL1* gene demonstrating red fluorescence; upon fusion of these genes in the Philadelphia chromosome, a yellow fusion signal is observed. However, probes of this type yield a relatively high number of false-positive fusion signals (2–6%) [16, 17] as a result of the close proximity and combination of target chromosomes in interphase nuclei, limiting their use to metaphase cells, which are typically more uncommon when scoring for mutations or detecting minimal residual disease. The next generation of *BCR-ABL1* single-fusion probes, single-fusion extra-signal (ES) probes, makes it possible to discriminate potentially false-positive cells. Extra-signal (ES) probes reduce the frequency of normal cells exhibiting an abnormal FISH pattern due to the random colocalization of probe signals in a normal nucleus [18]. The larger ES probe spans regions upstream and downstream of the *ABL* breakpoint, while the other probe flanks the breakpoint on the *BCR* gene. Extra-signal probes work on the same principle as their predecessor but the part of the DNA sequences recognized by one of the probes (*ABL1*) remains at the original site, giving rise to an extra red signal with diminished fluorescence intensity. Therefore, false positives can be distinguished from genuine fusion signals by the absence of the extra red signal for the 5′ *ABL1* sequences resulting in improved specificity.

3.3.2 Dual-Color, Dual-Fusion Probes

Dual-color dual-fusion probes greatly reduce the number of normal nuclei exhibiting abnormal signal patterns and are optimal for detecting low numbers of nuclei possessing a simple balanced translocation. Two differentially labeled large probes spanning regions upstream and downstream of the two translocation breakpoints on different chromosomes allow the simultaneous visualization of a fusion signal on both derivative chromosomes, significantly reducing the impact of false-negative results, a source of concern in single-fusion probes [19] (Fig. 5).

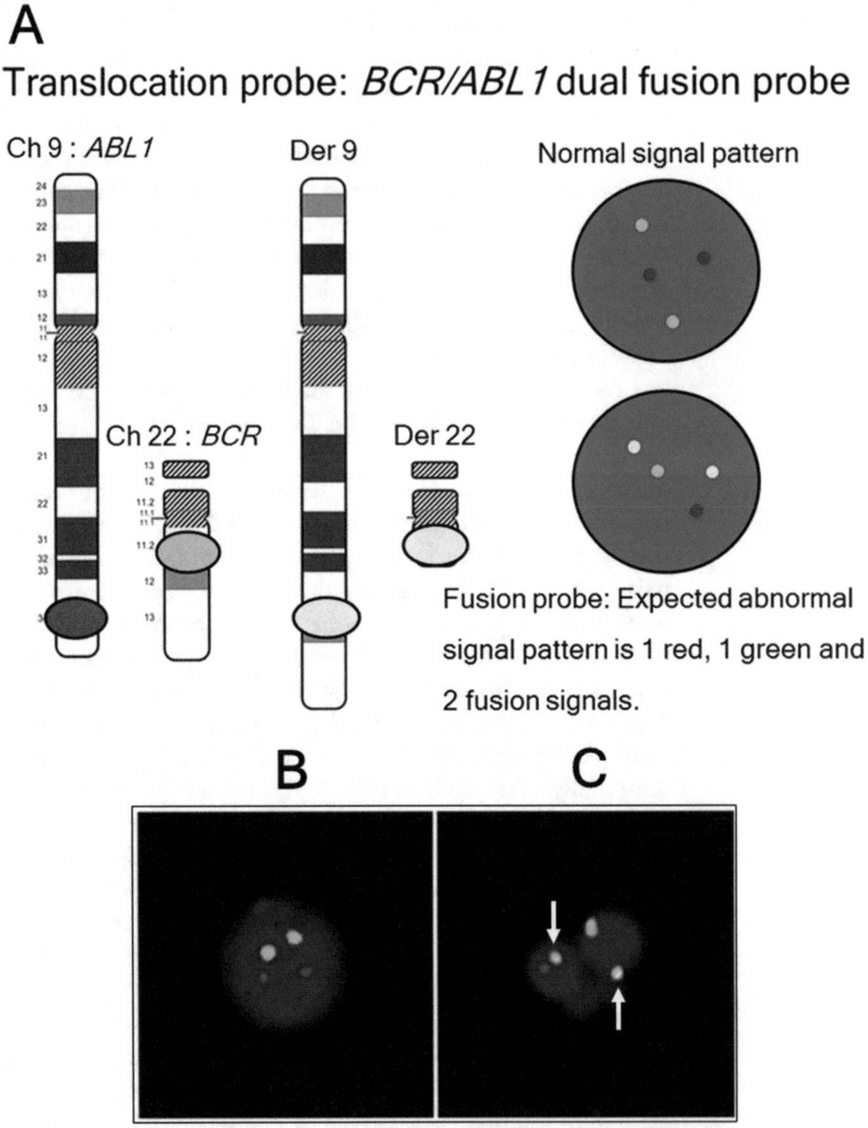

Fig. 5 (**a**) A schematic illustration of the *BCR-ABL1* dual-color, dual-fusion probe designed to detect the reciprocal translocation of the *ABL1* gene on chromosome 9q34 and the *BCR* gene on chromosome 22q11.2 by fluorescence in situ hybridization (FISH). (**b**) *BCR-ABL1* dual-color, dual-fusion probe hybridized to normal interphase cells as indicated by two orange and two green signals in each nucleus. (**c**) Interphase cells with translocation affecting the *BCR* and *ABL1* loci as indicated by one orange signal, one green signal, and two orange/green (*yellow*) fusion signals (*arrows*)

3.3.3 Dual-Color, Break-Apart Probes

Useful in cases where there may be multiple translocation partners associated with a known genetic breakpoint, this labeling scheme features two differently labeled probes that hybridize to targets on opposite sides of a breakpoint in one gene. Dual-color, break-apart rearrangement probes are essentially the reverse of the aforementioned dual-fusion probes. They consist of sequences flanking the gene disrupted by the rearrangement. The break-apart FISH technique was initially introduced as an innovative and simple experimental approach for the detection of all types of *MLL* gene translocations in ALL and AML, using only a single FISH test [20]. Probes are located in adjacent DNA regions spanning common breakpoints consisting of a 5′ centromeric portion of the *MLL* gene labeled in green and a largely 3′ telomeric portion of the *MLL* gene labeled in red. Two yellow fusion signals are observed in normal cells without disruption of the *MLL* gene, whereas separate red and green signals are observed where the sequences are separated as a result of a translocation (Fig. 6). In addition, the break-apart *MLL* probe allows for the assessment of the copy number to determine whether deletions, duplications, or amplifications of the gene have occurred. The sensitivity of this probe is exceedingly high with excellent specificity.

The break-apart FISH approach has several advantages over the more traditional fusion-signal FISH. First, the detection of a translocation is independent of the involved partner gene. This is particularly of great interest for target genes with multiple partner genes such as *MLL* and *ETV6*. Second, break-apart FISH in principle allows the identification of the partner chromosome if metaphase chromosomes are present on the slide. As a result of the translocation, one of the probes moves to the partner chromosome, der(partner), while the other probe remains on the der(target) chromosome. Therefore, the break-apart approach allows the detection of new partner chromosomes or chromosome regions involved in the translocation. Further molecular analysis can then be performed to identify the new partner gene, such as panhandle PCR or long-distance inverse PCR. Another advantage of break-apart FISH is the absence of the traditionally high levels of false-positivity as observed using the fusion-signal FISH approach.

3.3.4 Probes for Abnormal Copy Number (Deletion or Amplification) Detection

Locus-specific probes can also be used in combination with centromeric repeat probes to determine whether an individual is missing genetic material from a particular chromosome or how many copies of a gene exist within a particular genome. The optimal approach to determine if a gene is truly amplified is to have a probe set with both the locus-specific probe and the centromeric enumeration probe for the same chromosome. This procedure is used in various types of FISH testing such as Human epidermal growth factor receptor 2 (*HER2/neu*) (Fig. 7), Epidermal growth factor receptor

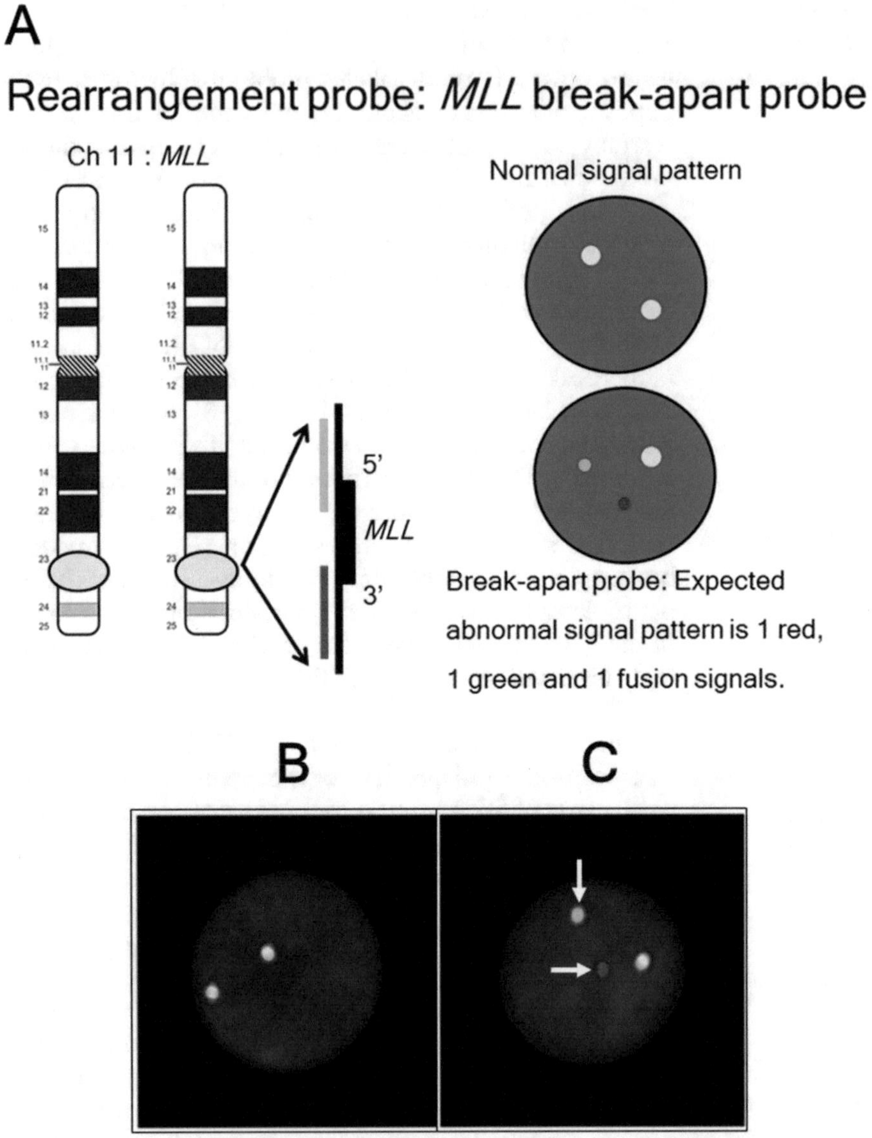

Fig. 6 (**a**) A schematic illustration of the *MLL* break-apart rearrangement probe consisting of the centromeric portion of the *MLL* gene breakpoint cluster region labeled with a green fluorochrome and the largely telomeric portion labeled with an orange fluorochrome. (**b**) *MLL* break-apart probe hybridized to normal interphase cells as indicated by two fusion signals in each nucleus (*arrows*). (**c**) Interphase nuclei hybridized with *MLL* break-apart probe showed a split signal pattern of *MLL* gene (*arrows*)

(*EGFR*), and Myelocytomatosis cellular oncogene (*MYC*). Amplification is usually determined by a comparison of the gene copy number to the number of centromeres in the same cell. The ratio of gene to centromere number is used frequently in reporting whether a tumor is amplified or deleted for a particular gene.

Some of the common uses of locus-specific probes in clinical cytogenetics are for the diagnosis of microdeletion and

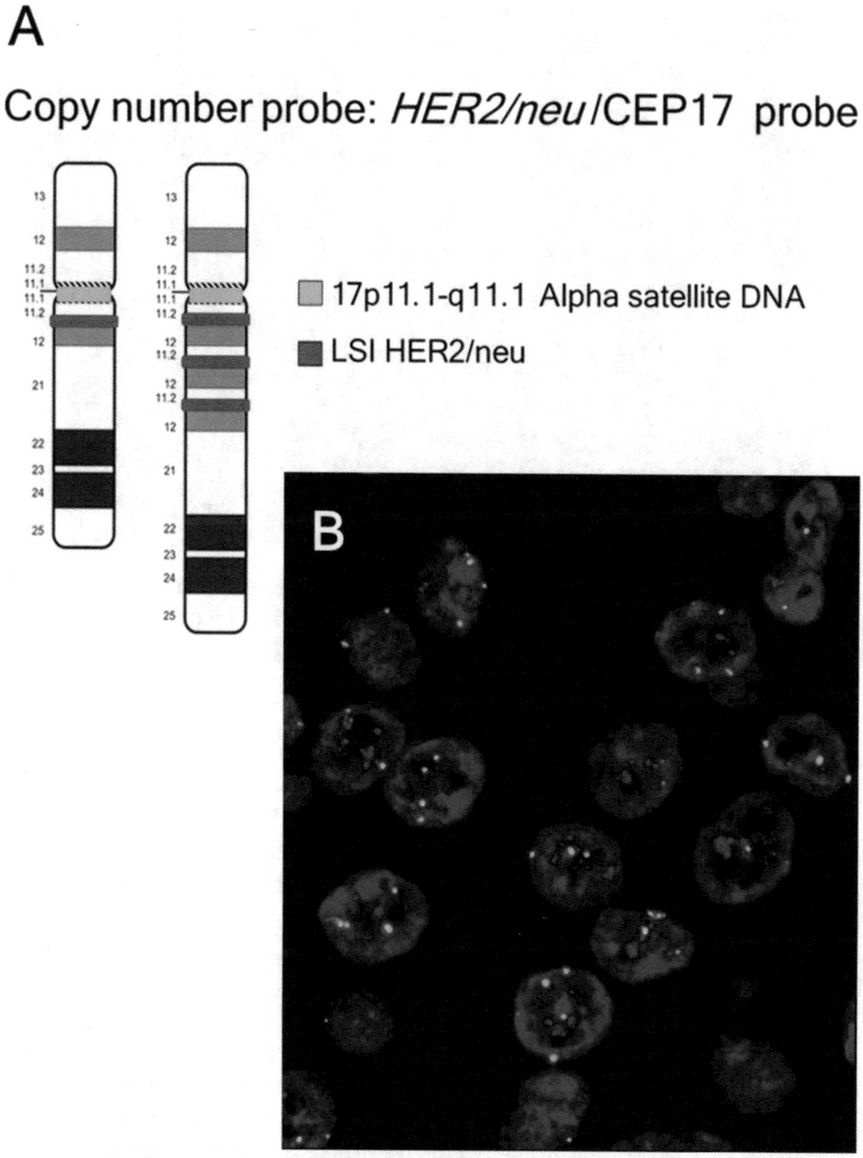

Fig. 7 (**a**) A schematic illustration of the human epidermal growth factor receptor 2 (*HER2/neu*) FISH probe containing two directly labeled fluorescent DNA probes. The *orange*-labeled *HER2/neu* probe covers the chromosome region 17q11-q12 and the *green*-labeled chromosome enumeration CEP17 probe covers the chromosome region 17p11.1-q11.1. (**b**) The ratio of *HER2* to CEP17 by FISH is used to determine *HER2* gene status in breast cancer. This ratio distinguishes increased *HER2* gene copy number secondary to *HER2* gene amplification from increased *HER2* gene copy number secondary to extra copies of chromosome 17. FISH-positive result is defined as a *HER2*/CEP17 ratio $\geq$2.0

microduplication syndromes. Microdeletion syndromes are a heterogeneous group of disorders brought about by the deletion of specific regions of chromosomal DNA causing haploinsufficiencies of important genes. These deletions are smaller than 5 megabase

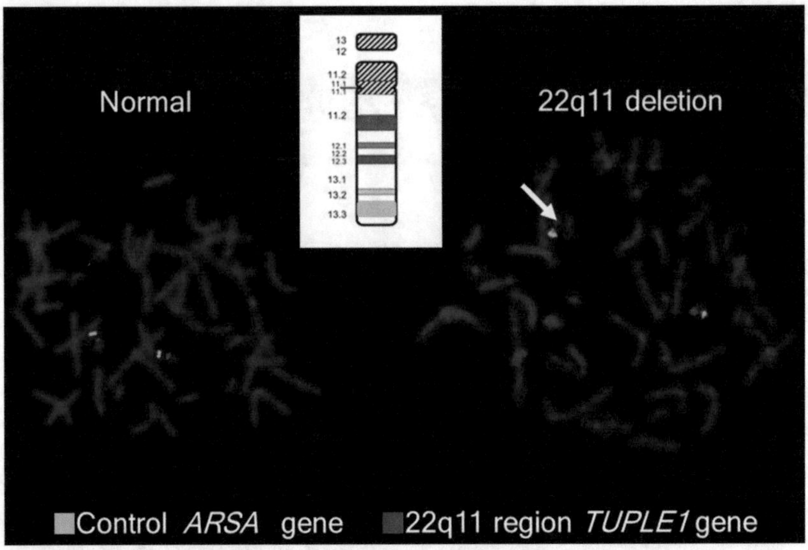

Fig. 8 Fluorescence in situ hybridization (FISH) analysis using the DiGeorge/VCF syndrome probe. Loss of red fluorescent signal of *TUPLE1* (22q11.2) gene was detected on one of the chromosome 22 (*arrow*). The *ARSA* (22q13.3) gene probe (*green*) was included as an internal control

pairs (Mb), spanning several genes that are too small to be detected by conventional cytogenetic methods or high resolution karyotyping (2–5 Mb). Nevertheless, FISH can resolve these submicroscopic deletions and has therefore become the method of choice for the diagnosis of these disorders [21, 22] (Fig. 8).

4 Advantages and Limitations of FISH

FISH allows very precise spatial resolution of morphological and genomic structures. The technique is rapid, simple to implement, and offers great probe stability. The entire chromosomes, chromosomal-specific regions, or single-copy unique sequences can be identified, depending on the probes used. The high sensitivity and specificity of FISH and the availability of a wide range of quality controlled probes are the main reasons for the widespread implementation of the technique. The use of FISH for cytogenetic analysis is widely accepted primarily due to the ease of use and the speed of analysis. Thousands of cells can be evaluated in a relatively short period of time increasing sample sizes and enhancing statistical power. Major advantages of FISH are that it can be performed on non-dividing interphase cells and the ease with which a large number of cells can be scored. The conventional cytogenetic analysis has a limited role in the detection of early relapse or minimal residual disease. FISH can be a valuable tool for monitoring the remission status when clonal chromosome abnormalities have been identified at diagnosis. Using FISH, the cytogenetic data can be obtained from poor samples that contain low cell yield and low mitotic activity of leukemic cells. The assessment of interphase nuclei from uncultured preparations allows for a rapid screening for specific chromosome rearrangements or numerical abnormalities associated with hematologic malignancies and monitoring therapeutic responses. The result is that FISH has become a quantitative test that requires a reference range to distinguish minimal residual disease from background noise. Along with the advantages of being able to analyze interphase cells comes one clear disadvantage, the inability to directly identify the chromosome and chromosomal regions targeted by the probe. Genetic changes that are detected by FISH are limited to position and copy number changes, nonrandom translocations, primarily losses (deletions), and, in some instances, gains (duplications) of the specific chromosomal regions for which the employed DNA probes are localized. FISH can only detect those abnormalities specifically targeted by the probe used and which are larger than the probe used. It is possible that very small deletions may not be detected by FISH. Moreover, FISH testing does not usually screen all chromosomes for changes; the cytogenetic data can be obtained only for the target chromosomes. Therefore, FISH is not a good screening tool for unusual chromosomal aberrations. In some cases, further characterization of abnormal cell populations by metaphase FISH or conventional cytogenetic methods is recommended.

When a new FISH probe is introduced in the laboratory, extensive validation is needed including specific validation of the probe itself (probe validation) and validation of the procedures utilizing the probe (analytical validation) [23]. FISH results should be interpreted within the broader context of these probe and analytical validations. It is important that each probe is evaluated in every laboratory on a series of normal controls for each tissue investigated.

References

1. Heim S, Mitelman F (eds) (2015) Cancer cytogenetics: chromosomal and molecular genetic aberrations of tumor cells, 4th edn. Wiley-Blackwell, New York
2. Rowley JD (1973) A new consistent chromosomal abnormality in chronic myelogenous leukaemia identified by quinacrine fluorescence and Giemsa staining. Nature 243:290–293. doi:10.1038/243290a0
3. Gozzetti A, Le Beau MM (2000) Fluorescence in *situ* hybridization: uses and limitations. Semin Hematol 37:320–333
4. Vardiman JW, Thiele J, Arber DA et al (2009) The 2008 revision of the World Health Organization (WHO) classification of myeloid neoplasms and acute leukemia: rationale and important changes. Blood 114(5):937–951
5. Richkind K (2012) The role of classical cytogenetics in hematologic diagnosis. In: Davis BH, Kottke-Marchant K (eds) Laboratory hematology practice. Wiley-Blackwell, Oxford, UK
6. Wan TS, Ma ES (2011) Molecular cytogenetics: an indispensable tool for cancer diagnosis. Chang Gung Med J 35(2):96–110
7. Kolialexi A, Tsangaris GT, Kitsiou S et al (2005) Impact of cytogenetic and molecular cytogenetic studies on hematologic malignancies. Anticancer Res 25(4):2979–2983

8. Amiel A, Arbov L, Manor Y et al (1997) Monoallelic p53 deletion in chronic lymphocytic leukemia detected by interphase cytogenetics. Cancer Genet Cytogenet 97(2): 97–100
9. Schröck E, du Manoir S, Veldman T et al (1996) Multicolor spectral karyotyping of human chromosomes. Science 273:494–497
10. Kakazu N, Ashihara E, Hada S et al (2001) Development of spectral colour banding in cytogenetic analysis. Lancet 357:529–530. doi:10.1016/S0140-6736(00)04051-4
11. NCI and NCBI (2001) SKY/M-FISH and CGH Database (2001). http://www.ncbi.nlm.nih.gov/sky/skyweb.cgi
12. Schröck E, Padilla-Nash H (2000) Spectral karyotyping and multicolor fluorescence in situ hybridization reveal new tumor-specific chromosomal aberrations. Semin Hematol 37(4):334–347
13. Cuneo A, Bigoni R, Roberti MG et al (1997) Detection of numerical aberrations in hematologic neoplasias by fluorescence in situ hybridization. Haematologica 82:85–90
14. Bishop R (2010) Applications of fluorescence in situ hybridization (FISH) in detecting genetic aberrations of medical significance. Biosci Horizons 3:85–95
15. Dewald GW, Schad CR, Christensen ER et al (1993) The application of fluorescent in situ hybridization to detect *Mbcr/abl* fusion in variant Ph chromosomes in CML and ALL. Cancer Genet Cytogenet 71(1):7–14
16. Chase A, Grand F, Zhang JG et al (1997) Factors influencing the false positive and negative rates of BCR-ABL fluorescence in situ hybridization. Genes Chromosom Cancer 18(4):246–253
17. Kowalczyk JR, Gaworczyk A, Winnicka D et al (2003) Fluorescence in situ hybridization *BCR/ABL* fusion signal rate in interphase nuclei of healthy volunteer donors: a test study for establishing false positive rate. Cancer Genet Cytogenet 142(1):51–55
18. Primo D, Tabernero MD, Rasillo A et al (2003) Patterns of *BCR/ABL* gene rearrangements by interphase fluorescence in situ hybridization (FISH) in *BCR/ABL*+ leukemias: incidence and underlying genetic abnormalities. Leukemia 17:1124–1129. doi:10.1038/sj.leu.2402963
19. Volpi EV, Bridger JM (2008) FISH glossary: an overview of the fluorescence in situ hybridization technique. Biotechniques 45(4):385–386
20. van der Burg M, Beverloo HB, Langerak AW et al (1999) Rapid and sensitive detection of all types of *MLL* gene translocations with a single FISH probe set. Leukemia 13(12):2107–2113
21. Shaffer LG (2001) Diagnosis of microdeletion syndromes by fluorescence in situ hybridization (FISH). Curr Protoc Hum. doi:10.1002/0471142905.hg0810s14
22. Test and Technology Transfer Committee, American College of Medical Genetics (2000) Technical and clinical assessment of fluorescence in situ hybridization: an ACMG/ASHG position statement. I. Technical considerations. Genet Med 2:356–361
23. Wolff DJ, Bagg A, Cooley LD, The Association for Molecular Pathology Clinical Practice Committee and the American College of Medical Genetics Laboratory Quality Assurance Committee et al (2007) Guidance for fluorescence in situ hybridization testing in hematologic disorders. J Mol Diagn 9(2):134–143. doi:10.2353/jmoldx.2007.060128

Chapter 9

Fluorescence In Situ Hybridization Probe Preparation

Doron Tolomeo, Roscoe R. Stanyon, and Mariano Rocchi

Abstract

The public human genome sequencing project utilized a hierarchical approach. A large number of BAC/PAC clones, with an insert size approximate from 50 kb to 300 kb, were identified and finely mapped with respect to the Sequence Tagged Site (STS) physical map and with respect to each other. A "golden path" of BACs, covering the entire human genome, was then selected and each clone was fully sequenced. The large number of remaining BACs was not fully sequenced, but the availability of the end sequence (~800–1000 bp) at each end allowed them to be very precisely mapped on the human genome.

The search for copy number variations of the human genome used several strategies. One of these approaches took advantage of the fact that fosmid clones, contrary to BAC/PAC clones, have a fixed insert size (~40 kb) (Kidd et al., Nature 453: 56–64, 2008). In this context, the ends of ~7 million fosmid clones were sequenced, and therefore it was possible to precisely map these clones on the human genome.

In summary, a large number of genomic clones (GC) are available for FISH experiments. They usually yield bright FISH signals and are extremely precious for molecular cytogenetics, and in particular cancer cytogenetics. The already-labeled probes available commercially are usually based on a combination of such GCs. The present chapter summarizes the protocols for extracting, labeling, and hybridization onto slides of DNA obtained from GC.

Key words FISH, Molecular cytogenetics, Probe labeling and hybridization

1 Introduction

To identify the appropriate genomic clones (GC), there are three main genome browsers where GCs are reported in detail. We usually use the UCSC genome browser (https://genome.ucsc.edu). The last assembly of the human genome (hg38) was released on 2013. BAC/PAC probes are present, but fosmid clones are not yet reported. We therefore refer to the previous public release, hg19 (2009). The genome browser can display several different kinds of data (tracks). In this context the most relevant tracks are BAC End Pairs, Fosmid End Pairs, Ref Seq Genes, and Segmental Duplications. They can be shown at different level of resolution: dense, squish, pack, and full. For each clone a specific sheet is available. The Segmental Duplication track is also of interest if a univocal signal is desired, as occurs in most cases.

Thomas S.K. Wan (ed.), *Cancer Cytogenetics: Methods and Protocols*, Methods in Molecular Biology, vol. 1541,
DOI 10.1007/978-1-4939-6703-2_9, © Springer Science+Business Media LLC 2017

The identified clones can be purchased from the BAC/PAC Resources Center (https://bacpac.chori.org). GCs have to be validated before use. We have done this for hundreds of clones as shown at our web site "Resources for Molecular Cytogenetics" (http://www.biologia.uniba.it/rmc/).

2 Materials

All solutions have to be prepared using ultrapure water and analytical-grade reagents.

2.1 Slide Pretreatment

1. Coplin jar holding 10 or 16 slides back to back.
2. FISH hybridizer or moist chamber (for hybridization).
3. 0.005% Pepsin/0.01 M HCl: Add 50 μL of 1% pepsin to 100 μl of 1 M HCl. Adjust volume up to 10 mL with double-distilled water.
4. 1× Phosphate-buffered saline (PBS): 137 mM NaCl, 2.7 mM KCl, 10 mM Na_2HPO_4, 2 mM KH_2PO_4. To prepare 10× PBS, dissolve 80 g of NaCl, 2 g of KCl, 14.4 g of Na_2HPO_4, and 2.4 g of KH_2PO_4 in 800 mL of double-distilled water. Adjust pH to 7.4 with HCl. Add double-distilled water up to a volume of 1 L and autoclave.

2.2 Post-Fixation

1. Post-fixation buffer: 1× PBS and 0.05 M $MgCl_2$. Add 5 mL of 10× PBS, 5 mL of 0.5 M $MgCl_2$, and 40 mL of double-distilled water in Coplin jar.
2. 4% Paraformaldehyde (PFA) solution: 1× PBS, 0.05 M $MgCl_2$, and PFA. Add 5 mL of 10× PBS, 5 mL of 0.5 M $MgCl_2$, 25 mL of 8% PFA, and adjust volume up to 50 mL with double-distilled water.
3. Ethanol series (70, 90, 100%).

2.3 Bacteria Culture

The antibiotic resistance of vectors can be found at http://www.biologia.uniba.it/rmc/0-1a_pagina/4-libraries.html.

1. Antibiotic solution: 200 mg/mL ampicillin, 50 mg/mL chloramphenicol and 50 mg/mL kanamycin.
2. LB agar-plates: Add 4 g of yeast extract, 8 g of NaCl, 8 g of tryptone, and 16 g of agar to ultrapure water and adjust volume up to 800 mL with ultrapure water. Autoclave, cool to approximately 55 °C, add antibiotics solution (if needed, 50 μL of ampicillin, 400 μL of chloramphenicol or 800 μL of kanamycin), and pour into petri dishes. Let harden, then invert and let them dry overnight at 37 °C. Store at 4 °C in dark.
3. LB medium: Add 4 g of yeast extract, 8 g of NaCl, and 8 g of tryptone to ultrapure water and adjust final volume up to

800 mL with ultrapure water. Autoclave and keep at room temperature. Before using add appropriate antibiotic solution (50 μL of ampicillin, 400 μL of chloramphenicol or 800 μL of kanamycin).

2.4 Probe Preparation

2.4.1 GC Extraction from Cultured Bacteria

1. Glucose-Tris–EDTA (GTE): 50 mM glucose, 25 mM Tris buffer (pH 8.0) and 10 mM EDTA.
2. Denaturation solution: 0.2 N NaOH and1 % SDS (freshly prepared).
3. 7.5 M Ammonium acetate.
4. Isopropanol.
5. 70% Ethanol.
6. TE buffer: 10 mM Tris–HCl and 1 mM EDTA (pH 7.5).
7. 100 μg/mL RNase: Dissolve pancreatic RNase at concentration of 100 μg/mL in 0.01 M sodium acetate (pH 5.2). Heat to 100 °C for 15 min. Allow it cool slowly to room temperature. Adjust the pH by adding 0.1 volume of 1 M Tris–HCl (pH 7.4). Dispense into aliquots and store at −20 °C.
8. DNA precipitation reagents: 3 M sodium acetate in absolute ethanol.

2.4.2 Probe Labeling by Nick-Translation: Direct Labeling

1. 10× Nick-translation buffer: 0.5 M Tris–HCl (pH 7.8–8.0), 50 mM $MgCl_2$ and 0.5 mg/mL BSA.
2. dACG mix (stock 0.5 mM).
3. dUTP-FluorX/ dUTP-Cy3/ dUTP-Cy5 (stock 1 mM).
4. 0.1 M Beta-mercaptoethanol.
5. DNA polymerase I (10 U/μL).
6. DNase I (2 U/μL).

2.4.3 Probe Labeling by Nick-Translation: Indirect Labeling (Biotin)

1. 10× Nick-translation buffer.
2. dACG mix (stock 0.5 mM).
3. Biotin-11-dUTP solution (1 mM).
4. 0.1 M Beta-mercaptoethanol.
5. DNA polymerase I (10 U/μL).
6. DNase I (2 U/μL).

2.4.4 DOP-PCR Labeling

1. Random primer 1 = TAGCTCTTGATCAGAGGNNNNS (20 μM).
2. Random primer 2 = AGTTGGTAGCTCTTGATCAGAGG (100 μM).
3. Taq polymerase (5 U/μL).
4. 10× PCR buffer: 200 mM Tris-HCl (pH 8.4) and 500 mM KCl.

5. 10 mM dNTP mix.
6. *N*-Tris[hydroxymethyl]methyl-3-aminopropanesulfonic acid (TAPS) (0.2 M, pH 8).
7. Biotin-16-dUTP (5-(*N*-[*N*-Biotinyl-ε-aminocaproyl-γ--aminobutyryl]-3-aminoallyl)-2′-deoxyuridine 5′-triphosphate, Bio-16-dUTP tetralithium salt).
8. Digoxigenin-11-dUTP.
9. W1 detergent (Polyoxyethylene ether W-1).

2.5 Probe Precipitation

1. 1 μg/μL Human Cot-1 DNA.
2. 10 mg/mL Salmon sperm DNA (SSD).
3. 3 M Sodium acetate (pH 5.0).
4. Cold (-20 °C) absolute ethanol.

2.6 Hybridization

1. 20× SSC: Dissolve 175.3 g of NaCl and 88.2 g of sodium citrate in 800 mL of water. Adjust pH to 7.0 with a 10 N NaOH, add double-distilled water up to 1 L and autoclave.
2. Hybridization mix (MIX FISH): Mix 5 μL of deionized formamide, 2 μL of 50% autoclaved dextran sulfate, 2 μL of double-distilled water and 1 μL of 20× SSC. Store at 4 °C, in a bottle wrapped with aluminum foil.

2.7 Post-Hybridization Washing and Staining

1. 20× SSC.
2. 50% Formamide in 2× SSC.
3. Blocking solution: 3% bovine serum albumin (BSA), 4× SSC, and 0.1% Tween 20.
4. Detection buffer: 1% BSA, 1× SSC, and 0.1% Tween 20.
5. Washing solution: 4× SSC and 0.1% Tween 20.
6. 100 μg/mL 4′,6-diamidino-2-phenylindole (DAPI): Dilute DAPI 1:500 in 2× SSC.
7. Antifade-mounting medium: Add 0.233 g of 1,4-diazabicyclo-(2.2.2)octane (DABCO), 800 μL of double-distilled water, 200 μL of 1 M Tris–HCl and 9 mL of glycerol. Store at 4 °C, in a bottle wrapped with aluminum foil.

3 Methods

3.1 Slide Aging

Prior to FISH procedures, slide are usually aged either by storing them for 5–7 days at room temperature, or incubating overnight at 65 °C or for 60–90 min at 90 °C. Freshly prepared slide without aging do not maintain chromosome morphology and nuclei/chromosomes are often lost during denaturing. Too old slides may become difficult to hybridize.

3.2 Slide Pretreatment

Incubate in moist chamber with 0.005% pepsin/0.01 M HCl at 37 °C for 30 min and rinse with 1× PBS.

3.3 Post-Fixation

All steps are carried out in a Coplin jar.

1. Prewash in post-fixation buffer at room temperature for 5 min.
2. Wash in post-fixation 4% PFA (*see* **Note 1**) solution at room temperature for 5 min.
3. Wash in 1× PBS at room temperature for 5 min. Dehydration in 70%, 90% and 100% ethanol (*see* **Note 2**) series and air-dry. It is possible to store slide in cold ethanol 100% for several weeks.

3.4 Bacterial Culture and DNA Extraction

Bacterial artificial chromosomes (BAC) were purchased from "BAC/PAC Resources Center" and are provided as "stabs" (small tubes containing bacterial cells in agar). They have to be grown as follows (*see* **Note 3**). This procedure is somewhat tedious.

3.4.1 DNA Extraction (Miniprep)

1. Grow bacteria in 5 mL of bacterial medium containing the right antibiotic in 50-mL falcon tubes for 16–20 h.
2. Centrifuge at 3166 × *g* for 7 min.
3. Discard the supernatant and resuspend pellet completely with 300 μL of GTE.
4. Transfer the cell suspension into 2-mL Eppendorf tubes.
5. Add 600 μL of denaturation solution (freshly prepared) and mix by inverting several times (do not vortex), but DO NOT lyse for >5 min. The lysate should appear viscous.
6. Add 500 μL of 7.5 M ammonium acetate and mix immediately by inverting several times (do not vortex). Leave on ice for 10 min and invert several times during the incubation period.
7. Centrifuge at 17,000 × *g* for 20 min.
8. Pour the supernatant into fresh 2-mL Eppendorf tubes; the supernatant is most often not clear and centrifuge the supernatant again at 17,000 × *g* for 10 min.
9. Pour the supernatant into fresh 2-mL Eppendorf tubes.
10. Add 700 μL of isopropanol and mix by inverting several times.
11. Centrifuge at 17,000 × *g* for 20 min.
12. Discard the supernatant and the pellet should be barely visible.
13. Wash the pellet with 500 μL of 70% ethanol.
14. Centrifuge at 17,000 × *g* for 5 min.
15. Discard the supernatant but do not let the pellet dry.
16. Resuspend the pellet in 100 μL of TE by taping the tubes.
17. Treat with RNase at 37 °C for 30 min.

18. Precipitate the DNA with 1/10 volume of sodium acetate and three volume of ethanol.
19. Incubate at −20 °C for 20 min.
20. Centrifuge at 17,000 ×*g* for 15 min and discard supernatant.
21. Wash with 70% ethanol.
22. Resuspend in TE (appropriate volume).
23. Check on gel for concentration, against a ladder. Store at 4 °C.
24. Before labeling, centrifuge at 17,000 ×*g* for 15 min.

3.4.2 DNA Extraction with BioRad Kit

The above described miniprep protocol is tedious. There are several kits, from different companies, that allow a quick and more efficient DNA extraction. We report here the kit we use in our lab (BioRad kit, with minor modifications) (*see* **Note 4**).

1. Grow bacteria in 10 mL of bacterial medium containing the right antibiotic in 50-mL falcon tubes for 16–20 h.
2. Centrifuge at 3166 ×*g* for 7 min.
3. Discard supernatant and resuspend the pellet in 200 μL of Resuspension Buffer.
4. Transfer the pellet in 2-mL Eppendorf tube.
5. Add 250 μL of Lysis Buffer.
6. Gently resuspend the cells by inverting the tube.
7. Add 250 μL of Neutralization Buffer and gently resuspend by inverting the tube.
8. Centrifuge at 17,000 ×*g* for 5 min. In the meanwhile, prepare a new 2-mL Eppendorf tube with the elution column and mix well the Matrix Solution.
9. Aspirate the supernatant and transfer it to the elution column.
10. Add 200 μL of Matrix Solution and mix by pipetting.
11. Centrifuge at 17,000*g* for 30–60 s and discard the eluate.
12. Wash with 500 μL of Wash Buffer and centrifuge at 17,000 ×*g* for 30–60 s.
13. Discard the eluate again and repeat **step 12**.
14. Transfer the elution column to a 1.5-mL Eppendorf tube. Add 150 μL of double-distilled water and leave at room temperature for few min.
15. Centrifuge at 17,000 ×*g* for 1 min.
16. Add 150 μL of double-distilled water and leave at room temperature for few min.
17. Centrifuge at 17,000 ×*g* for 2 min. The final volume is now 300 μL.
18. Check on gel for concentration, against a marker. Store at 4 °C.

3.5 Probe Labeling (See Note 5, Important!)

The DNase I should be calibrated to give fragments of 100–500 bp; so dilute DNase I (2 U/μL) 1:1000, i.e., 1 μL of 2 U/μL DNAase in 1 mL of double-distilled water and store on ice.

3.5.1 Direct Labeling with Cy3 or Fluorescein or Cy5 by Nick-Translation

Add to a microfuge tube, on ice:

1. 1 μg of DNA.
2. 5 μL of 10× nick-translation buffer.
3. 1 μL of dACG.
4. 0.5 μL of dUTP-Cy3 (or dUTP-fluorescein or dUTP-Cy5).
5. 0.25 μL of DNA polymerase I.
6. 10 μL of DNase I dilution.
7. Add sterile double-distilled water up to total final volume of 50 μL.
8. Incubate at 15 °C for 2 h.
9. Stop reaction on ice.

3.5.2 Indirect Labeling with Biotin by Nick-Translation

Add to a microcentrifuge tube, on ice:

1. 1 μg of DNA.
2. 5 μL of 10× nick-translation buffer.
3. 5 μL of dACG.
4. 2.5 μL of Biotin-11-dUTP.
5. 0.25 μL of DNA polymerase I.
6. 10 μL of DNAse I dilution.
7. Add sterile double-distilled water up to total final volume of 50 μL.
8. Incubate at 15 °C for 2 h.
9. Stop the reaction on ice.

3.6 DOP-PCR of DNA from GCs with a Random-Primer-Set (See Note 6)

Ensure the pipettes are set aside for PCR use only. We suggest using a hot-start polymerase.

3.6.1 Primary PCR

1. For a 50 μL reaction assemble the following reagents:
   5 μL of 10× PCR buffer, 1 μL of dNTP mix, 2.0 μL of Random primer 1, 1.0 μL of Taq polymerase, 50–100 ng of GC DNA and Add sterile double-distilled water up to total final volume of 50 μL.
2. Place on a PCR block and run the following cycling program:
   94°C for 7 min; (94 °C for 1 min; 15 °C for 3 min; 22 °C for 45 s; Ramp at 0.1 °C/s to 40 °C; 40 °C for 10 s; 72 °C 1.5 min) for 5 cycles; 72 °C 4 min; pause at 4 °C.

3. Add 1 μL of Random Primer 2 and 0.5 μL of Taq polymerase.
4. Place on a PCR block and run the following cycle:

   94°C for 2 min; (94 °C for 1 min; 45 °C for 1.5 min; 72 °C for 1 min) for 5 cycles; 72 °C 5 min; pause at 4 °C.
5. Run 5 μL of PCR product on a 1% agarose gel with ethidium bromide to check the size of PCR product. You should have a product in the range of 200 bp to 2 kb.

3.6.2 Secondary DOP-PCR (Labeling)

1. For a 50 μL reaction assemble the following reagents:

   5 μL of 10× TAPS buffer, 5 μL of dNTPs (2:2:2:1 i.e., 1/2 dTTP), 1.3 μL of Biotin-16-dUTP (or dig-11-dUTP or FITC-dUTP), 1 μL of Random Primer 2, 5 μL of W1 detergent, 0.6 μL of Taq polymerase, 200 ng (about 2 μl) of primary GC PCR product, and add sterile double-distilled water up to total final volume of 50 μL.
2. Place on a PCR block and run the following cycles:

   94°C for 2 min; (94 °C for 1 min; 55 °C 1 min; 70 °C for 1 min 40 s) for 31 cycles; 72 °C for 7 min; pause at 4 °C.
3. Run 3–5 μL of secondary PCR product on a 1% agarose gel with ethidium bromide to check the size of PCR product. If the product is a large smear (>700 bp) it will need cutting down, either by sonication or by DNase I treatment.

3.7 Precipitation of Labeled Probes (See Note 7)

1. Precipitate labeled DNA (50 μL) with:

   4 μL of human Cot-1 DNA (per each probe if in cohybridization; not for repeated sequences, i.e., alphoid DNA), 3 μL of SSD (standard amount per slide, not per probe), 1/10 volume of 3 M sodium acetate (pH 5.0) and three volume of cold (−20 °C) absolute ethanol.
2. Leave at −80 °C for 15 min or at −20 °C for 30 min.
3. Spin for at 17,000 ×*g* for 10–15 min and discard supernatant.
4. Dry completely the pellet on a Savant centrifuge for few min.
5. Dissolve the pellet in an appropriate volume of MIX FISH (10 μL per half slide and 15 μL per entire slide) by vortexing for 15 min.

3.8 Hybridization by Simultaneous Denaturation of Probes and Target DNA on Slide (See Note 8)

1. Apply hybridization mix to slide, avoiding air bubbles.
2. Cover with 24 mm × 24 mm (half slide) or 24 mm × 50 mm (entire slide) clean coverslip; seal with rubber cement.
3. Incubate in a FISH hybridizer at 68 °C for 2 min and then 37 °C overnight.

3.9 Post-Hybridization Washing and Staining

IMPORTANT: Do not allow slide to dry throughout the experiment! All washing steps are done in Coplin jar. The washes stringency is based on the complementary level between probes and sample DNA sequences.

3.9.1 Direct-Labeled Probe

1. High-stringency washes: Remove coverslips and wash 3 times for 5 min each in a prewarmed solution of 0.1× SSC in Coplin jar placed in 60 °C shaker water bath with low speed.
2. Low-stringency washes: Remove coverslips and wash three times for 5 min each in prewarmed solution 50 % formamide/2× SSC in Coplin jar in 37 °C shaking water bath with slow speed. Wash three times for 5 min each in prewarmed 2× SSC at 42 °C.

3.9.2 Indirect-Labeled Probes and Cohybridization with Direct Probe

1. Blocking step: Apply 200 μL of blocking solution per slide, cover with 24 mm × 50 mm coverslip, transfer the slide in a dark moist chamber, and then incubate at 37 °C for 30 min.
2. Detection step: Dilute stock solution of avidin-Cy3 (1:300) or avidin-FITC (1:300) or streptavidin-DEAC (1:100) in detection buffer. Let coverslips slide off, apply 100 μL of detection solution per slide and cover with 24 mm × 50 mm coverslips. Transfer the slide in a dark moist chamber. Incubate at 37 °C for 30 min.
3. Washing: Remove the coverslips, rinse the slide three times for 5 min each in prewarmed washing solution 4× SSC/0.1 % Tween 20 in 42 °C water bath.

3.10 Counterstain with DAPI and Slide Assembly

Immerse slide in Coplin jar (wrapped with an aluminum foil) containing counterstain solution at room temperature for 5 min. Apply few drop of antifade-mounting medium and cover with 24 mm × 50 mm coverslip and slide can be stored at 4 °C for weeks in dark.

3.11 Image Handling

Many companies provide a microscope image acquisition set up which includes a software for image handling. Adobe Photoshop™ can do the basics of image handling: pseudocoloring, merging of images, etc. The description of the sequence of commands would be too long for the purposes of this book. Repetitive command sequences, fortunately, can be recorded in a macro (Action in Photoshop), and they can be grouped in a file. This file is a document we freely distribute. It can be downloaded from http://www.biologia.uniba.it/Actions/. Unzip the file and place it in the Photoshop folder. Further details can be requested to mariano.rocchi@uniba.it.

4 Notes

1. Paraformaldehyde promotes covalent links between amino acid residual in proteins.
2. Alcohols were chosen with the idea that they would replace the water in cells, and allow heating of proteins without changing chromosome morphology.
3. Before setting up bacterial cultures, it is better to stick the bacteria on an agar plate (with the appropriate antibiotic) and then set up the 10 mL culture from a single colony.
4. We use BioRad Quantum Prep Plasmid Miniprep kit for plasmids. Perhaps the efficiency of the BAC/PAC-specific kit is higher, but it is far more expensive.
5. The dUTP Cy3, fluorescein, or Cy5 conjugates are expensive. There are protocols for "do it yourself" protocols, as the one described in [2]. Alternatively, you can download a protocol (pdf) from http://derisilab.ucsf.edu/data/pdfs/amino-allyl-protocol.pdf. We use these reliable protocols for many years.
6. If a small amount of DNA is available, it can be amplified and labeled using DOP-PCR.
7. The amount of probe depends on the type of probe: 20–50 ng for repetitive DNA (alphoid sequences, in that case it is not necessary to add Cot-1 DNA); 500–600 ng for GC probes (BACs, PACs, fosmids); 1000 ng for very small probes (PCR products).
8. Alternatively, the probe and target DNA denaturation can be done separately. Slide can be denatured in a Coplin jar. However this protocol uses large quantity of formamide (toxic), and is preferably avoided.

References

1. Kidd JM, Cooper GM, Donahue WF et al (2008) Mapping and sequencing of structural variation from eight human genomes. Nature 453:56–64
2. Henegariu O, Bray-Ward P, Ward DC (2000) Custom fluorescent-nucleotide synthesis as an alternative method for nucleic acid labeling. Nat Biotechnol 18:345–348

Chapter 10

Fluorescence In Situ Hybridization Probe Validation for Clinical Use

Jun Gu, Janice L. Smith, and Patricia K. Dowling

Abstract

In this chapter, we provide a systematic overview of the published guidelines and validation procedures for fluorescence in situ hybridization (FISH) probes for clinical diagnostic use. FISH probes—which are classified as molecular probes or analyte-specific reagents (ASRs)—have been extensively used in vitro for both clinical diagnosis and research. Most commercially available FISH probes in the United States are strictly regulated by the U.S. Food and Drug Administration (FDA), the Centers for Disease Control and Prevention (CDC), the Centers for Medicare & Medicaid Services (CMS) the Clinical Laboratory Improvement Amendments (CLIA), and the College of American Pathologists (CAP). Although home-brewed FISH probes—defined as probes made in-house or acquired from a source that does not supply them to other laboratories—are not regulated by these agencies, they too must undergo the same individual validation process prior to clinical use as their commercial counterparts. Validation of a FISH probe involves initial validation and ongoing verification of the test system. Initial validation includes assessment of a probe's technical specifications, establishment of its standard operational procedure (SOP), determination of its clinical sensitivity and specificity, development of its cutoff, baseline, and normal reference ranges, gathering of analytics, confirmation of its applicability to a specific research or clinical setting, testing of samples with or without the abnormalities that the probe is meant to detect, staff training, and report building. Ongoing verification of the test system involves testing additional normal and abnormal samples using the same method employed during the initial validation of the probe.

Key words Validation, Fluorescence in situ hybridization, FISH, Probe, Sensitivity, Specificity, Cutoff value, Normal range, BETAINV function

1 Introduction

Accredited cytogenetic and molecular genetics laboratories use fluorescence in situ hybridization (FISH) probes extensively to make clinical diagnoses, and under United States law, these laboratories must validate their FISH probes before use. The U.S. Food and Drug Administration (FDA) regulates the manufacture of commercial FISH probes, while the Centers for Medicare & Medicaid Services (CMS) and the Centers for Disease Control and Prevention (CDC) regulate the testing methodology through their Clinical

Thomas S.K. Wan (ed.), *Cancer Cytogenetics: Methods and Protocols*, Methods in Molecular Biology, vol. 1541, DOI 10.1007/978-1-4939-6703-2_10, © Springer Science+Business Media LLC 2017

Laboratory Improvement Amendments (CLIA). Thus, it is mandated in the United States that all FISH probes must be validated before clinical use in an accredited clinical diagnostic laboratory. Guidelines for FISH probe validation have been published by the American College of Medical Genetics (ACMG) and the College of American Pathologists (CAP). The Clinical and Laboratory Standards Institute (CLSI) has produced similar guidelines (International Organization for Standardization (ISO) 15189). Currently, the responsibility of FISH probe validation rests with each accredited laboratory, and the details of the validation procedures adapted by these laboratories can vary. The major steps for FISH test validation include assessment of a probe's technical specifications, establishment of its standard operational procedure (SOP), determination of its clinical sensitivity and specificity, development of its cutoff, baseline, and normal reference ranges, gathering of analytics, confirmation of its applicability to a specific research or clinical setting, testing of samples with or without the abnormalities that the probe is meant to detect, staff training, and report building. Documentation of the validation should be maintained for laboratory accreditation and reaccreditation purposes. Based on available guidelines and regulations, this chapter provides a systematic overview of FISH probes and their validation for use in clinical diagnosis.

1.1 Guidelines

Home-brew FISH probes are not currently regulated by the FDA, although the FDA requires the inclusion of the following disclaimer on all reports of in-house tests using them: "*This test was developed and its performance characteristics determined by [Laboratory Name]. It has not been cleared or approved by the U.S. Food and Drug Administration.*" [1]. In contrast, the FDA does control the manufacture of molecular probes (called analyte-specific reagents or ASRs), which are classified as Class I, II, or III according to the level of oversight necessary to expect that they are reasonably effective and safe. While the majority of the probes in use are Class I—meaning that they are not required to undergo premarket approval—those in Class II or III, including FISH in vitro diagnostic devices, must be authorized by the FDA before they can be marketed in the United States. According to the CLIA'88, FISH probes that the FDA approves as Class II or III devices must only be used by clinical laboratories qualified to perform high-complexity testing. Such laboratories must document that the assay's performance characteristics are the same as or better than those stated by the probe manufacturer in the package insert. Clinical laboratories must also maintain documentation of subsequent biannual calibrations of the test system. The ACMG, the CAP, and the CLSI have also produced guidelines for FISH probe validation. The ACMG requires laboratories to validate FISH probes by establishing their clinical sensitivity and specificity, cutoff values, baseline reference ranges, and normal ranges. The organization published its first position statement on the use of interphase FISH in prenatal diagnosis in 1993 [2]. The first description of validation methods for FISH tests was made by Schad in 1995 [3]. The preclinical validation of FISH recommended by Wiktor et al. was widely accepted [4]. The ACMG has also published guidelines relevant to FISH probe validation in constitutional and oncologic clinical cytogenetic analysis [5–8]. The CAP emphasizes the documentation of FISH probe validation in CYG.42700 of its Cytogenetic Checklist, and in CYG.42900 indicates that written procedures for establishing normal cutoff values and records from cutoff-value studies should be maintained for interphase FISH tests. In CYG.43250, CAP requires that there be a system in place to ensure FISH probe colocalization, which can be accomplished by using metaphase cells in an interphase cell analysis or by including an internal or external target that could give a positive signal for each hybridization. In CYG.48399, CAP provides guidelines for FISH validation in formalin-fixed, paraffin-embedded (FFPE) tissues. The National Committee on Clinical Laboratory Standards (NCCLS) published its first FISH validation guidelines in 2004 [9] and, after being renamed as the Clinical and Laboratory Standards Institute, published guideline ISO 15189 for probe validation. In August 2013, CLSI also made recommendations for FISH probe and test validation in an updated version of regulation MM07-A2 for clinical laboratory FISH methods [10], and this new version of MM07-A2 fully agreed with the FISH recommendations from the ACMG. Table 1 summarizes the guidelines produced by the agencies that regulate FISH test validation.

1.2 Work Flow Chart

Figure 1 gives an overview of the work flow for FISH test validation. Steps 1 and 2 are preclinical evaluations, step 3 is the major part of the clinical evaluation, and step 4 deals with the post-validation work required before a test can be put into clinical use.

2 Assessment of FISH Probe Technical Specifications

2.1 Types of FISH Probes

Commonly used FISH probes include chromosome-painting probes, repetitive-sequence probes, and locus-specific probes. Locus-specific probes include those with dual-color/single-fusion, dual-color/extra-signal, dual-color/dual-fusion, triple-color/dual-fusion, and dual-color/break-apart designs. The use of control probes with each type of FISH probe design is essential to reduce the number of false-positive and false-negative results.

2.2 Hybridization Adequacy

A probe's slide hybridization adequacy should be evaluated before determining its analytic sensitivity and specificity. Slide hybridization adequacy is determined by assessing the probe's signal intensity, background, and localization validation on metaphase cells. The specimen's target viewing area should be located using low-power objective lens with a DAPI filter and should have a minimum of

Table 1
FISH test validation and verification guidelines

FDA (1996)	ACMG (2009)	CLSI (2013)	CAP (2015)
Code of Federal Regulations, Title 21 (21 CFR) 21 CFR §809 Regulates in vitro diagnostic products for human use 21 CFR §809.30(e) ASR disclaimer 21 CFR §809.30(f) Order restriction for in-house tests	Standards and Guidelines for Clinical Genetics Laboratories, Section E (Clinical Cytogenetics) E9.1.1 Types of molecular probes E9.2.1.1 Validation of unique sequence FISH probes not approved of Class II or III ASR kits E9.4 Target tissues E9.7.3.1 ASR disclaimer E10.1.7 Interphase FISH validation E10.3.1 Database collection E10.3.2 Reportable reference ranges E11.2 Multitarget FISH probe validation	International Organization for Standardization (ISO) Quality Document 15189, Molecular Methods (MM) MM07-A2-7 Production of new FISH probes MM07-A2-8.3 Test sensitivity and specificity MM07-A2-8.4.1 The hybridization optimization process MM07-A2-8.4.3 Establishing normal cutoff values MM07-A2-8.4.4 FISH performed on selected cells or cell populations subjected to enrichment procedures MM07-A2-8.4.5 FISH on FFPE MM07-A2-8.6 Controls	Cytogenetics Standards (CYG) CYG.42700 FISH probe validation CYG.42900 Interphase FISH cutoff values CYG.43000 FISH scoring CYG.43200 FISH controls CYG.43250 FISH probe intended target CYG.43600 ASR disclaimer CYG.48399 HER2 (ERBB) assay validation

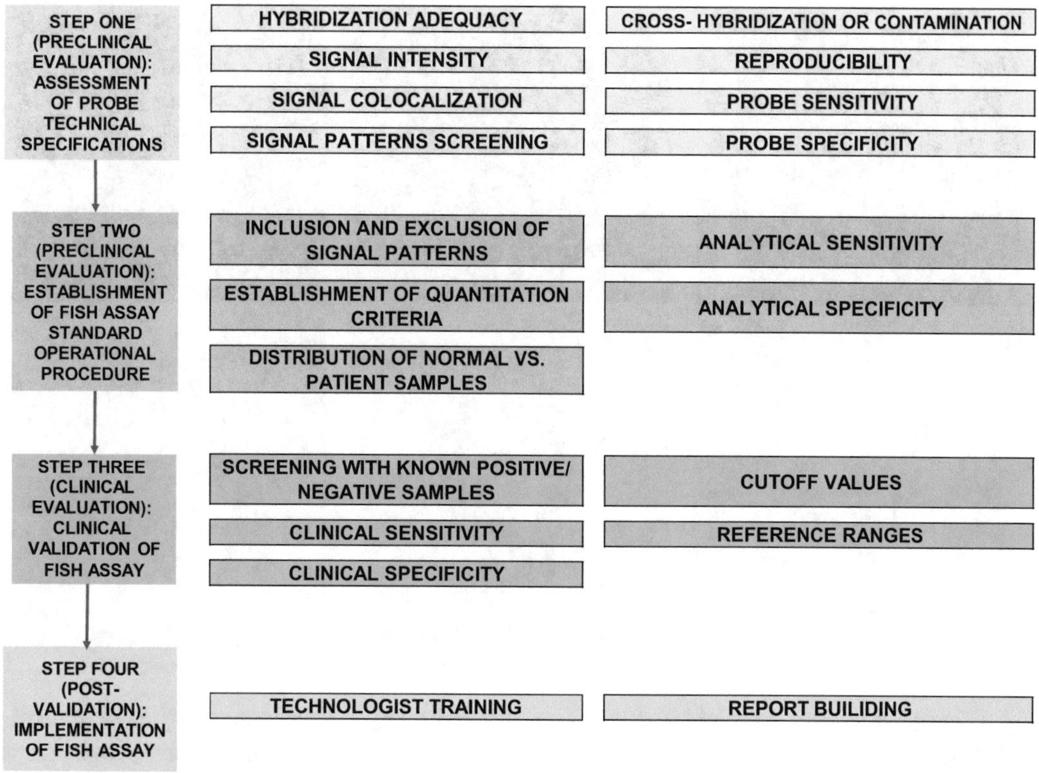

Fig. 1 FISH probe validation flowchart

50 interphase nuclei in order to pass the initial hybridization adequacy assessment. The specimen is classified as uninformative if it fails the hybridization adequacy assessment. Generally, hybridization efficiency should be 98% or higher for chromosome enumeration probes.

2.3 Signal Colocalization

The goal of signal colocalization is to demonstrate that the test probe only hybridizes to the intended target, i.e., without cross-hybridization. A 60× or 100× objective lens with corresponding filters should be used to check anticipated signal patterns on metaphase cells from five normal male individuals. Although ACMG recommends evaluating a minimum of five metaphases to confirm localization [8], autosomal locus validation typically requires 20 metaphases, and sex chromosome locus validation typically requires 40 [10]. To determine chromosomal localization, standard chromosome analysis should be performed on the sample on which the FISH probe will be used. Either karyotyping (using inverted DAPI images from a computer imaging system) (Fig. 2) or sequential staining (FISH on G-banded slides) may be employed [11].

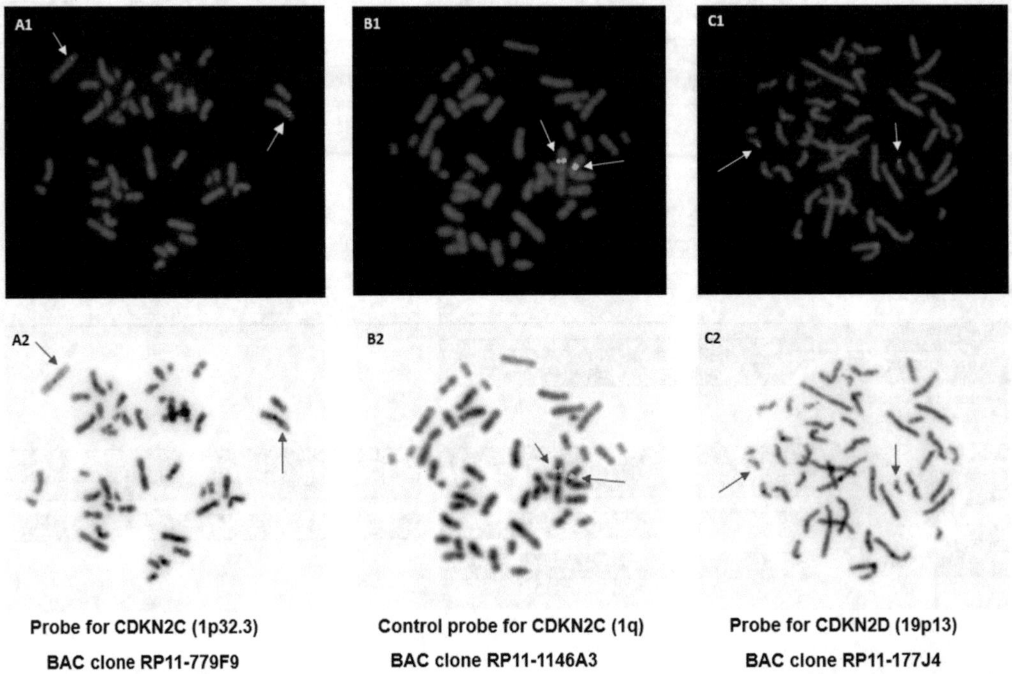

Fig. 2 Colocalization of home-brewed FISH probes from bacterial artificial chromosome (BAC) clones on normal metaphases. *Top panels*: *arrows* pointing to the anticipated signals on chromosomes. *Bottom panels*: *arrows* pointing to the anticipated signals on inverted DAPI stain

The main steps of sequential G-band FISH are as follows:

1. Locate and photograph the G-banded cells on the slide.
2. De-oil the slide by soaking it in xylene or a xylene substitute for 1 min.
3. Rinse the slide twice in fresh 3:1 methanol:acetic acid fixative for 5 min each time. (Note: It is very important to rinse the slide until it is clean. Otherwise, denaturation and hybridization will not be successful.)
4. Dry the slide. Incubate it in 2× saline sodium citrate buffer at 37 °C for 30 min. Then, co-denature the slide and probe at 72 °C for 2 min and incubate it at 37 °C overnight in a humidified chamber.
5. Relocate the G-banded cells on the slide and capture the FISH image.
6. Superimpose the G-banded image with the FISH image to locate the control signal.

Chromosomal localization may also be confirmed by using both known positive and negative control samples. The use of positive and negative control slides validates abnormal results found in single signal probe hybridizations. In any case, a cell should not be counted if the proper control signal pattern is not observed.

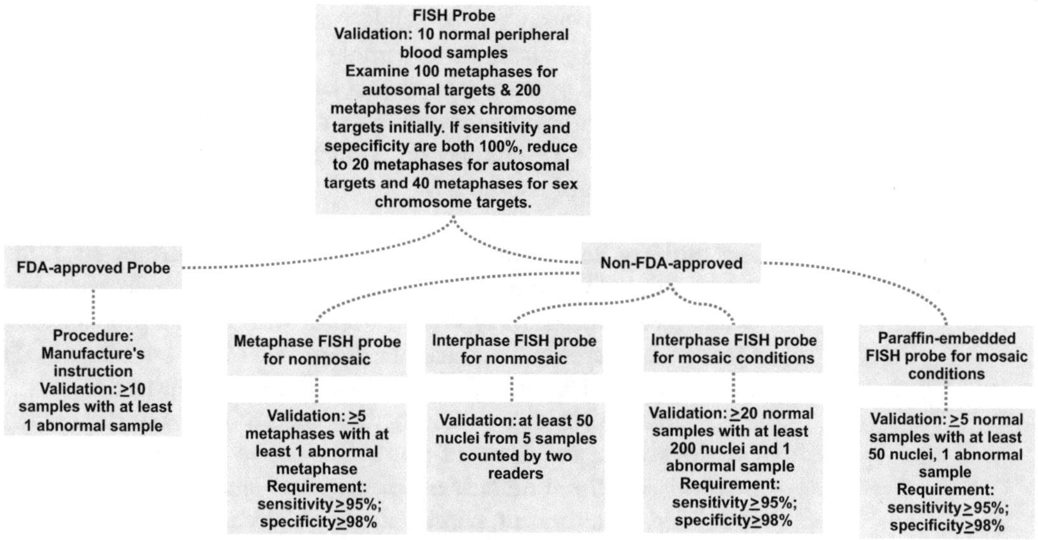

Fig. 3 FISH probe sensitivity and specificity determination

2.4 Probe Sensitivity and Specificity

Probe sensitivity measures how frequently a probe hybridizes to its intended genomic target. It is calculated as the percentage of correct targets detected out of the total number of intended targets presented. Minimum probe sensitivity should be 95%. Probe specificity measures how frequently a target detected by a probe is truly the intended genomic target by design. It is calculated as the percentage of correct targets detected out of the total number of targets detected. Minimum probe specificity should be 98%. Probe sensitivity and specificity are different in different types of samples, e.g., suspensions or FFPE tissues. A brief overview of probe sensitivity and specificity determination, based on ACMG and CLSI recommendations [8, 10], is summarized in Fig. 3. During the initial step of probe validation, probe sensitivity and specificity should be measured for the type of sample on which the assay will be used, and the results should be documented for inspection purposes. If a probe does not achieve a minimum sensitivity of 95% and specificity of 98%, the preparation of the samples and/or the FISH protocol should be optimized. Probe sensitivity and specificity must be remeasured after optimization. If the above-mentioned probe sensitivity and specificity requirements are not met after remeasurement, the FISH test should not be introduced into clinical use.

2.5 Cross-Hybridization and Contamination Issues

Any possible cross-hybridization inherent to a probe, as well as contaminations with other DNA sequences, should be identified and documented. Examine metaphases using the signal colocalization method described in Subheading 2.3 should be simple and effective. Probes with significant cross-hybridization or contamination should not be used.

2.6 Reproducibility

Intra- and inter-assay reproducibility should be demonstrated and documented in at least three samples. Intra-assay reproducibility can be achieved by testing triplicates of three or more samples on a single day. Inter-assay reproducibility can be done by testing duplicates of 3 or more samples on 2 different days. Variation of the results should not exceed 5%.

2.7 Establishment of FISH Assay SOPs

Establishing and optimizing a SOP is very important to FISH probe validation, and the SOP should be strictly followed when dealing with different types of samples with special preparations. Qualified, accredited clinical laboratories must establish SOPs based on the laboratory FISH procedure used in-house or the FISH manufacturer's recommendations. SOPs vary depending on the source and type of the FISH probe and should include methods for the modification of prepared slides, pretreatment of the slides, denaturation conditions, probe hybridization, and post-wash in order to maximize signal intensity and minimize background noise. It is also necessary to check fluorescent imaging equipment to make sure all components are working properly, since incompatible fluorescent filter cubes, misaligned mercury light bulbs, and incorrect fluorescent microscope settings can all contribute to weak signaling for FISH assays. In some cases, the design of the probe or the method of fluorescent labeling contributes to weak signals.

2.8 Inclusion and Exclusion of Signal Patterns

Because there are currently no standardized criteria for signal pattern inclusion and exclusion, accredited laboratories—whether using manual signal quantitation or FISH spot-counting software—must set up criteria for evaluating signal patterns and frequencies when validating clinical FISH tests. Depending on the probe design, there is usually more than one signal pattern that is considered abnormal and/or indicative of a chromosome abnormality. For example, dual-color, dual-fusion probes can give either a single fusion signal or dual fusion signals, both of which could be counted as patterns positive for an abnormality. In a break-apart probe assay, either a separated red and green signal pattern or a single-color signal outside the gene of interest (caused by the deletion of the other color signal that is mapped to the region of the gene of interest) is considered positive. Twenty to 30 known-positive samples by another gold-standard test should be used to screen for different positive signal patterns and their frequencies. Rare signal patterns seen in less than 10% of the known-positive samples should be excluded from future signal quantitation.

2.9 Establishment of Quantitation Criteria

Quantitation criteria should be established for each clinical FISH assay during validation. Such criteria include the eligibility of cells for signal quantitation and the definition of positive and negative signal patterns. Clustered cells with too much overlap that interferes with signal quantitation should not be used. Validated positive and negative signal patterns should be specified on a FISH signal quantitation record sheet. Similar criteria should be established for FISH assays quantitated by automated FISH spot counters. The effectiveness of quantitation criteria could be evaluated by clinical sensitivity and specificity measurements.

2.10 Establishment of Analytical Sensitivity and Specificity

Analytical sensitivity and specificity evaluate the relationship between abnormal cells and abnormal signal patterns regardless of presence or absence of disease. Analytical sensitivity is defined as the percentage of cells with abnormal signal patterns that a FISH test reliably detects. Analytical specificity is defined as the percentage of cells with normal signal patterns that a FISH test identifies correctly. Analytical sensitivity and specificity should be no less than 95 % for a good FISH assay, although greater discriminatory power may be needed to distinguish mosaicism. The ACMG guidelines recommend the use of 200 unique genomic targets for analytical sensitivity and specificity establishment. Such unique genomic targets are defined as the same sequence from each of the separable metaphase chromatids that will hybridize with the unique sequence probe. By this definition, a metaphase has four unique genomic targets when the target sequence is away from the centromere and clearly separable. Fifty cells are required for this type of analysis. On the other hand, a metaphase has two unique genomic targets if the target sequence is located near the centromere that could result in two non-separable hybridization signals. Such analysis would require 100 cells instead (ACMG, E9.2.1.1). Cells should be from five chromosomally characterized individuals (Choosing aneuploidy cell lines can maximize the number of targets). Pooling of cells from these five individuals is acceptable as long as all cells have the same number of potential targets and comparable mitotic indices. If discordance is present, test the individual cell lines separately. All internal validation data should be fully documented.

3 Clinical Validation of FISH Assays

3.1 Use of Controls

Standard control probes or samples should be used to detect errors or technical failures during the three phases of the clinical validation process. The goal in the pre-analytic phase is to determine whether the correct probe was used; the goal in the analytic phase is to verify that the counting criteria are followed correctly; and the goal in the post-analytic phase is to determine whether the assay's performance is satisfactory. Qualitative FISH tests are used in most nonmosaic situations, while quantitative FISH tests are designed to evaluate tumor burden or levels of mosaicism. Different control strategies should be considered for qualitative and quantitative FISH tests. Positive samples are useful as quality control indices during the clinical validation phase, and untreated patient samples are preferred because the percentage of abnormal cells may drop below the defined threshold level after treatment. It is also helpful to use control samples with different concentrations of positive cells in order to ensure the analytical sensitivity of quantitative FISH tests. Commercial, chromosome-specific, centromeric, or telomeric probes are commonly used as control probes for home-brewed, loci-specific probes either on the same or on different chromosomes. A common source of control samples is extra sampling materials, such as positive cell pellets in fixative and cell lines that are positive for the tested abnormalities [12]. Known positive or negative samples are confirmed by other testing to be with or without a particular genetic abnormality. FISH probe validation should include at least one positive sample during the process of technical specification assessment. Negative samples used for clinical validation should be confirmed by other tests as being truly negative for the abnormality that the FISH probe is meant to detect.

3.2 Clinical Sensitivity and Specificity

Clinical sensitivity and specificity evaluate the relationship between disease status and a positive FISH test. Clinical sensitivity is defined as the percentage of positive cases that a FISH test identifies and that are confirmed as positive by a gold standard test. Clinical specificity is defined as the percentage of negative cases that a FISH test identifies and that are confirmed to be free of disease by a gold standard test. Gold standard tests useful in clinical validations of FISH tests include pathologic evaluations or, in the case of many genetic disorders, G-band karyotyping. A gold standard test that is a validated alternative method of confirming positive and negative cases—performed either in the same laboratory or in a reference laboratory—should be used on the same set of samples for comparison. For example, if immunohistochemistry (IHC) staining is used as an alternative validation method, a positive FISH test should correspond to a positive IHC staining test. Criteria for concordance should be maintained as a part of the laboratory's validation records, and the degree of concordance between the two methods should be documented. Any major changes to or modifications of SOPs warrant revalidation of the assay (Fig. 4). Hajdinjak's evaluation of clinical sensitivity and specificity using the UroVysion FISH probe kit for bladder cancer provides a good model of FISH test validation [13]. In addition, clinical studies supporting the validity of FISH assays and published in peer-reviewed journals can be very helpful in this regard.

3.3 Determination of Reference Ranges

Determining a reference range for interphase FISH assays is necessary for both constitutional and acquired abnormalities. The reference range is defined as the range of FISH test values in 95% of individuals who are free of the genetic condition relevant to the FISH test [14]. Healthy individuals should be recruited and tested

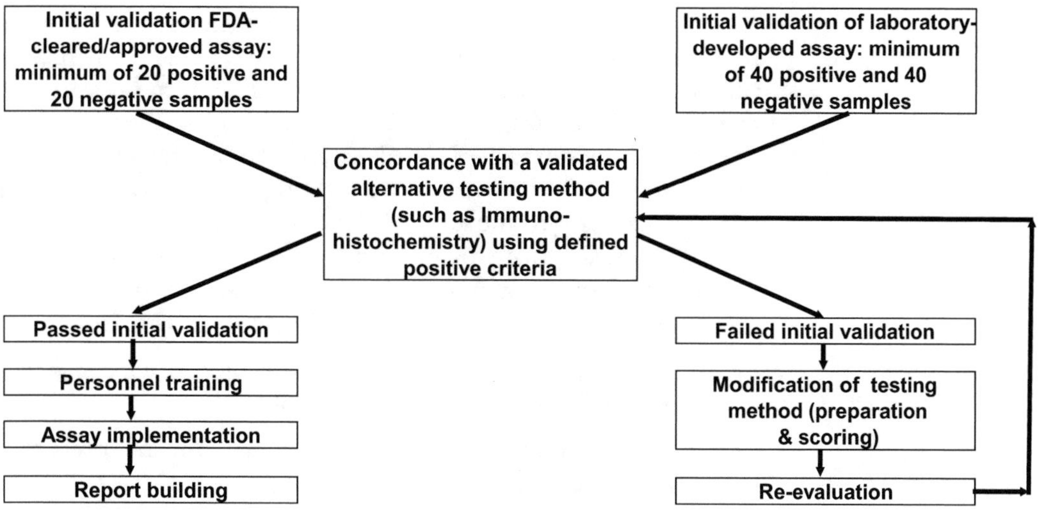

Fig. 4 Formalin-fixed paraffin-embedded tissue assay validation flowchart

to determine the appropriate reference range, and a database should be developed to store this information. Based on the CLSI's recommendations (CLSI 8,4.3), samples should be collected from at least 20 individuals without the clinical condition the FISH test is intended to diagnose. Based on the design of the FISH probe, all anticipated signal patterns should be sorted into either positive or negative signal pattern groups. Single and double fusions, break-apart signals, and gains and losses of individual probe signals within critical regions should be counted as positive signal patterns. A minimum of 200 suspension-harvested interphase cells per sample should be tested when validating FISH assays intended to detect acquired or mosaic abnormalities, and this number may be reduced to 50 interphase cells for FISH assays intended to detect constitutional microdeletions or microduplications. Samples that meet the established FISH scoring criteria should be stored in a database of reference ranges. Database samples should be tested in the same manner that will be used for patient samples [10]. A 95 % confidence interval should be calculated for each probe signal pattern in the database. Samples that do not meet the established FISH-testing criteria should not be included in the database.

3.4 Establishing Normal Cutoff Values

When used to test normal samples, interphase FISH probes may identify cells with abnormal signal patterns. Specifically, a small percentage of cells with a single fusion signal pattern may be observed in a normal sample due to the random overlapping of two different color signals. Because of the possibility of such false-positive results, establishing normal cutoff values is an essential step in validating quantitative interphase FISH assays. The normal cutoff value is defined as the maximum number of interphase cells with an abnormal signal pattern observed in a normal sample. Cutoff values must be established for each signal pattern and tissue type unless it can be proven that there is no significant difference between the data sets obtained from the different sample types. Tests based on the ratio of the number of signals discovered by one probe to the number of signals discovered by a second probe—such as ratio of erb-b2 receptor tyrosine kinase 2 (*ERBB2*) signals to centromeric 17 signals, when both probes were tested on either FFPE or non-FFPE tissues—do not need to have multiple cutoff values.

Steps for establishing normal cutoff values are as follows:

1. Set up a database by creating a spreadsheet (such as the Microsoft Excel example shown in Table 2).
2. Collect 20–30 karyotypically normal samples for the database.
3. Perform FISH testing.
4. For each sample, 2 technologists analyze half of the sample each.
5. Enter data into the spreadsheet.
6. For each abnormal signal pattern, identify the sample with the greatest number of false-positive cells.
7. For each abnormal signal pattern, calculate the normal cutoff values using the statistical method of your choice.

The ACMG recommends using 500 nuclei from each of 20 normal samples (total 10,000 nuclei) for most interphase FISH validation studies. In our validation study described in Table 2, we demonstrated the use of 200 nuclei from each of 64 karyotypically normal individuals (unpublished data using more than 10,000 nuclei). Our data indicated that the greatest number of false-positive cells [7] was found in sample 8 (Lab ID: FISH10-008), which showed the greatest variation within a single fusion signal pattern (1O1G1F) when compared to double-fusion patterns (1O1G2F). Gaussian distributions, inverse beta functions, and binomial distributions are among the most frequently used methods of calculating normal cutoff values [4, 15–17]. Although there is no consensus on the ideal method of calculating the normal cutoff value, it is widely agreed that most interphase FISH test data follow a binomial distribution [4]. Theoretically the most accurate method for FISH tests cutoff value determination should be the binomial treatment of the data, which could be done using Microsoft Excel's CRITBINOM function (*n*,*p*,*pr*), where *n* = the number of cells scored from each sample, *p* = the probability of a positive cell, and *pr* = 0.95 (the confidence limit). An example of normal cutoff values calculated by Microsoft Excel's CRITBINOM function (*n*,*p*,*pr*) for single fusion signal pattern is demonstrated in Table 2. As Ciolino suggested, FISH data can also be treated as a Gaussian distribution when the DeMoivre-Laplace Theorem is

Table 2
Build a spread sheet for cutoff values determination using BETAINV & CRITBINOM function

			Type of sample	# Cells	2 0	1 0, 1 G	1 0, 1 G	3 0	2 0	Cyto	Techs	Date
#	Lab ID	Indication		Scored	2 G	1 Fusion	2 Fusion	2 G	3 G	Results		
1	FISH10-0001	Anemia	BM	200	192	5	0	2	1	46,XX[20]	TECH1/TECH2	Apr-10
2	FISH10-0002	Thrombocytopenia	BM	200	196	1	0	1	2	46,XX[20]	TECH1/TECH2	Apr-10
3	FISH10-0003	Pancytopenia	BM	200	195	4	0	0	1	46,XX[20]	TECH1/TECH2	Apr-10
4	FISH10-0004	Thrombocytopenia	BM	200	197	2	0	0	1	46,XY[20]	TECH1/TECH2	Apr-10
5	FISH10-0005	Thrombocytopenia	BM	200	196	3	0	1	0	46,XX[20]	TECH1/TECH2	Apr-10
6	FISH10-0006	Anemia	BM	200	193	6	0	0	1	46,XY[20]	TECH1/TECH2	Apr-10
7	FISH10-0007	Pancytopenia	BM	200	193	4	0	0	4	46,XY[20]	TECH1/TECH2	Apr-10
8	FISH10-0008	Neutropenia	BM	200	192	7	0	1	1	46,XX[20]	TECH1/TECH2	Apr-10
9	FISH10-0009	Eosinophilia	BM	200	195	5	0	0	0	46,XY[20]	TECH1/TECH2	Apr-10
57	FISH11-0018	Anemia	BM	200	197	3	0	0	0	46,XY[20]	TECH3/TECH4	May-11
58	FISH11-0019	Anemia	BM	200	193	3	0	1	3	46,XY[20]	TECH3/TECH4	May-11
59	FISH11-0020	Thrombocytopenia	BM	200	196	3	0	0	1	46,XX[20]	TECH3/TECH4	May-11
60	FISH11-0021	Thrombocytopenia	BM	200	196	3	0	0	1	46,XX[20]	TECH3/TECH4	Jun-11
61	FISH11-0022	Pancytopenia	BM	200	196	4	0	0	0	46,XY[20]	TECH3/TECH4	Jun-11
62	FISH11-0023	Anemia	BM	200	195	3	0	1	1	46,XY[20]	TECH3/TECH4	Jun-11

(continued)

Table 2
(Continued)

#	Lab ID	Indication	Type of sample	# Cells Scored	2 O 2 G	1 O, 1 G 1 Fusion	1 O, 1 G 2 Fusion	3 O 2 G	2 O 3 G	Cyto Results	Techs	Date
63	FISH11-0024	Increased WBC	BM	200	196	2	0	1	1	46,XX[20]	TECH3/TECH4	Jul-11
64	FISH11-0025	Pancytopenia	BM	200	195	4	0	0	1	46,XX[20]	TECH3/TECH4	Jul-11
			Total	12,800	12,456	232	0	39	73			
				$p=232/12,800=0.018$								
		Maximum number of false-positive cells				7	0	2	4			
		pr (one-sided confidence level)				0.95	0.95	0.95	0.95			
		α (Max. # of false-positive cells + 1)				8	1	3	5			
		β (# of cells analyzed)				200	200	200	200			
		BETAINV(pr,α,β)				0.0626[a]	0.0149	0.0308	0.0443			
		CRITBINOM(n,p,pr) = CRITBINOM (200,0.018,0.95)				14[b]						

[a]Using BETAINV function, a sample contains more than 6% of cells with single fusion is considered as positive.
[b]Using CRITBINOM function, a sample contains more than 14 cells with single fusion out of 200 cells counted is considered as positive.

applied [17]. In such an instance, the Gaussian distribution approximates a binomial distribution when the number of cells scored from each sample (n) is large enough and the number of cells scored times the probability of a single fusion signal ($n \times p$) is significantly larger than one [18]. For example, using the data in Table 2, one could easily calculate the mean and standard deviation (SD) needed for the determination of the cutoff value. In this illustration, the cutoff value could be set at a SD of 1.65 times above the mean, based on a one-sided confidence limit of 95 %. Table 3 is an example of normal cutoff values calculated by Microsoft Excel's BETAINV function (pr,α,β), where $pr=0.95$, $\alpha=$the maximum

Table 3
Normal cutoff value table calculated by BETAINV function assumed a binomial distribution[a]

Maximum number of false-positive cells	Number of cells counted						
	50	100	200	300	400	500	5000
0	5.816%	2.951%	1.487%	0.994%	0.746%	0.597%	0.060%
1	8.967%	4.611%	2.338%	1.566%	1.178%	0.943%	0.095%
2	11.617%	6.044%	3.084%	2.070%	1.558%	1.249%	0.126%
3	13.985%	7.356%	3.775%	2.539%	1.913%	1.534%	0.155%
4	16.154%	8.585%	4.431%	2.986%	2.251%	1.807%	0.183%
5	18.169%	9.751%	5.060%	3.416%	2.578%	2.070%	0.210%
6	20.055%	10.866%	5.667%	3.833%	2.896%	2.327%	0.236%
7	21.832%	11.936%	6.258%	4.240%	3.206%	2.578%	0.262%
8	23.514%	12.968%	6.833%	4.638%	3.510%	2.823%	0.288%
9	25.110%	13.966%	7.394%	5.027%	3.808%	3.065%	0.313%
10	26.629%	14.932%	7.943%	5.410%	4.102%	3.303%	0.338%
11	28.079%	15.870%	8.482%	5.787%	4.391%	3.538%	0.363%
12	29.465%	16.781%	9.010%	6.157%	4.676%	3.770%	0.388%
13	30.792%	17.667%	9.529%	6.522%	4.958%	3.999%	0.412%
14	32.065%	18.531%	10.038%	6.883%	5.236%	4.225%	0.436%
15	33.287%	19.372%	10.540%	7.238%	5.511%	4.450%	0.460%
16	34.463%	20.193%	11.033%	7.589%	5.783%	4.672%	0.484%
17	35.594%	20.994%	11.519%	7.936%	6.052%	4.892%	0.508%
18	36.684%	21.777%	11.998%	8.278%	6.319%	5.110%	0.531%
19	37.735%	22.542%	12.470%	8.617%	6.583%	5.326%	0.555%

[a]BETAINV(pr,α,β) where $pr=0.95$, $\alpha=$Max. # of false-positive cells + 1, and $\beta=$# of cells counted (assume # of cells counted is much bigger than the # of false-positive cells in a sample)

number of false-positive cells + 1, and β = the number of cells analyzed (assuming that the number of cells analyzed is much bigger than the number of false-positive cells in a sample). The BETAINV function can be problematic as a means of determining double-fusion reference ranges because false-positive double-fusion signal patterns usually are not presented in samples from normal individuals [19]. For this reason, the probability of finding double-fusion signal patterns in normal samples, as calculated using the BETAINV function, might not be as accurate as anticipated. It should be emphasized that the cutoff value is an arbitrary estimate that could lead to either false-positive or false-negative results, so borderline-positive interphase FISH tests should be interpreted with caution. Once the cutoff value has been established, more normal and abnormal cases should be assessed to ensure that they fall within the correct range. There should also be a continuous quality-monitoring mechanism in place to ensure the established cutoff value is still applicable as recommended by ACMG.

3.5 Implementing FISH Assays

FISH assays should be implemented only after they have been validated and the laboratory procedure manual has been updated. Assay performance, such as clinical sensitivity and specificity, should be evaluated periodically for quality assurance purposes.

3.5.1 Training Technologists

All technologists who will perform the FISH assay should be trained on how to handle and prepare specimens, perform FISH hybridizations and post washes, quantitate FISH signals, and prepare results for reporting. Technologists should pass a competency test before performing these tasks independently. Interpersonal scoring variations for tests conducted on the same sample should not exceed 5 %. Any competency test failures require further investigation, and the technologists' reasons for failure should be documented. Re-training may be necessary.

3.5.2 Building Reports

Report templates should be built into the laboratory information system (LIS) for each validated FISH test. Reports should include brief descriptions of specimen collection, quality assessments, sample preparations, quantitation methods, reference ranges, and cutoff values. Use the International System for Human Cytogenomic Nomenclature (ISCN) to report results and provide explanations. Be sure to include standardized disclaimers at the end of the report according to FDA regulations and to check the accuracy of all Current Procedural Terminology (CPT) codes for technical and professional charges. Any modifications of the original reports in the LIS system should be reflected in an addendum report.

3.5.3 Conducting Ongoing Verifications of the Test System

To meet the ACMG's requirement for continuous monitoring of quality, perform and document biannual FISH test calibrations to maintain a high quality level. Periodic testing of known normal or abnormal samples should be included in the assay monitoring process. The sensitivity and specificity of each new lot of samples must be equal to or better than those of the previous lot. Any quality issues causing out-of-reportable-range results are subject to immediate investigation and correction. Additional normal samples should be tested and added to the normal database over time, especially in the event of equipment or staff changes [8]. Finally, having professional statisticians continually assess the normal database's distribution of samples is not required by any regulation or guideline, but including this step is useful in determining when adjustments to cutoff values and reference ranges are needed.

Acknowledgement

We thank Laura L. Russell, Scientific Editor at the Department of Scientific Publications, the University of Texas MD Anderson Cancer Center for her excellent editorial assistance.

References

1. FDA (1996) Federal register. http://www.federalregister.gov/agencies/food-and-drug-administration. Accessed 6 Jan 2016
2. American College of Medical Genetics (1993) Prenatal interphase fluorescence in situ hybridization (FISH) policy statement. Am J Hum Genet 53(2):526–527
3. Schad CR, Dewald GW (1995) Building a new clinical test for fluorescence in situ hybridization. Appl Cytogenet 21:1–4
4. Wiktor AE, Van Dyke DL, Stupca PJ et al (2006) Preclinical validation of fluorescence in situ hybridization assays for clinical practice. Genet Med 8(1):16–23. doi:10.109701.gim.0000195645.00446.61
5. American College of Medical Genetics (2000) Technical and clinical assessment of fluorescence in situ hybridization: an ACMG/ASHG position statement. I. Technical considerations. Genet Med 2(6):356–361
6. Wolff DJ, Bagg A, Cooley LD et al (2007) Guidance for fluorescence in situ hybridization testing in hematologic disorders. J Mol Diagn 9(2):134–143. doi:10.2353/jmoldx.2007.060128
7. Saxe DF, Persons DL, Wolff DJ et al (2012) Validation of fluorescence in situ hybridization using an analyte-specific reagent for detection of abnormalities involving the mixed lineage leukemia gene. Arch Pathol Lab Med 136(1):47–52. doi:10.5858/arpa.2010-0645-SA
8. Mascarello JT, Hirsch B, Kearney HM et al (2011) Technical standards and guidelines: fluorescence in situ hybridization. Genet Med 13(7):667–675. doi:10.1097/GIM.0b013e3182227295
9. National Committee for Clinical Laboratory Standards (NCCLS) (2004) Fluorescence In Situ Hybridization Methods for Medical Genetics: Approved Guideline. NCCLS Document MM7-A. [ISBN1-56238-524-0]. NCCLS, 940 West Valley Road, Suite 1400, Wayne, Pennsylvania 19087–1898 USA
10. Clinical and Laboratory Standards Institute (CLSI) (2013) Fluorescence In Situ Hybridization Methods for Clinical Laboratories; Approved Guideline—Second Edition. CLSI document MM07-A2 [ISBN 1-56238-885-1] Clinical and Laboratory Standards Institute, 940 West Valley Road, Suite 2500, Wayne, Pennsylvania 19087-1898 USA
11. Zhao L, Hayes K, Glassman A (1998) A simple efficient method of sequential G-banding and fluorescence in situ hybridization. Cancer Genet Cytogenet 103(1):62–64
12. Stupca PJ, Meyer RG, Dewald GW (2005) Using controls for molecular cytogenetic testing in clinical practice. J Assoc Genet Technol 31(1):4–8
13. Hajdinjak T (2008) UroVysion FISH test for detecting urothelial cancers: meta-analysis of diagnostic accuracy and comparison with

urinary cytology testing. Urol Oncol 26(6): 646–651.doi:10.1016/j.urolonc.2007.06.002

14. Kearney HM, Thorland EC, Brown KK et al (2011) American College of Medical Genetics standards and guidelines for interpretation and reporting of postnatal constitutional copy number variants. Genet Med 13(7):680–685. doi:10.1097/GIM.0b013e3182217a3a
15. Dewald G, Stallard R, Alsaadi A et al (2000) A multicenter investigation with D-FISH BCR/ABL1 probes. Cancer Genet Cytogenet 116(2):97–104
16. Thall PF, Jacoby D, Zimmerman SO (1996) Estimating genomic category probabilities from fluorescent in situ hybridization counts with misclassification. J R Stat Soc C-Appl 45(4):431–446
17. Ciolino AL, Tang ME, Bryant R (2009) Statistical treatment of fluorescence in situ hybridization validation data to generate normal reference ranges using Excel functions. J Mol Diagn 11(4):330–333. doi:10.2353/jmoldx.2009.080101
18. Papoulis A (1980) Citation classic – probability, random-variables, and stochastic-processes. Cc/Eng Tech Appl Sci 19:14
19. Dewald GW, Wyatt WA, Juneau AL et al (1998) Highly sensitive fluorescence in situ hybridization method to detect double BCR/ABL fusion and monitor response to therapy in chronic myeloid leukemia. Blood 91(9):3357–3365

Chapter 11

Fluorescence In Situ Hybridization on Tissue Sections

Alvin S.T. Lim and Tse Hui Lim

Abstract

Formalin-fixed paraffin-embedded (FFPE) tissues are typically the specimens available for FISH analysis of solid tissues, particularly of tumor specimens. Occasionally, tissue cores constructed as tissue microarrays from several patients are presented for simultaneous evaluation. FFPE sections can also be prepared from cell blocks derived from cell suspensions. The interphase fluorescence in situ hybridization assay employs specific nucleic acid sequences (probes) that target complementary sequences of interest to detect gains or losses of genes/gene loci or a fusion gene within the tissue. In this chapter, we describe the protocols utilized in our laboratory and include slide deparaffinization, pretreatment, protease treatment, hybridization, washing, and counterstaining. This protocol can be applied to all of the earlier FFPE preparations. In general, the assay takes 3 consecutive days to complete, although a more rapid assay can be performed.

Key words Formalin-fixed paraffin-embedded tissues, Fluorescence in situ hybridization, Probes

1 Introduction

Tissue specimens retrieved for histology purposes can typically be preserved either as formalin-fixed paraffin-embedded (FFPE) tissues or as frozen tissues. Both preparations can preserve specimen integrity well and have their particular advantages and disadvantages. For the most part, FFPE preparations are much more widely utilized because of its convenience, cost effectiveness, and superior morphology. The tissues need to be preserved in 10% neutral-buffered formalin (NBF), and in particular for *ERBB2* detection, be fixed for between 6 and 72 h and the cold ischemia time (the time between specimen removal from the body and tissue fixation) is recommended to be <1 h [1, 2]. A delay may result in tissue decay and autolysis, which may affect the quality of the fluorescence in situ hybridization (FISH) signals [3]. The tissues are then dehydrated and embedded in paraffin wax into a paraffin block. Microtome sections of 4–5 μm thickness are then made and these sections are mounted onto positively charged slides for subsequent investigations with various stains and other DNA tests. NBF

Thomas S.K. Wan (ed.), *Cancer Cytogenetics: Methods and Protocols*, Methods in Molecular Biology, vol. 1541,
DOI 10.1007/978-1-4939-6703-2_11, © Springer Science+Business Media LLC 2017

fixation is appropriate because the induced protein–protein and protein–nucleic acid cross-links have a high efficacy for tissue preservation and preservation of the tissue architecture [4]. However, progressive formation of cross-linking network leads to a loss of probe accessibility to the intended target, high background autofluorescence, truncated nuclei, overlapping cells, and a low level hybridization efficiency, therein the importance of avoiding overfixation through prolonged exposure to formalin [5]. The pre-treatment steps described in this chapter are essential to circumventing much of these problems. Because of tumor heterogeneity, it is imperative that a pathologist marks out the tumor regions on the unstained sections/biopsies, or an accompanying hematoxylin and eosin (H&E) slide with the tumor region circumscribed is made available to the laboratory, so that the FISH probes are applied solely to tumor regions on the unstained slide and the analysis is performed only within this region.

2 Materials

Prepare working solutions using ultrapure water (prepared by purifying deionized water to attain a sensitivity of 18 MΩcm with the total oxidizable carbon ≤5 ppb). Prepare and store all reagents at room temperature (unless otherwise indicated). Disposal of all waste materials should follow the waste disposal regulations and reagents are handled according to the Material Safety Data Sheet.

2.1 Slide Deparaffinization

1. Xylene (*see* **Note 1**).
2. Ethanol: Absolute ≥99.5 % (*see* **Note 2**).
3. Laboratory heating slide warmer.
4. Diamond-tipped glass scribe.
5. Metal forceps.

2.2 Pretreatment

1. 0.2 N HCl (*see* **Note 3**).
2. 20× saline sodium citrate (SSC): 3 M NaCl, 0.3 M sodium citrate, pH5.3 (*see* **Note 4**).
3. 2× SCC: Dilute 20× SSC by mixing 100 mL of 20× SSC with 900 mL of purified water. Store in a 1-L glass bottle.
4. 1 M sodium thiocyanate (*see* **Note 5**).
5. Water bath at 80 ± 1 °C.
6. Coplin jars.

2.3 Protease Treatment

1. 0.5 % protease (pepsin with activity range of 1:3000–1:3500) (*see* **Note 6**).
2. Protease buffer: 0.01 N HCl (*see* **Note 7**).
3. Light-proof box (*see* **Note 8**).

4. Water bath at 45 ± 1 °C.
5. 2× SSC: Dilute 20× SSC by mixing 100 mL of 20× SSC with 900 mL of purified water. Store in a 1-L glass bottle.
6. Ethanol: 70, 85 % and absolute ≥99.5 % (*see* **Note 9**).
7. Coplin jars.

2.4 Hybridization

1. Microscope slide glass coverslip (*see* **Note 10**).
2. Microcentrifuge.
3. Rubber cement.
4. Automated slide thermal cycler (*see* **Note 11**).
5. Metal forceps.

2.5 Washing

1. Posthybridization wash buffer: 2× SSC, 0.1 % Igepal CA-630 (*see* **Note 12**).
2. Water bath at 75 ± 1 °C.
3. Glass coplin jars.
4. Metal forceps.
5. Digital timer.

2.6 Counterstaining

1. Antifade mounting medium with 4′,6-diamidino-2-phenylindole (DAPI).
2. Metal forceps.
3. Nail vanish.
4. Microscope slide box with lid or slide folders.

3 Methods

Carry out all procedures at room temperature or otherwise specified.

3.1 Slide Deparaffinization

For optimal FISH assays, the tissues are fixed in 10% neutral-buffered formalin with the fixation duration ranging from 6 to 72 h. Avoid exposing the specimens to strong acids (decalcifying agents), strong bases, and extreme heat as such conditions can lead to damaged DNA resulting in FISH failures. The tissue sections should be about 5 ± 1 μm thick and be mounted on positively charged glass slides. Inappropriate glass slides can result in tissue loss. For each FISH assay, at least 2 paraffin section-mounted slides are needed in case a repeat hybridization is required.

1. Bake the FFPE sections overnight at 56 °C on a slide warmer. Insufficient baking can result in tissue loss or degraded tissue morphology.

2. Immerse the slide in the first coplin jar containing xylene for 10 min at room temperature (*see* **Note 13**).
3. Repeat this step twice using xylene each time.
4. Dehydrate the slide in absolute ethanol for 10 min at room temperature.
5. Air dry the slide (*see* **Note 14**) and mark the intended targeted area with a diamond-tipped glass scribe pen on the underside of the slide.

3.2 Slide Pretreatment

1. Immerse the slide in a coplin jar containing 0.2 N HCl for 20 min.
2. Immerse the slide in a coplin jar containing purified water for 3 min.
3. Immerse the slide in a coplin jar containing 2× SSC for 3 min.
4. Immerse the slide in a glass coplin jar containing 1 M sodium thiocyanate at 80 °C for 30 min (*see* **Note 15**).
5. Immerse the slide in a coplin jar containing purified water for 1 min.
6. Immerse the slide in a coplin jar containing 2× SSC for 10 min.

3.3 Protease Treatment

1. Remove the slide and blot off the excess buffer on a paper towel.
2. Add a few drops of protease solution to the tissue section using a plastic pasteur pipette and seal with a plastic paraffin film.
3. Place the slide in a humidified box at 45 °C and incubate for 1 to 2 h (*see* **Note 16**).
4. Immerse the slide in a coplin jar containing 2× SSC for 10 min.
5. Dehydrate the slide through an ethanol series (70, 85, 100% approximately 40 mL in each coplin jar) for 1 min in each jar. Air dry or blow dry the slide.

3.4 Hybridization

1. Vortex the vial containing the probe mixture and pulse spin the vial with a microcentrifuge.
2. Apply 1–3 μL of probe mixture to the slide and overlay with a glass coverslip (*see* **Note 10**). Ensure no air bubbles are trapped under the coverslip (*see* **Note 17**).
3. Seal the edges of the coverslip with rubber cement.
4. Program the automated slide thermal cycler by setting the denaturation temperature at 80 °C for 4 min, followed by hybridization temperature at 37 °C for up to 16 h. Start the hybridization program after placing the slide on the instrument.

3.5 Slide Washing

1. Pour 50 mL of the posthybridization wash buffer into a glass coplin jar and place it inside a water bath. Cover the jar with the lid. Allow the jar to warm up from room temperature to 75 °C. The water level in the water bath should be above the level of the wash solution in the jar.
2. Prepare another coplin jar containing posthybridization wash buffer at room temperature.
3. When the water bath has reached its set temperature, carefully remove the slide from the slide thermal cycler. Peel off the rubber cement from the coverslip with a pair of forceps. Wet the slide by dipping it briefly in the posthybridization wash buffer at room temperature. Remove the coverslip by gently sliding it off the slide to avoid damaging the tissue. Do not allow the slide to dry until washing is completed.
4. Place the slide into the coplin jar containing posthybridization wash buffer at 75 °C and gently agitate for 1–3 s. Replace the lid. Remove the slide after 1–2 min and then transfer the slide to the second coplin jar containing posthybridization wash buffer for 1 min. Discard the wash solution after use.
5. Remove the slide and air dry or blow dry under dim lighting at room temperature.

3.6 Counterstaining

1. Apply approximately 10 μL of DAPI counterstain and mount a 22 mm × 22 mm glass coverslip over the hybridization area.
2. Seal with nail varnish and allow the sealant to dry completely.
3. Place the slide in a light-proof box. Perform analysis with an epi-illumination fluorescence microscope using appropriate filter sets.
4. Store the hybridized slide at 4 °C or −20 °C, protected from light.

4 Notes

1. Use a glass coplin jar to hold the xylene solution. Prepare three coplin jars of xylene prior to deparaffinization and label the jars according to the sequence of use. After use, close the jar with the glass cover and wrap with paraffin film. Keep the jars inside a fume hood. The xylene solution can be reused several times until the solution becomes cloudy with excessive use. An alternative clearing agent is Hemo-De solution.
2. Use a plastic coplin jar to hold the ethanol. Keep the jar inside a fume hood with the lid tightly screwed on. The ethanol can be reused up to 2 weeks until the solution becomes diluted or cloudy due to excessive use.

3. Dilute 1 N HCl solution to 0.2 N HCl by mixing 200 mL of 1 N HCl with 800 mL of purified water. Store the reagent in a glass bottle at room temperature. Discard the working 0.2 N HCl solution after each use.
4. To prepare the 20× SSC, weigh 175.3 g of NaCl and 88.2 g of trisodium citrate, mix thoroughly and make it to 1 L with purified water. Adjust pH to 5.3 with HCl.
5. Dilute 8 M sodium thiocyanate solution (pH 5–8) to a working solution of 1 M by diluting 100 mL of 8 M sodium thiocyanate with 700 mL of purified water. Store the working solution at 4 °C. Discard the solution after use.
6. Dissolve 250 mg of protease in 50 mL of protease buffer. Aliquot 1 mL of protease solution into microcentrifuge tubes. Store the aliquots at −20 °C. Do not thaw and freeze the solution repeatedly.
7. To prepare the protease buffer, dilute 2.5 mL of 0.2 N HCl in 47.5 mL of purified water.
8. Line any light-proof box with a moist tissue and cover the box tightly after placing the slide inside. Let the box float inside the water bath that is set at 45 °C.
9. To prepare 70% ethanol, mix 350 mL of absolute ethanol with 150 mL of purified water. To prepare 85% ethanol, mix 425 mL of absolute ethanol with 75 mL of purified water. Store the solution in tightly capped glass bottles. Aliquot the solution into plastic coplin jars. The volume should be sufficient to cover the tissue sections. Store the solution in tightly capped coplin jars at 4 °C to minimize evaporation. The ethanol solution can be reused for up to 2 weeks until the solution becomes diluted or cloudy due to excessive use.
10. The size of the microscope slide glass coverslip used will depend on the area of the marked tumor region. This can range from a 12 mm round coverslip to a 22 mm × 22 mm square coverslip. The amount of probe to be applied will depend on the size of the coverslip. For a 12 mm round coverslip, 1 μL of probe will be sufficient. At least 3 μL of probe is required for a 22 mm × 22 mm coverslip. An insufficient amount of probe can result in weak signals or an uneven signal distribution.
11. An automated denaturation and hybridization system for slides is preferred as it provides consistent and reproducible heating temperatures with ease of use. Refer to the instrument operator manual for instructions on instrument use. Alternatively, a slide warmer with adjustable temperature settings can be used for denaturation followed by hybridization at 37 °C in an incubator.

12. Mix 100 mL of 20× SSC solution with 850 mL of purified water in a 1-L glass bottle. Add 1 mL of Igepal CA-630 and bring the volume up to 1 L with purified water. Let the solution stand overnight for the detergent to dissolve completely before use. Store the posthybridization wash solution at room temperature. Discard the wash solution after each use.
13. The coplin jars can easily accommodate up to eight slides each time when the slides are placed back to back. The solution must be sufficient to cover the tissue entirely.
14. To facilitate fast drying of the glass slide, a handheld blow dryer is preferred to air drying.
15. Over-pretreatment can result in tissue loss or degraded tissue morphology. Conversely, under-pretreatment can result in weak or no signals. The pretreatment time can be extended for sections that are thicker or sections that are over-fixed in formalin.
16. Inadequate protease digestion can result in weak or no signals. Conversely, protease overdigestion can lead to tissue loss or morphology degradation.
17. Air bubbles trapped under the glass coverslip can lead to uneven probe distribution which can cause signal intensity variation across the tissue section. Apply the coverslip by first touching the surface of the probe mixture with it and then using a pair of metal forceps to squeeze the air bubbles, if any, out of the coverslip by gently tapping on the coverslip.

References

1. Wolff AC, Hammond ME, Hicks DG et al (2007) American Society of Clinical Oncology/College of American Pathologists guideline recommendations for human epidermal growth factor receptor 2 testing in breast cancer. Arch Pathol Lab Med 131:18–43
2. Wolff AC, Hammond ME, Hicks DG et al (2013) Recommendations for human epidermal growth factor receptor 2 testing in breast cancer: American Society of Clinical Oncology/College of American Pathologists clinical practice guideline update. J Clin Oncol 31:3997–4013. doi:10.1200/JCO.2013.50.9984
3. Petersen BL, Sorensen MC, Pedersen S et al (2004) Fluorescence in situ hybridization on formalin-fixed and paraffin-embedded tissue: optimizing the method. Appl Immunohistochem Mol Morphol 12(3):259–265
4. Müller S, Matthiesen SH, Nielsen KV (2009) Preparation of FFPE tissue slides for solid tumor FISH analysis. In: Kumar GL, Rudbeck L (eds) Education guide. Immunohistochemical (IHC) staining methods, 5th edn. Dako North America, Carpinteria, CA
5. Sommerlad C, Mehraein Y, Giersberg M et al (2002) Formalin-fixed and paraffin-embedded tissue sections. In: Rautenstrauss BW, Liehr T (eds) FISH technology. Springer, Berlin, Heidelberg

Chapter 12

Cytoplasmic Immunoglobulin Light Chain Revelation and Interphase Fluorescence In Situ Hybridization in Myeloma

Sarah Moore, Jeffrey M. Suttle, and Mario Nicola

Abstract

The cytogenetic analysis of plasma cell myeloma (PCM) allows stratification of patients so that prognosis may be determined and appropriate therapeutic options can be discussed. Owing to the patchy nature of the disease in the bone marrow (BM), the low proliferative activity of plasma cells and the cryptic nature of some PCM-associated cytogenetic changes, karyotypic analysis in this disease should be augmented with targeted interphase fluorescence in situ hybridization (FISH). Immunofluorescent revelation of cytoplasmic immunoglobulin light chains, together with interphase FISH (cIg-FISH), allows the identification of plasma cells within a sample so that they may be scored preferentially. This is particularly useful in situations where there are only a small percentage of plasma cells in a sample. Where an underlying myeloid disease is suspected the cIg-FISH-negative cells can be scored separately. Two methods are provided in this chapter: the technique for cIg-FISH in fresh PCM BM samples and a procedure for use in fixed cytogenetics preparations.

Key words Plasma cell myeloma, Cytoplasmic light chains, Fluorescence in situ hybridization, cIg-FISH, Prognosis, Plasma cell

1 Introduction

Plasma cell myeloma (PCM) is an incurable malignancy characterized by the accumulation of monoclonal plasma cells and, in some patients, leads to cytopenias, bone resorption (lytic bone lesions, hypercalcemia), the production of a monoclonal protein (paraprotein), and renal impairment [1]. It has a heterogeneous clinical course with a corresponding range of genetic and other prognostic markers. PCM can advance from the premalignant condition of monoclonal gammopathy of undetermined significance (MGUS) in which the monoclonal protein is present, but there are <10% plasma cells in the bone marrow. End-organ damage is not evident in this stage. Frank PCM can also be preceded by smoldering myeloma (SM) and this is an indolent, asymptomatic form of the

Thomas S.K. Wan (ed.), *Cancer Cytogenetics: Methods and Protocols*, Methods in Molecular Biology, vol. 1541, DOI 10.1007/978-1-4939-6703-2_12, © Springer Science+Business Media LLC 2017

disease with 10–30% plasma cells in the bone marrow. In turn, PCM can evolve into an even more aggressive entity known as plasma cell leukemia (PCL) in which end-organ damage is evident and there are circulating malignant plasma cells.

PCM is an incurable disease with a mean survival of 3–4 years, but it is highly heterogeneous in that some patients die very early while others will remain alive up to 10 years later [1]. It is this large range in clinical outcomes that has driven the search for prognostic disease markers. These began with the Durie-Salmon system [2], which is mostly a measure of tumor burden and which considers the severity of anemia, calcium level, kidney function, presence or absence of bone lesions, and the quantity of abnormal proteins. It is a staging system and lacks prognostic strength. The International Staging System (ISS) [3] measured the peripheral blood (PB) β2-microglobulin and albumin levels and was revised (ISS-R) [4] to include acquired genetic changes in the risk assessment. These acquired changes remain the best indicator of disease aggressiveness despite their lack of consideration of constitutional genetic changes and other factors such as age and comorbidities [5–8].

The treatment for PCM is highly dependent on the stage of the disease and the risk stratification [9, 10]. For some elderly patients with advanced disease palliative care may be appropriate, while for others the aim is to prolong survival while maintaining quality of life. Unfortunately genomic studies of PCM are not straightforward; plasma cells are difficult to culture, perhaps because PCM is a malignancy affecting a more differentiated class of cells with a low proliferative rate, but also because plasma cells may die in culture. Particularly in the early stages of the disease the malignant plasma cells are anchorage dependent and rely on interaction with the bone marrow stroma and extracellular matrix [11]. Cytogenetic culture (i.e., without a 'feeder layer') often results in growth of only karyotypically normal cells. As the disease progresses plasma cells are less reliant on their environment, may switch on autocrine cytokine production or constitutive activation of signaling pathways, and are free to proliferate in a stromal-independent manner [11]. This latter situation is commonly associated with increased tumor burden, disease progression, and ability to give rise to karyotypic abnormalities in culture. To increase the number of patients in whom cytogenetic abnormalities are detectable at all stages of PCM it is necessary to examine nondividing cells and this is achievable by interphase FISH. Since the proportion of malignant plasma cells may be low (particularly in MGUS and SM) it is recommended [1, 12, 13] to use plasma cell selection, either real or virtual, prior to FISH analysis. Plasma cell selection may be undertaken by flow sorting or by bead separation, but these procedures are expensive and not available to most laboratories. Common to all malignant plasma cell populations is high surface expression of CD138 and cytoplasmic expression of Ig-Kappa or Ig-Lambda light chains. CD138 (Syndecan-1) may be a less useful marker since it is lost from the cells surface over time [14]. Cytoplasmic revelation of immunoglobulin light chains (by staining with goat anti-human kappa or lambda light chain conjugated with 7-amino-4-methylcoumarin-3-acetic acid (AMCA)), together with 2-color interphase FISH (cIg-FISH) allows the identification of plasma cells within a sample so that they may be scored preferentially [15–17]. Immunostaining can be enhanced by the application of a secondary anti-goat immunoglobulin also conjugated with AMCA.

Recommendations for the FISH probes to be used are made according to their demonstrated prognostic utility. To this end it is considered useful to use dual fusion translocation probes for MMSET: *IGH-FGFR3* to detect the cryptic t(4;14)(p16;q32) and *IGH-MAF* to detect t(14;16)(q32;q23); and deletion probes for *TP53* (del17p). These probe sets identify very high-risk genetic features. Laboratories are encouraged to add to these probe sets as is required with, for example, probes for hyperdiploid PCM (which would include an odd-numbered chromosome such as chromosome 15 or 19 with a probe for 5q) and a deletion 1p/gain 1q probe set for identifying changes associated with disease progression. The *IGH-CCND1* dual fusion translocation probes may also be considered since this translocation is seen in almost all cases of IgM PCM. It may also help to distinguish this type of PCM from lymphoplasmacytic leukemia (Waldenstrom's macroglobulinemia). Some laboratories use *IGH* break-apart probes to identify patients with *IGH* rearrangements and reflex to *IGH-FGFR3*, *IGH-MAF*, and *IGH-CCND1* in positive cases. This can provide cost savings in terms of probe use.

The cIg-negative cells can also be examined in the event that an underlying myeloid disease is suspected. Myelodysplastic syndrome can arise post-therapy for PCM [18] and demonstration of 5q- or 7q- in the cIg-negative cell population would be instructive.

The cIg-FISH utilizes immunofluorescence for the immunoglobulin light chains that are produced by B-cells. The two methods provided later are for different purposes. The first method incorporates the use of paraformaldehyde as a fixative. It is most useful when fresh PCM samples are received by the laboratory and can be preceded by a density gradient separation step to enrich for mononuclear cells (MNC). The MNC can then either be transferred to a microscope slide by cytospin or spread onto a slide in the manner of blood film preparation. This technique may be the more robust of the two methods.

The second method is applicable to cytogenetic preparations and it is recommended that an additional, preferably direct harvest is performed and set aside for this purpose. This technique fits well into the routine operation of a diagnostic cytogenetics laboratory.

These techniques have similar steps and an overview is provided in Fig. 1.

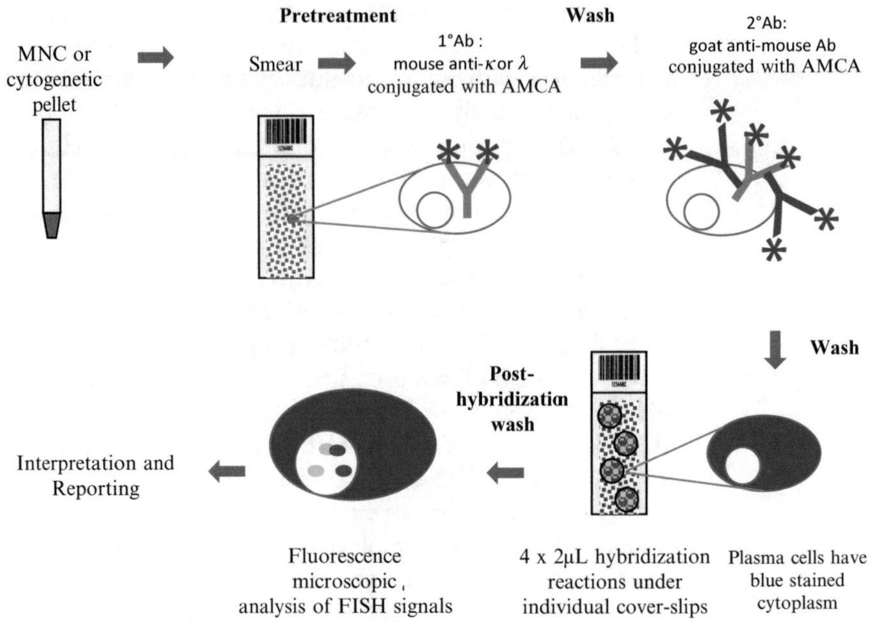

Fig. 1 Overview of the cIg-FISH procedure. A smear of cells is made on a microscope slide and pretreatments are performed as described in the method. Primary antibody (Ab) (mouse anti-k or λ conjugated with AMCA) is applied to stain the cytoplasmic immunoglobulin light chain. After washing steps the secondary Ab (goat anti-mouse Ab conjugated with AMCA) is applied and this amplifies staining. Multiple hybridizations can be performed on a single cell smear

2 Materials

Universal precautions should be used throughout the procedure and personal protective clothing (laboratory gown, safety glasses, and gloves) should be worn at all times. For all chemicals the material safety data sheet (MSDS) should be consulted and chemicals should be used under conditions appropriate to their possible harm. All solutions are made with reverse osmosis (RO) water (*see* **Note 1**).

2.1 cIg-FISH on Fresh Bone Marrow Samples

2.1.1 Slide Preparation

1. 10-mL sterile disposable pipettes.
2. Density gradient medium for the isolation of mononuclear cells.
3. SepMate 50-mL tube (Stemcell Technologies, Canada) (*see* **Note 2**).
4. 50-mL plastic centrifuge tubes.
5. 1× Phosphate buffered saline (PBS).
6. PBS/2 mM EDTA (pH 7.2), store at 2–8 °C.
7. Bench top centrifuge.
8. Glass microscope slides (*see* **Note 3**).

9. 95% ethanol: Add 50 mL RO water to 950 mL of 100% ethanol. Mix well store at room temperature in a stoppered bottle.
10. Phase contrast microscope.

2.1.2 cIg Light Chain Immunofluorescence

1. Three Coplin jars.
2. 2× Saline sodium citrate (SSC), pH 7–7.5.
3. 1× PBS.
4. NP40.
5. 1× PBD: 1× PBS (pH 7.2) and 0.1% NP40.
6. 1–10 μL air displacement pipette.
7. 20–100 μL air displacement pipette.
8. 22 mm × 50 mm coverslip.
9. Primary antibody (Ab):
   (a) AMCA anti-human Lambda chain (α-λ), store at 4–8 °C.
   (b) AMCA anti-human Kappa (α-k) chain, store at 4–8 °C.
10. Secondary Ab: AMCA anti-goat Ig (α-goat H+L), store at 4–8 °C.
11. Ab diluent: 1× PBS/1% bovine serum albumin/0.1% NP40. Sprinkle 1 g of BSA onto the surface of 100 mL of sterile PBS in a wide mouthed sterile bottle. Do not mix, but allow the BSA to soak into the PBS. Once fully dissolved adjust the pH to 7.2 and add 100 μL NP40. Warm slightly to aid mixing of the NP40 then store at 4–8 °C in 1 mL aliquots.
12. Humidified chamber: Place absorbent paper towel in the bottom of a lidded plastic container and just moisten it with 2× SSC (*see* **Note 4**).

2.1.3 Fixation and Permeabilization Prior to FISH

1. Seven Coplin jars.
2. 1× PBS.
3. NP40.
4. 1× PBD: 1× PBS (pH 7.2) and 0.1% NP40.
5. 2× SSC, pH 7–7.5.
6. 70% ethanol: Add 300 mL RO water to 700 mL of 100% ethanol. Mix well store at room temperature in a stoppered bottle.
7. 80% ethanol: Add 200 mL RO water to 800 mL of 100% ethanol. Mix well store at room temperature in a stoppered bottle.
8. Absolute (100%) ethanol. Stored at room temperature in a stoppered bottle.
9. Proteinase K: 20 μg/mL proteinase K in 2× SSC. Store in 500 μL aliquots at −20 °C.

10. 2% paraformaldehyde (PFA): Warm 450 mL of RO water with 10 drops of 2 M NaOH to 65–70 °C on a heating block with magnetic stirrer in a fume hood. Turn off heat, but continue stirring and add 10 g of PFA. Cool to room temperature and add 50 mL of 10× PBS. Store at −20 °C in 40 mL aliquots (*see* **Note 5**).
11. 22 mm × 50 mm coverslip.
12. Humidified chamber: Place absorbent paper towel in the bottom of a lidded plastic container and just moisten it with 2× SSC (*see* **Note 4**).

2.2 cIg-FISH on Carnoy-fixed Cytogenetic Preparations

2.2.1 Slide Preparation

1. Bench top centrifuge.
2. 10-mL polypropylene screw top centrifuge tubes.
3. 100% methanol.
4. 2-mL disposable plastic dropping pipettes.
5. Glass microscope slides (*see* **Note 3**).
6. Phase contrast microscope.
7. 96% ethanol: Add 40 mL of RO water to 960 mL of 100% ethanol. Mix well store at room temperature in a stoppered bottle.

2.2.2 Antigen Retrieval and cIg Light Chain Immunofluorescence

1. Six Coplin jars.
2. Antigen Retrieval Buffer (10 mM citrate buffer): Dissolve 1 g of citric acid and 1.45 g of trisodium citrate in 500 mL of water. Adjust pH to 6.0 with NaOH and make volume up to 1 L.
3. Water bath set to 95 °C.
4. 1× PBS.
5. 70% ethanol: Add 300 mL of RO water to 700 mL of 100% ethanol. Mix well store at room temperature in a stoppered bottle.
6. 80% ethanol: Add 200 mL of RO water to 800 mL of 100% ethanol. Mix well store at room temperature in a stoppered bottle.
7. 96% ethanol: Add 40 mL of RO water to 960 mL of 100% ethanol. Mix well store at room temperature in a stoppered bottle.
8. 1–10 μL air displacement pipette.
9. 20–100 μL air displacement pipette.
10. Primary Ab:

    AMCA anti-human Lambda chain (α-λ), store at 4–8 °C; AMCA anti-human Kappa (α-k) chain, store at 4–8 °C; Secondary Ab: AMCA anti-goat lg (H + L), store at 4–8 °C.

11. Humidified chamber: Place absorbent paper towel in the bottom of a lidded plastic container and just moisten it with 2× SSC (*see* **Note 4**).

2.3 FISH Hybridization and Washing for Both Methods

1. Two Coplin jars.
2. Fluorescently labeled commercially prepared probes, e.g., *IGH-FGFR3*, *IGH-MAF*, *TP53/D17Z1*, 1p/1q (*see* **Notes 6** and **7**).
3. Microfuge.
4. Solvent resistant marker pen.
5. 12 mm circular coverslip.
6. Fine-pointed forceps.
7. Rubber cement and nail polish.
8. 80 °C heating block and 37 °C humidified chamber OR FISH hybridizer.
9. Water bath set at 72 °C.
10. 0.4× SSC/0.3 % NP40 prewarmed to 72 ± 1 °C.
11. 2× SSC/0.1 % NP40.
12. Antifade solution without DAPI, store at 4–8 °C.

2.4 Analysis and Reporting for Both Methods

1. Fluorescence microscope equipped with appropriate filter sets (*see* **Note 8**), camera, and imaging software.
2. Immersion oil for fluorescence microscopy.
3. Laboratory recording sheets.

3 Methods

3.1 cIg-FISH on Fresh BM Samples

This method is NOT for cytogenetics preparations but is suitable for bone marrow that has been collected within 8 h. An advantage over the method given in Subheading 3.2 is that mononuclear cell selection will increase the percentage of plasma cells in the sample. The morphology of cells that have undergone this technique is shown in Fig. 2.

3.1.1 Preparation of Slides

1. Pipette 15 mL of density gradient medium into the central hole of the SepMate tube (*see* **Note 3**).
2. In a 50-mL centrifuge tube dilute fresh BM 1:2–4 with PBS/2 mM EDTA (pH 7.2) to a volume of 34 mL and mix by inversion.
3. Add the diluted BM to the SepMate tube by pipetting it down the side of the tube.

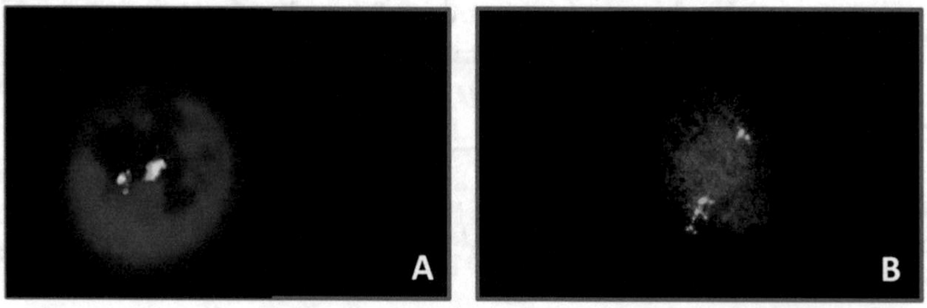

Fig. 2 The cIg-FISH on fresh bone marrow using an *IGH* dual color break-apart probe. (**A**) A cIg-positive plasma cell demonstrating a normal signal pattern. Note the aqua ring around a largely unstained nucleus. (**B**) A cIg-negative cell showing normal *IGH* signals. The background has been enhanced so that the nuclear borders are visible

4. Centrifuge the tube at 1200 × *g* for 10 min with the brake on (*see* **Note 9**).
5. Tip the contents of the SepMate tube above the barrier, i.e., MNC plus plasma (invert <2 s) into a new 50-mL plastic centrifuge tube and add PBS to make the volume up to 50 mL.
6. Centrifuge the MNC at 250 × *g* for 10 min.
7. Remove the supernatant by aspiration and resuspend the cells in PBS to 50 mL.
8. Centrifuge the MNC at 250 × *g* for 10 min.
9. Remove supernatant by aspiration to the desired cell density.
10. Add a small drop of the resuspended cells to the end of a methanol cleaned dry glass microscope slide.
11. Using a second clean slide scrape the cells down the slide using a single smooth light motion (as if preparing a blood film) (*see* **Note 10**).
12. Make 2–4 smears and air dry.
13. Fix the slides in 95% ethanol for 5 min then air dry (*see* **Notes 11** and **12**).

3.1.2 cIg Light Chain Immunofluorescence

1. Prewarm a Coplin jar of PBD and a Coplin jar of 2× SSC to 37 °C.
2. Assemble two Coplin jars containing 1× PBD at room temperature.
3. Make 1/10 dilution of appropriate primary Ab and secondary Ab in Ab diluent. 50 μL is needed for each slide (*see* **Note 13**).
4. Place the slide in the Coplin jar of 1× PBD at 37 °C for 5 min.
5. Add 50 μL of diluted primary Ab to the slide and cover with a 22 mm × 50 mm coverslip. Incubate in the dark for ≥20 min at ambient temperature in a humidified chamber.
6. Flick the coverslip off to waste (*see* **Note 14**).

7. Wash slides in the two Coplin jars of 1× PBD at room temperature for 2 min each.
8. Flick the slide dry and wipe the back of the slide with a tissue.
9. Add 50 μL of diluted secondary Ab to the slide and cover with a 22 mm × 50 mm coverslip. Incubate in the dark for ≥20 min at ambient temperature in a humidified chamber.
10. Flick the coverslip off to waste (*see* **Note 14**).
11. Wash slides in the two Coplin jars of 1× PBD at room temperature for 2 min each.
12. Flick the slide dry and wipe the back of the slide with a tissue.
13. Air dry the slides in dark.

3.1.3 Fixation and Permeabilization Prior to FISH

1. Assemble two Coplin jars containing 1× PBD at room temperature, one Coplin jar containing 2× SSC at room temperature, and one Coplin jar containing 2× SSC prewarmed to 37 °C.
2. Assemble three Coplin jars containing 70 % ethanol, 80 % ethanol, and 100 % ethanol.
3. Thaw Proteinase K at room temperature.
4. Thaw an aliquot of 2 % PFA at room temperature and keep it in dark. When thawed transfer to a Coplin jar.
5. Treat slides in 2 % PFA at room temperature for 5 min.
6. Wash slides twice in 1× PBD for 2 min each.
7. Put 50 μL of Proteinase K on each slide and cover with a 22 mm × 50 mm coverslip. Incubate at room temperature in a humidified chamber for 15 min.
8. Wash slides in a Coplin jar of 1× PBD for 2 min.
9. Wash slides in a Coplin jar of 2× SSC for 2 min.
10. Incubate slides in a Coplin jar of 2× SSC at 37 °C for 30 min.
11. Dehydrate slides through an ethanol series (70, 80, 100 % for 1 min each)
12. Air dry the slides in dark.

3.1.4 FISH Hybridization and Washing

1. Prepare the FISH probes according to the manufacturer's instructions (dilute with hybridization buffer if necessary) (*see* **Notes 15** and **16**).
2. Mark four well-spaced areas on the underside of the slide with a solvent-resistant marker.
3. Apply 2 μL of probe to the first area and cover it with a 12 mm diameter circular glass coverslip. Remove any bubbles from under the coverslip by applying pressure with fine-pointed forceps.
4. Seal the coverslip with rubber cement.
5. Apply 2 μL of the next probe to the second area and seal it.

6. Continue until four different probes have been applied to each of the 4 different marked areas (*see* **Note 17**).
7. When the rubber cement has completely set put the slide into the FISH hybridizer or onto the heating block and co-denature cellular and probe DNA at 80 °C for 5 min, followed by hybridization at 37 °C overnight in the FISH hybridizer or in a prewarmed humidified chamber in an incubator.
8. Next day prewarm a Coplin jar of 0.4× SSC/0.3% NP40 to 73 ± 1 °C in the water bath.
9. Remove the rubber cement and each 12 mm circular coverslip using fine-pointed forceps.
10. Wash slides in 0.4× SSC/0.3%NP40 at 72 °C for 2 min (*see* **Note 18**). Then rinse slides in a Coplin jar with 2× SSC/0.1% NP40 at room temperature for 30 s.
11. Air dry slides lying on their long side in the dark.
12. Apply a small amount of antifade mounting medium to the slide, cover with a 22 mm × 50 mm coverslip, blot to remove excess mountant and to remove air bubbles, and then seal the edge of the coverslip to the slide using a very fine bead of rubber cement or nail polish (*see* **Notes 19** and **20**).

3.1.5 Analysis and Reporting

1. Apply a small drop of microscopy oil to each of the hybridization areas on the slide.
2. Using the 20× oil immersion objective and the AMCA filter establish the focal plane and assess cIg-AMCA staining of plasma cells (*see* **Notes 21–23**).
3. Using the 100× oil immersion objective assess AMCA positive (and negative) cells for FISH signal patterns (*see* **Notes 24** and **25**).
4. Each of two analysts should independently count the hybridization signals for each probe set in 50 AMCA positive cells (*see* **Note 26**). The AMCA-negative cells should be checked to ensure that they show a negative (normal) FISH result. This provides an inbuilt control of all aspects of the procedure.
5. If both analysts results are either above or below established cut-offs then the counts are added together to give a count out of 100. If the analysts' counts are discordant then a third analyst should score the hybridization signals in 50 cells and the 2 concordant results should be added together to give the result.
6. In the case of possible non-PCM disease (e.g. MDS) 50–100 AMCA negative cells may be scored by each of two analysts.
7. Capture at least two images of representative cells of each clone using imaging software.

8. Cutoffs should be established by individual laboratories (*see* **Note 26**), but as a guide conservative cutoffs (10% for dual fusion or break-apart probes and 20% for numerical abnormalities) are recommended [12].
9. Reports should contain the method used in plasma cell identification, the probes used, and the number of normal and abnormal cells scored for each abnormality. Reports should also contain an interpretative comment that clearly indicates the significance of the results [12].

3.2 cIg-FISH on Carnoy-fixed Cytogenetic Preparations

This procedure is for use on samples that have been through a routine cytogenetic harvest and have undergone three changes of fresh cold 3:1 methanol:acetic acid (Carnoy's fixative). It is best to use a direct harvest or a 24-h culture for this procedure to reduce the amount of plasma cell degradation that may occur in culture. It is advisable to check the percentage of plasma cells in the original sample since this procedure works best on samples with at least 20% plasma cells. The advantage of this procedure is that it fits well in the routine cytogenetics laboratory work flow. The morphology of cells that have undergone this technique is shown in Fig. 3.

3.2.1 Slide Preparation

1. Pellet the Carnoy-fixed cytogenetic cell preparation by centrifuging at $250 \times g$ for 10 min in a bench top centrifuge and carefully remove the supernatant by aspiration.
2. Resuspend the pellet in 100% methanol (room temperature) to a volume of 10 mL.
3. Pellet the cells by centrifuging at $250 \times g$ for 10 min in a bench top centrifuge and carefully remove the supernatant by aspiration.
4. Resuspend the pellet in 100% methanol (room temperature) to an appropriate cell density such that when the suspension is dropped onto a clean dry slide phase contrast microscopy reveals approximately 100–150 cells per low power (100×) view. Adjust the volume of methanol if required.

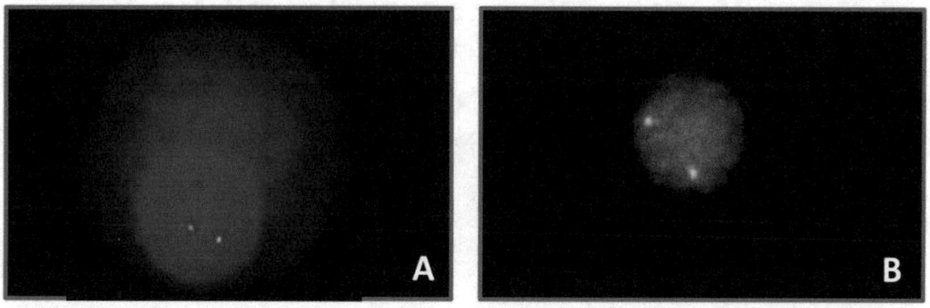

Fig. 3 The cIg-FISH on Carnoy-fixed cytogenetic preparations with an *IGH* dual color break-apart probe. (**A**) A cIg-positive plasma cell with an *IGH* rearrangement. Note the aqua halo that is a feature of this method. (**B**) A cIg-negative cell showing normal *IGH* signals. The background has been enhanced so that the nuclear borders are visible

5. Drop the adjusted cell suspension onto a fresh clean dry slide and while cells are drying (as indicated by Newton's rings) gently add 1–2 drops of 96% ethanol to the slide.
6. Allow slides to dry air dry.

3.2.2 Antigen Retrieval and cIg Light Chain Immunofluorescence

1. Preheat a Coplin jar containing antigen retrieval buffer in the water bath until the buffer reaches 95 °C.
2. Assemble the humidified chamber and prewarm it to 37 °C in an incubator.
3. Assemble two Coplin jars containing 1× PBS at room temperature.
4. Assemble three Coplin jars containing 70% ethanol, 80% ethanol, and 96% ethanol, respectively.
5. Make a 1/10 dilution of appropriate primary Ab and a 1/20 dilution of the secondary Ab in 1× PBS. 50 μL is needed for each slide (*see* **Note 13**).
6. Perform antigen retrieval by incubation in antigen retrieval buffer in the water bath at 95 °C for 10 min.
7. Remove the Coplin jar containing the slide from the water bath and leave on the bench to cool for 30 min.
8. Remove the slide from the buffer, flick dry, and place immediately into a Coplin jar containing 1× PBS for 2 min.
9. Transfer the slide to a second Coplin jar containing 1× PBS for 2 min.
10. Flick the slide dry and wipe the back of the slide with a tissue.
11. Add 50 μL of primary Ab to the slide and cover with a 22 mm × 50 mm coverslip.
12. Lie the slide flat in the humidified container at 37 °C for 1 h.
13. Flick the coverslip off to waste (*see* **Note 14**).
14. Wash twice in 1× PBS for 2 min each, flick dry and wipe back of slide.
15. Add 50 μL of secondary Ab (AMCA-rabbit anti-goat Ab) to slide and coverslip with a 22 mm × 50 mm coverslip.
16. Return to the humidified chamber at 37 °C for 1 h.
17. Flick the coverslip off to waste (*see* **Note 14**).
18. Wash twice in 1× PBS for 2 min each.
19. Dehydrate in graded alcohol series 70, 80, 96% ethanol for 2 min each.
20. Dry slide on its long side in the dark.

3.2.3 FISH Hybridization, Washing, Analysis, and Reporting

FISH hybridization, washing, analysis, and reporting are described in Subheadings 3.1.4 and 3.1.5.

4 Notes

1. RO water is water prepared by reverse osmosis. If this is not available distilled water is a suitable substitute.
2. Leucoprep tubes (Greiner) are a suitable alternative. The use of these barrier tubes simplifies density gradient MNC separation.
3. Soak glass microscope slides for at least 15 min in 100% methanol in Coplin jar in a fume cupboard. Before use remove the slide from the methanol and scrub the slide with clean lint-free tissue until dry.
4. In moistening the paper towel for the humidified chamber ensure that it is not over wet. There should be no runoff if the chamber is tipped.
5. WARNING: do not continue heating the solution once PFA has been added or explosion could result.
6. There are many probe manufacturers; examples are Vysis, MetaSystems, CytoCell, DAKO, Empire Genomics, etc.
7. If a second malignancy is suspected, e.g. myelodysplastic syndrome (MDS), then probe sets appropriate to that diagnosis should be used.
8. The following filters are appropriate: for AMCA use excitation/emission filter set of 344/446, for Texas red labeled probes use excitation/emission 595/615; for Cy3 or spectrum Orange labeled probes use excitation/emission 559/588, and for FITC or Spectrum Green labeled probes use excitation/emission 497/524. A red/green dual bandpass filter can be used for simultaneous visualization of red and green probes. A red/green/blue triple bandpass filter can be used for simultaneous visualization of red and green probes and AMCA cIg staining. The single band pass filter sets give the brightest fluorescence signals.
9. To calculate revolutions per min the following equation can be used where g is the relative centrifugal force, R is the radius of the rotor in centimeters, and S is the speed of the centrifuge in revolutions per minute. $g = (1.118 \times 10^{-5})\ R\ S^2$
10. Adjust the cell density, volume of the cell drop, and pressure of the scraper until phase contrast microscopy reveals approximately 100–150 cells per low power (100×) view.
11. Once dry, slides can be wrapped in aluminum foil and store at −20 °C.
12. Before use remove the slides from freezer and allow to warm to ambient temperature while still wrapped in foil.
13. Once the technique has been established it may be practical to use a mixture of α-k and α-λ primary antibodies so that it is not

necessary to identify which light chain is expressed in every patient. Use 5 μL of each Ab and add 90 μL of Ab diluent. While establishing the method use α-k on one slide and α-λ on another to test for specificity of Ig staining.

14. If the coverslip doesn't come off easily dip the slide into Coplin jar of 1× PBD (fresh BM method) or 1× PBS (Carnoy-fixed method) at room temperature and then try again.
15. Before removing probe from the vial it is essential to pulse spin in a microfuge at maximum speed and then to mix the vial contents by flicking the bottom of the tube with a finger.
16. Caution: hybridization buffer contains formamide which is a teratogen.
17. Do not allow the hybridization areas to overlap or the signals will be uninterpretable.
18. Wash four slides at a time because the wash solution will fall to the desired temperature. If fewer than four slides are being washed then add blank slides to make the number up to four. If there are more than four slides to wash then wash them in batches of four, allowing the wash solution time to regain temperature in between batches.
19. Mount slides in antifade (without DAPI because AMCA is blue).
20. Seal the coverslip well because microscopy oil under the coverslip will quench fluorescent signal.
21. Plasma cells may have distinctive morphology. They tend to be large and mononuclear and the nucleus may be eccentric and surrounded by cytoplasm [19].
22. cIg AMCA staining may be absent if:
    (a) There are few or no plasma cells in the sample either because there were none in the original sample, or because there was too long (≥8 h) between sample collection and cIg-FISH slide preparation. In these situations a new specimen will be required.
    (b) There was a problem with primary or secondary Ab staining. In this situation new slides can be thawed for use. Be sure to add the primary Ab before the secondary Ab and ensure that all washing solutions are at the correct concentration, pH, and temperature. Be sure that the isotype-specific Ab was used, i.e., α-k in a kappa chain restricted PCM or α-λ in a lambda chain restricted PCM.
23. cIg-AMCA staining may be nonspecific if:
    (a) Washes were not performed or not performed correctly, or if Ab concentrations were too high. In either situation the assay should be repeated on the spare slides.

(b) Background has resulted from nonspecific Ab staining. Consider using 5 % fetal calf serum or 1 % BSA in the Ab diluent.

(c) All nuclei appear aqua then check that DAPI wasn't added to the antifade.

24. FISH signals may be weak if:

    (a) Slides were not adequately denatured. Ensure that slides reach 80 °C during denaturation and that this temperature is held for 5 min. Higher temperature or time (in 1 °C intervals) may be tried.

    (b) Probe was not sufficiently centrifuged and mixed prior to application.

    (c) Probe was not applied.

    (d) Posthybridization washing was too stringent (concentration of SSC was too low or temperature was too high).

25. FISH signals may be nonspecific or background may be high if:

    (a) Microscope slides were not sufficiently clean. Clean slides according to Note 3.

    (b) Wash solutions are incorrect (concentration of SSC is too high, or temperature is too low). Ensure that four slides are always washed together and that temperature of wash solution is regained in between batches.

    (c) The probe was too concentrated. Dilute probes according to the manufacturer's recommendations.

    (d) The probe mix may have dried out during hybridization. Ensure that the coverslip is completely sealed with rubber cement.

26. Use of the Excel CRITBINOM statistical function (Microsoft) is recommended for measurement of uncertainty of interphase FISH procedures and to establish sensitivity cutoff values [20].

References

1. Fonseca R, Bergsagel PL, Drach J et al (2009) International Myeloma Working Group molecular classification of multiple myeloma: spotlight review. Leukemia 23(12):2210–2221
2. Durie BGM, Salmon SE (1975) A clinical staging system for multiple myeloma. Cancer 36:842–854
3. Greipp PR, San Miguel J, Durie BGM et al (2005) International Staging System for multiple myeloma. J Clin Oncol 23:3412–3420
4. Palumbo A, Avet-Loiseau H, Oliva S et al (2015) Revised International Staging System for Multiple Myeloma: a report from International Myeloma Working Group. J Clin Oncol 33(26):2863–2869
5. Fonseca R (2003) Many and multiple myeloma(s). Leukemia 17:1943–1944
6. Sawyer JR (2011) The prognostic significance of cytogenetics and molecular profiling in multiple myeloma. Cancer Genet 204(1):3–12
7. Debes-Marun CS, Dewald GW, Bryant S et al (2003) Chromosome abnormalities clustering and its implications for pathogenesis and prognosis in myeloma. Leukemia 17(2):427–436

8. Fonseca R, Blood E, Rue M et al (2003) Clinical and biologic implications of recurrent genomic aberrations in myeloma. Blood 101(11):4569–4575
9. Lonial S, Boise LH, Kaufman J (2015) How I treat high risk myeloma. Blood 126(13):1536–1543
10. Mateos M-V, San Miguel JF (2013) How should we treat newly diagnosed multiple myeloma patients? American Society of Hematology Educ Program. pp 488–495
11. Caligaris-Cappio F, Gregoretti MG, Merico F et al (1992) Bone marrow microenvironment and the progression of multiple myeloma. Leuk Lymphoma 8(1-2):15–22
12. Ross FM, Avet-Loiseau H, Ameye G et al (2012) Report from the European Myeloma Network on interphase FISH in multiple myeloma and related disorders. Haematologica 97(8):1272–1277
13. Put N, Lemmens H, Wlodarska I et al (2010) Interphase fluorescence in situ hybridization on selected plasma cells is superior in the detection of cytogenetic aberrations in plasma cell dyscrasia. Genes Chromosomes Cancer 49(11):991–997
14. Grigoriadis G, Whitehead S (2010) CD138 shedding in plasma cell myeloma. Br J Haematol 150(3):249
15. Drach J, Angerler J, Schuster J et al (1995) Interphase fluorescence in situ hybridization identifies chromosomal abnormalities in plasma cells from patients with monoclonal gammopathy of undetermined significance. Blood 86:3915–3921
16. Ahmann GJ, Jalal SM, Juneau AL et al (1998) A novel three-colour, clone-specific fluorescence in situ hybridisation procedure for monoclonal gammopathies. Cancer Genet Cytogenet 101:7–11
17. Gole L, Lin A, Chua C et al (2014) Modified cIg-FISH protocol for multiple myeloma in routine cytogenetic laboratory practice. Cancer Genet 207(1-2):31–34
18. Kobayashi Y, Nakayama M, Uemura N et al (1999) Analysis of myelodysplastic syndrome clones arising after multiple myeloma: a case study by correlative interphase cytogenetic analysis. Jpn J Clin Oncol 29(8):374–377
19. Hartmann L, Biggerstaff JS, Chapman DB et al (2000) Detection of Genomic abnormalities in multiple myeloma. The application of FISH analysis in combination with various plasma cell enrichment techniques. Am J Clin Pathol 136:712–720
20. Ciolino AL, Tang ME, Bryant R (2009) Statistical treatment of fluorescence in situ hybridization validation data to generate normal reference ranges using excel functions. J Mol Diagn 11(4):330–333

Chapter 13

Quantitative Fluorescence In Situ Hybridization (QFISH)

Ivan Y. Iourov

Abstract

Fluorescence in situ hybridization (FISH) has a wide spectrum of applications in current molecular cytogenetic and cancer research. This is a unique technique that can be used for chromosomal DNA analysis in all cell types, at all stages of the cell cycle, and at molecular resolution. Recent developments in microscopy and imaging systems have allowed quantification of digital FISH images (quantitative FISH or QFISH) and have provided a new way for molecular cytogenetic analysis at single-cell level. QFISH can be applied for studying chromosome imbalances in interphase nuclei or metaphase spreads, measuring relative DNA content at chromosomal loci and identifying parental origin of homologous chromosomes. Here, a QFISH protocol suitable for the majority of DNA probes using the popular US National Institute of Health developed ImageJ software is described.

Key words Chromosome abnormalities, DNA probes, Fluorescence in situ hybridization, Interphase, Nucleus, Quantification, QFISH

1 Introduction

Quantitative fluorescence in situ hybridization (QFISH) is an approach combining fluorescence in situ hybridization (FISH) and digital quantification of microscopic images. It has been shown to be applicable for a variety of purposes in molecular cytogenetics studies [1–4]. QFISH represents an important part of studying somatic chromosomal mosaicism and molecular cytogenetic detection of chromosomal variations in interphase nuclei [5–9]. Furthermore, QFISH using DNA or peptide nucleic acids (PNA) probes has been successfully employed for the in situ quantification of telomeric DNA repeats [1, 10, 11]. This technique is then subsequently developed for distinguishing the two homologous human chromosomes of parental origin at single cell level [12, 13]. Strikingly, QFISH are found to be an important and indispensable tool in cancer research nowadays. In this context, these applications have been proven to enhance the efficiency for the detection of chromosome instability and quantification of gene amplification or correlation of the size of noncoding repeated sequences during disease progression [7, 11,

Thomas S.K. Wan (ed.), *Cancer Cytogenetics: Methods and Protocols*, Methods in Molecular Biology, vol. 1541, DOI 10.1007/978-1-4939-6703-2_13, © Springer Science+Business Media LLC 2017

14–16]. Additionally, these approaches have also been used for the discrimination and quantification of microorganisms in microbiology studies [17].

To enhance the precision of molecular cytogenetic analysis of human chromosomes, QFISH is generally employed to discriminate "real" genomic/chromosomal change from false-positive signal appearance. For example, chromosome loss in interphase nuclei can be differentiated from signal overlapping using QFISH [3–9, 18]. Furthermore, QFISH allows visualization of small copy number variations in situ [19]. Thus, chromosome instability analysis seems to be benefitted from QFISH [3–9, 15, 16, 18, 19]. Finally, QFISH has enabled developing more sophisticated FISH-based approaches, i.e., interphase chromosome-specific multicolor banding (ICS-MCB) [20, 21] and 3-dimensional (3-D) profiling of FISH signals [22], which enable analyses of somatic genome variations and nuclear genome organization at chromosomal (supramolecular) level [20–22]. Here, a detailed QFISH protocol from cell suspension preparation for interphase FISH [23], basic FISH procedures [3, 5–9] and quantitation of FISH signals using ImageJ software [24] is presented.

2 Materials

The standard molecular biological and cytogenetic equipment, including standard solutions (ethanol, methanol, formamide, formaldehyde, etc.), are not mentioned. Only specialized items are listed below (*see* **Note 1**).

1. 20× Saline sodium citrate (SSC).
2. Antifade solution.
3. Biotinylated antiavidin.
4. Phosphate buffered saline (PBS): Mix equal parts of 0.5 M Na_2HPO_4 and 0.5 M NaH_2PO_4 (pH 7.0), aliquot and store at −20 °C.
5. Rubber cement.
6. Carnoy's fixative: Methanol:glacial acetic acid = 3:1 (v/v), freshly prepared and store at −20 °C.
7. Working DAPI (4,6-diamidino-2-phenylindol · 2HCl) solution: 5 mL of DAPI stock solution in 100 mL of 4× SSC/0.2 % Tween, freshly prepared before use.
8. Denaturation buffer: 70 % deionized formamide, 10 % distilled water, 10 % 20× SSC, and 10 % phosphate buffer (v/v), freshly prepared before use.
9. Hybridization buffer: Add 2 g of dextran sulfate to 10 mL of 50 % deionized formamide/2× SSC/50 mM phosphate buffer at 70 °C for 3 h, aliquot and store at −20 °C.

10. Pepsin solution: Mix 50 μL of 10 % pepsin stock solution (w/v) to HCl solution (mix 1 mL of 1 M HCl with 99 mL of distilled water), pre-warmed at 37 °C for 20 min in Coplin jar; freshly prepared before use.
11. Chromosome-enumeration DNA probes (*see* **Note 2**) labeled with specific chromosomal loci for satellite DNA sequences [3–9].

3 Methods

3.1 Cell Suspension Preparation (See Note 3)

1. Rinse a piece of 3 mm^3 tissue with 0.9 % NaCl and transfer to a homogenizer glass tube.
2. Homogenize the tissue using teflon pestle.
3. Add 2 mL of PBS and continue homogenize until present of a liquid-like substance.
4. Transfer the homogenized tissue to another tube.
5. Add 1 mL of 60 % glacial acetic acid and incubate at room temperature for 3–5 min.
6. Add 9 mL of Carnoy's fixative (−20 °C) and centrifuge at 1000 × *g* for 5 min at room temperature.
7. Discard the supernatant and add 9 mL of Carnoy's fixative (−20 °C). Centrifuge at 1000 × *g* for 8 min at room temperature.
8. Repeat **step 6** at least three times.
9. Resuspend the cell pellet and transfer to a 2-mL tube (*see* **Note 4**).
10. Place 20–100 μL of the suspension on a microscope slide and air dry at room temperature for 15–20 min.

3.2 Slide Pretreatment

1. Put slides in 100 mL of 1× PBS at room temperature and slowly shake in a shaker for 2 min.
2. Put slides in pepsin solution at 37 °C for 5–10 min in Coplin jar.
3. Repeat **step 1** twice.
4. Put slides in 100 mL of formalin buffer at room temperature and slightly agitate for 10 min.
5. Repeat **step 1** twice.
6. Dehydrate slides in 70, 90, and 100 % ethanol series for 3 min each and air dry.

3.3 FISH

1. Place 5 μL of DNA probe on the pretreated slide and cover with 18 mm × 18 mm coverslip.
2. Denature the slides at a hotplate at 72–77 °C for 5–7 min.
3. Seal the coverslip's edges with rubber cement.

4. Place the slides in a humidified chamber at 37 °C overnight.
5. Wet the coverslip's edges with distilled water and remove coverslip gently using forceps to pick up the solidified rubber cement.
6. Wash slides in 50% formamide/2× SSC at 42 °C for 10 min.
7. Wash slides in 2× SSC/Tween20 at 42 °C for 15 min.
8. Add 24 μL of DAPI solution and cover with a coverslip.

3.4 Quantification of FISH Signals

1. Capture FISH images using a charge-coupled-device (CCD) camera mounted on a fluorescence microscope and equipped with a set of specific filters used for FISH (i.e., DAPI-, FITC-, Cy3-, etc.), a 100× (or 63×) objective and a software either incorporated into imaging system or purchased separately for imaging.
2. Capture FISH images using separate filters set specific for each fluorochrome and separately saved in 8-bit black and white images.
3. Load each FISH image into ImageJ software (https://imagej.nih.gov/ij/) [24] (*see* **Note 5**).
4. The area containing FISH signals is selected using "rectangular" selection tool.
5. The selected area is attributed to the first lane using "Select First Lane"—Analyze/Gels/Select First Lane or simply press Ctrl + 1 (*see* **Note 6**).
6. To obtain the Plot of image containing the graph depicting intensity profiles (*see* **Note 7**), "Plot profile" is used—Analyze/Plot Profile or simply press Ctrl + K.
7. To remove the grid from the Plot of image, Threshold is used (Image/Adjust/ Threshold… or Ctrl + Shift + T).
8. To define the borders of the graph corresponding to a signal (to select area to be measured), a line is to be drawn by "straight" for suggesting a line and Draw -Edit/Draw or simply press Ctrl + D.
9. The area resulting from the previous step is selected by Wand (tracing) tool.
10. The selection is measured using Measure–Analyze/Measure or simply press Ctrl + M.
11. Numerical values of area or perimeter are output in a separate window.
12. The numerical values of different signals from the same image (*see* **Note 8**) are compared (Fig. 1).

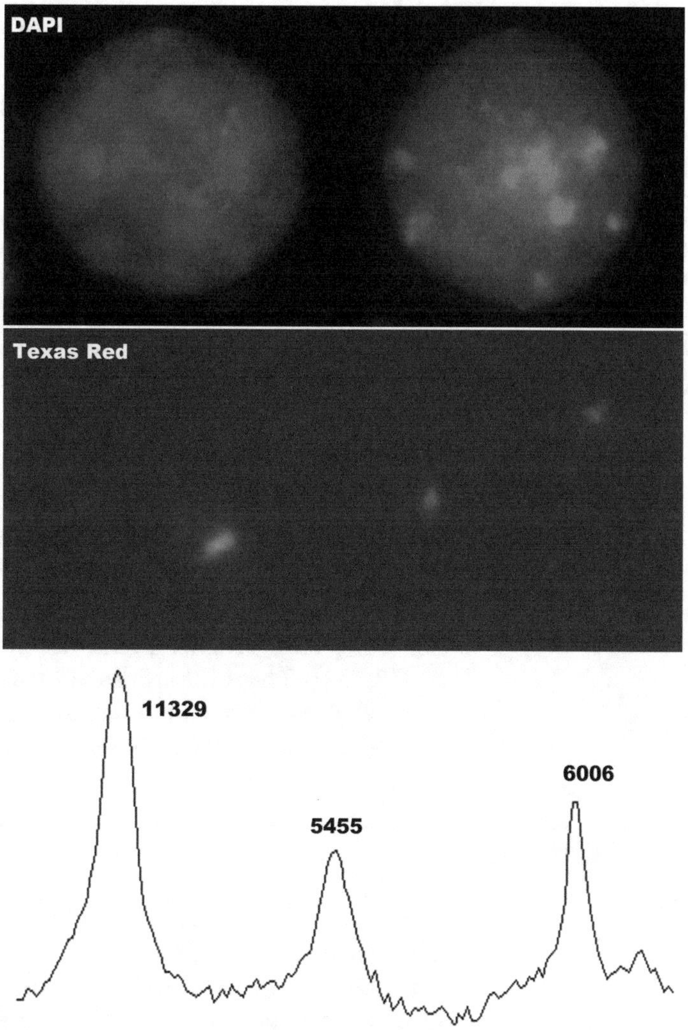

Fig. 1 QFISH with chromosome-enumeration DNA probe for chromosome X allows differentiating false-positive chromosome loss (monosomy) and signal overlap. A nucleus with one signal for chromosome X-specific probe (*left*) representing juxtaposition of two signals of a chromosome X-specific probe (relative intensity is 11,329 pixels), and a nucleus (*right*) with two signals of chromosome X-specific probe (relative intensities are 5455 and 6006 pixels). Single signal intensity in the left nucleus is nearly twice compared with signal intensities in the right nucleus

4 Notes

1. Some of the chemicals used are toxic, e.g., formaldehyde and formamide. These substances are to be collected and treated as hazardous waste after use.
2. DNA probes are either commercially available FISH probes or home-brewed FISH probes; current QFISH protocol is

independent of the chemical/physical properties and sequence specificity of DNA probes.

3. A step-by-step protocol of cell suspension preparation is given in [23].
4. Cell suspensions can be stored at −20 °C for at least 1 year.
5. This software allows quantification or intensity measuring of digital microscopic images. However, QFISH protocol is likely to become more widely used when free software for fluorescence signal quantitation is available. Currently, ImageJ seems to be one of the most popular free software used for similar research purposes [24].
6. To obtain better signal appearance with reduced background, "Threshold" can be used (Image/Adjust/Threshold... or Ctrl + Shift + T).
7. It is to note that FISH signal intensity is proportional to the DNA content in chromosomal loci painted by FISH [3, 12, 22].
8. In QFISH, relative intensities are usually measured in pixels [3, 22]. These intensities are used to be compared between each other. Still, additional calculations can be made to convert these values to other units.

Acknowledgements

The article is dedicated to Ilia V. Soloviev. I would like to express my gratitude to Prof. Svetlana G Vorsanova and Prof. Yuri B Yurov for helping in the preparation of this chapter. This work was supported by the Russian Science Foundation (Grant #14-35-00060).

References

1. Poon SS, Lansdorp PM (2001) Quantitative fluorescence in situ hybridization (Q-FISH). Curr Protoc Cell Biol 18:18.4. doi:10.1002/0471143030.cb1804s12
2. Truong K, Gibaud A, Dupont JM et al (2003) Rapid prenatal diagnosis of Down syndrome using quantitative fluorescence in situ hybridization on interphase nuclei. Prenat Diagn 23(2):146–151. doi:10.1002/pd.558
3. Iourov IY, Soloviev IV, Vorsanova SG et al (2005) An approach for quantitative assessment of fluorescence in situ hybridization (FISH) signals for applied human molecular cytogenetics. J Histochem Cytochem 53(3):401–408. doi:10.1369/jhc.4A6419.2005
4. Vorsanova SG, Yurov YB, Iourov IY (2010) Human interphase chromosomes: a review of available molecular cytogenetic technologies. Mol Cytogenet 3:1. doi:10.1186/1755-8166-3-1
5. Yurov YB, Iourov IY, Vorsanova SG et al (2007) Aneuploidy and confined chromosomal mosaicism in the developing human brain. PLoS One 2(6):e558. doi:10.1371/journal.pone.0000558
6. Yurov YB, Iourov IY, Vorsanova SG et al (2008) The schizophrenia brain exhibits low-level aneuploidy involving chromosome 1. Schizophr Res 98(1-3):139–147. doi:10.1016/j.schres.2007.07.035, http://dx.doi.org/

7. Iourov IY, Vorsanova SG, Liehr T et al (2009) Increased chromosome instability dramatically disrupts neural genome integrity and mediates cerebellar degeneration in the ataxia-telangiectasia brain. Hum Mol Genet 18(14):2656–2669. doi:10.1093/hmg/ddp207
8. Iourov IY, Vorsanova SG, Liehr T et al (2009) Aneuploidy in the normal, Alzheimer's disease and ataxia-telangiectasia brain: differential expression and pathological meaning. Neurobiol Dis 34(2):212–220. doi:10.1016/j.nbd.2009.01.003
9. Yurov YB, Vorsanova SG, Liehr T et al (2014) X chromosome aneuploidy in the Alzheimer's disease brain. Mol Cytogenet 7(1):20. doi:10.1186/1755-8166-7-20
10. Wan TS, Martens UM, Poon SS et al (1999) Absence or low number of telomere repeats at junctions of dicentric chromosomes. Genes Chromosomes Cancer 24(1):83–86. doi:10.1002/(SICI)1098-2264(199901)24:1<83::AID-GCC12>3.0.CO;2-C
11. Kawano Y, Ishikawa N, Aida J et al (2014) Q-FISH measurement of hepatocyte telomere lengths in donor liver and graft after pediatric living-donor liver transplantation: donor age affects telomere length sustainability. PLoS One 9(4), e93749. doi:10.1371/journal.pone.0093749
12. Vorsanova SG, Iourov IY, Beresheva AK et al (2005) Non-disjunction of chromosome 21, alphoid DNA variation, and sociogenetic features of Down syndrome. Tsitol Genet 39(6):30–36
13. Weise A, Gross M, Mrasek K et al (2008) Parental-origin-determination fluorescence in situ hybridization distinguishes homologous human chromosomes on a single-cell level. Int J Mol Med 21(2):189–200. doi:10.3892/ijmm.21.2.189
14. Rodenacker K, Aubele M, Hutzler P et al (1997) Groping for quantitative digital 3-D image analysis: an approach to quantitative fluorescence in situ hybridization in thick tissue sections of prostate carcinoma. Anal Cell Pathol 15(1):19–29. doi:10.1155/1997/790963
15. Truong K, Guilly MN, Gerbault-Seureau M et al (1998) Quantitative FISH by image cytometry for the detection of chromosome 1 imbalances in breast cancer: a novel approach analyzing chromosome rearrangements within interphase nuclei. Lab Invest 78(12):1607–1613
16. Stevens R, Almanaseer I, Gonzalez M et al (2007) Analysis of HER2 gene amplification using an automated fluorescence in situ hybridization signal enumeration system. J Mol Diagn 9(2):144–150. doi:10.2353/jmoldx.2007.060102
17. Zhou Z, Pons MN, Raskin L et al (2007) Automated image analysis for quantitative fluorescence in situ hybridization with environmental samples. Appl Environ Microbiol 73(9):2956–2962. doi:10.1128/AEM.02954-06
18. Amakawa G, Ikemoto K, Ito H et al (2013) Quantitative analysis of centromeric FISH spots during the cell cycle by image cytometry. J Histochem Cytochem 61(10):699–705. doi:10.1369/0022155413498754
19. Harutyunyan T, Hovhannisyan G, Babayan N et al (2015) Influence of aflatoxin B1 on copy number variants in human leukocytes in vitro. Mol Cytogenet 8:25. doi:10.1186/s13039-015-0131-x
20. Iourov IY, Liehr T, Vorsanova SG et al (2006) Visualization of interphase chromosomes in postmitotic cells of the human brain by multicolour banding (MCB). Chromosome Res 14(3):223–229. doi:10.1007/s10577-006-1037-6
21. Iourov IY, Liehr T, Vorsanova SG et al (2007) Interphase chromosome-specific multicolor banding (ICS-MCB): a new tool for analysis of interphase chromosomes in their integrity. Biomol Eng 24(4):415–417
22. Iourov IY, Vorsanova SG, Yurov YB (2008) Fluorescence intensity profiles of *in situ* hybridization signals depict genome architecture within human interphase nuclei. Tsitol Genet 42(5):3–8
23. Iourov IY, Vorsanova SG, Pellestor F et al (2006) Brain tissue preparations for chromosomal PRINS labeling. Methods Mol Biol 334:123–132. doi:10.1385/1-59745-068-5:123
24. Schneider CA, Rasband WS, Eliceiri KW (2012) NIH Image to ImageJ: 25 years of image analysis. Nat Methods 9(7):671–675. doi:10.1038/nmeth.2089

Chapter 14

High Resolution Fiber-Fluorescence In Situ Hybridization

Christine J. Ye and Henry H. Heng

Abstract

High resolution fiber-Fluorescence in situ hybridization (FISH) is an advanced FISH technology that can effectively bridge the resolution gap between probe hybridizing on DNA molecules and chromosomal regions. Since various types of DNA and chromatin fibers can be generated reflecting different degrees of DNA/chromatin packaging status, fiber-FISH technology has been successfully used in diverse molecular cytogenetic/cytogenomic studies. Following a brief review of this technology, including its major development and increasing applications, typical protocols to generate DNA/chromatin fiber will be described, coupled with rationales, as well as technical tips. These released DNA/chromatin fibers are suitable for an array of cytogenetic/cytogenomic analyses.

Key words DNA fiber-FISH, Chromatin fiber-FISH, Halo FISH, Stretched chromatin fiber-FISH, Free chromatin-FISH

1 Introduction

Despite the fact that free chromatin and defective mitotic figures (DMFs) were initially identified over 30 years ago for the purpose of analyzing high order chromosomal structures, it was the desire and requirement of high resolution FISH technology for physical mapping that introduced and promoted the development of fiber-FISH methodology [1–5]. The rationale of applying FISH detection on released chromatin fibers is straightforward: (1) Experimentally released chromatin fibers are less condensed than native chromosomes and even interphase chromatin, and different degrees of decondensation can be achieved based on the releasing conditions; (2) The distance between hybridized targets can be measured on stretched linear DNA/chromatin fiber so that quantitative measurements can be acquired.

The free chromatin FISH was initially introduced to improve the resolution of interphase FISH and meiotic chromatin FISH [6, 7]. The idea was quickly appreciated by different groups and various protocols were developed within a short period [8–14]. Modified protocols were established carrying different names,

Thomas S.K. Wan (ed.), *Cancer Cytogenetics: Methods and Protocols*, Methods in Molecular Biology, vol. 1541, DOI 10.1007/978-1-4939-6703-2_14, © Springer Science+Business Media LLC 2017

including free DNA FISH, DNA halo FISH, extended chromatin/DNA FISH, direct visual hybridization (DIRVSH), molecular combing or DNA/chromosome combing, and quantitative DNA fiber-FISH. Despite these different names, the major difference among these protocols is the means of releasing/preparing chromatin or DNA fibers on microscopic slides prior to probe hybridization. A variety of high-resolution FISH methods have been collectively referred to as high-resolution fiber FISH [15, 16]. The key consideration of selecting a protocol depends on the mapping resolution, target coverage, involvement of chromatin structure such as DNA/protein codetection, data interpretation, and available equipment/materials/reagents. For example, DNA fibers are better for the highest resolution mapping within a small region of the genome. In contrast, the term "chromatin fiber" describes chromatin released from the nucleus without striping most chromatin proteins; these fibers generally correspond to 30-nm structures. With a certain degree of preserved high order structure, released chromatin fibers offer an advantage in chromatin structural studies covering a relatively larger mapping region.

The introduction of fiber-FISH methodologies has greatly advanced the analyses of human, animal, and plant genomes, as well as lower eukaryote genomes, such as fungi and protozoan parasites [17–21]. Examples include: the sequencing gap estimation for the Human Genome Project; the study of copy number polymorphism among different individuals [22]; the determination of order and orientation of groups of genes/ESTs or DNA fragments [23]; the quantification of the sizes of duplicated or amplified fragments of special genes, chromosomal regions, or integrated foreign inserts [24, 25]; the identification or exclusion of genes or chromosomal regions defined by particular genetic markers [26]; the comparison of evolutionary conserved genomic regions among various species or cell lines [27, 28]; the illustration of multiple repetitive sequences within particular genomic regions and the direct visualization of genome organization [29]; the length measurement of telomeres or centromeres for the study of chromosomal packaging both in mitotic and meiotic cells [30–32]; and the study of DNA replication status and repair processing combined with codetection of DNA repair proteins [33]. Equally important, fiber-FISH has successfully applied to analyze genetic aberrations of human diseases, such as mapping translocation breakpoints [34, 35]; determining the number and orientation of duplicated genes that are responsible for Pelizaeus-Merzbacher disease [36]; developing probe sets covering many critical chromosomal regions involving diseases, which are essential for disease diagnosis when translocation or deletion/duplication occurs [37, 38] and illustrating the copy number variation among individual [22].

Realizing it is the entire set of chromosomes not just the individual genes defining the blueprint and function of cells, the karyotype represents an independent type of genetic coding, which preserves the topological relationship for gene interaction for a given species [39–41]. Therefore, the cancer cytogenetic analysis becomes increasingly important as genome heterogeneity is the key driver of cancer evolution [42, 43]. Such knowledge calls for the departure from gene-centric concepts to a novel genome theory where the molecular cytogenetic and cytogenomic analyses are essential [44, 45]. In particular, the systematic characterization of various types of chaotic genomes becomes a priority, and fiber-FISH will play an increasingly important role.

In this chapter, a number of protocols are provided for each type of fiber preparation to serve the purpose of diverse applications. Even though different reagents are used in variable protocols, they all share the goal of releasing high quality chromatin/DNA fiber using less complicated procedures. By comparing different protocols, readers can easily identify key steps and even modify them for their own experiments.

2 Materials

2.1 Chromatin Fiber Preparation

2.1.1 Releasing Chromatin Fibers with Alkaline Buffer

1. Trypsin/EDTA solution.
2. Alkaline buffer: Mix solutions A and B in 1:1 ratio before use. Solution A: 1 mM sodium borate, adjusted to pH 10 with NaOH. Solution B: 0.8% (w/v) KCl.
3. Fixative: 3:1 (v/v) methanol/glacial acetic acid (freshly prepared).
4. 15-mL screw-cap polystyrene tubes.
5. Centrifuge.
6. Microscope slides, chilled 5–10 min on ice or at −20 °C prior to use.
7. Phase-contrast microscope.
8. Giemsa solution.

2.1.2 Inducing Chromatin Fibers from Cultured Lymphocytes by Drug Treatment

1. Human peripheral blood.
2. Complete RPMI culture medium with 15% fetal bovine serum (FBS), 2% (v/v) phytohemagglutinin (PHA), 5 U/mL heparin, and antibiotics.
3. 10 mg/mL ethidium bromide or 10 mg/mL 5-bromodeoxyuridine (BrdU) or 5 mg/mL m-AMSA (*N*-[4-(9-acridinylamino)-3-methoxyphenyl] methanesulfonamide). 5 mg/mL m-AMSA: Dissolve 10 mg/mL m-AMSA in dimethylsulfoxide and dilute with 1 volume of distilled water. Filter to sterilize and store at 4 °C.

4. 0.4% KCl.
5. Carnoy's fixative: 3:1 (v/v) methanol/glacial acetic acid, freshly prepared before use.
6. 15-mL screw-cap polystyrene tubes.
7. Centrifuge.
8. Microscope slides, chilled 5–10 min on ice or at −20 °C prior to use.
9. Phase-contrast microscope.
10. 37 °C CO_2 incubator.

2.2 DNA Fiber Preparation

2.2.1 Preparing DNA Fibers Using Alkaline Treatment Followed by Mechanical Stretching

1. Alkaline solution: 0.07 M NaOH/ethanol (5:2, v/v).
2. 1× Phosphate buffered saline (PBS).
3. 0.4% KCl.
4. Carnoy's fixative: 3:1 (v/v) methanol/glacial acetic acid, freshly prepared before use.
5. Methanol.
6. 70, 95, and 100% ethanol.
7. Microscope slides.
8. 25 mm × 75 mm × 1 mm glass microscope slides.

2.2.2 Preparing DNA Fibers Using Chemical Lysis and Gravity

1. 1× PBS.
2. Lysis buffer: Mix 2.5 mL of 20% (w/v) SDS, 10 mL of 0.5 M EDTA, 20 mL of 1 M Tris–HCl (pH 7.4), 67.5 mL of distilled water. Store at room temperature and stable for >1 year.
3. Carnoy's fixative: 3:1 (v/v) methanol/glacial acetic acid, freshly prepared before use.
4. Microscope slides.

2.2.3 Preparing DNA Fiber from Halo Preparation

1. 1×, 2×, 5×, and 10× PBS.
2. Cytoskeleton (CSK) buffer: 10 mM PIPES (piperazine-N,N′-bis(2-ethanesulfonic acid) (pH 6.8), 100 mM NaCl, 0.3 M sucrose, 3 mM $MgCl_2$, and 0.5% Triton® X-100.
3. Ice.
4. 2 M NaCl buffer: 2 M NaCl, 10 mM PIPES (piperazine-*N,N′*-bis(2-ethanesulfonic acid) (pH 6.8), 10 mM EDTA, 0.1% digitonin, 0.05 mM spermine, 0.125 mM spermidine, 1 mg/mL aprotinin, 1 mg/mL leupeptin, and 1.2 mM phenylmethylsulfonyl fluoride.
5. 10%, 30%, 70%, and 95% ethanol.
6. Microscope slides.
7. Coplin jar.
8. Slide warmer.

9. Cytospin.
10. Clinical centrifuge.

2.3 FISH Detection

2.3.1 DNA Probe Preparation

1. Biotin-Nick Translation Mix: 1 vial (160 μL) with 5× concentrated stabilized reaction buffer in 50 % glycerol (v/v) and DNA Polymerase I, DNase I, 0.25 mM dATP, 0.25 mM dCTP, 0.25 mM dGTP, 0.17 mM dTTP, and 0.08 mM Biotin-16-dUTP. For Dig labeling, use Dig-Nick Translation Mix (Roche).
2. Stop buffer: 0.5 M EDTA, pH 8.0.
3. 70 and 100 % ethanol.
4. Nick column (or homemade Sephadex G50 column).
5. Equilibration buffer: 10 mM Tris–HCl (pH 7.5) with 1 mM EDTA.
6. Salmon sperm DNA (10 μg/μL) (100–500 bp fragments generated by sonicating).
7. 3 M sodium acetate.
8. 15 °C water bath.

2.3.2 Probe/Slide Denaturation, Hybridization, and Post-Washing

1. 20× saline sodium citrate (SSC): 3 M NaCl and 300 mM sodium citrate.
2. Hybridization solution I (for non-repetitive DNA probes): 50 % deionized formamide, 10 % dextran sulfate in 2× SSC.
3. Hybridization solution II (for repetitive DNA probes): 65 % formamide, 10 % dextran sulfate in 2× SSC.
4. Sonicated genomic DNA (100–1000 bp) or Cot-1 DNA.
5. 100 μg/mL RNase: Dilute 2 mg/mL RNase stock (DNase-free) in 2× SSC, freshly prepared.
6. Denaturation solution for slides: 70 % deionized formamide in 2× SSC.
7. 70 % (v/v) ethanol, ice-cold.
8. 100 and 90 % (v/v) ethanol, room temperature.
9. 22 mm × 40 mm coverslips, no. 1.
10. Rubber cement.
11. 25-mL plastic slide mailers.
12. Polyethylene Coplin jars.
13. Moist chamber.
14. Hybridization washing solution A (for non-repetitive DNA probes): 50 % formamide in 2× SSC.
15. Hybridization washing solution B (for repetitive DNA probes): 65 % formamide in 2× SSC.
16. Water baths at 37, 42, 70, and 75 °C.
17. 37 °C incubator.

2.3.3 FISH Signal Detection

1. Preavidin block solution: 3 mL of 20× SSC (pH 7.0), 600 μL of 25% (w/v) BSA, 3 mL of 25% (w/v) nonfat dry milk, 8.4 mL of distilled water. Mix well, and centrifuge at 1800×*g* for 5 min to clarify. Use a 0.45 μm filter to sterilize and store at 4 °C up to 6 months in 1-mL aliquots.
2. Fluorescein-avidin DN solution: 5 μg/mL fluorescein-avidin DN in 4× SSC/1% (w/v) BSA.
3. 4× SSC/0.1% (v/v) Triton X-100.
4. PN buffer: 100 mM Na_2HPO_4, 50 mM NaH_2PO_4, and 0.1% NP-40 (v/v).
5. NGS/PN solution: 4% (v/v) normal goat serum (NGS) in PN buffer. Store 1-mL aliquots at 4 °C.
6. 5 μg/mL biotinylated anti-avidin D antibody in NGS/PN solution.
7. 10 μg/mL mouse anti-digoxigenin antibody in NGS/PN solution.
8. 10 μg/mL digoxigenin-labeled polyvalent anti-mouse Ig $F(ab')_2$ fragment in NGS/PN solution.
9. 25 μg/mL rhodamine-conjugated anti-digoxigenin Fab fragment in NGS/PN solution.
10. DAPI: 0.2 mg/mL of stock solution in distilled water. Store at 4 °C in dark.
11. Antifade mounting medium.

2.3.4 Image and Analyses

Epifluorescence microscope with triple-band-pass filter and 60×, 100× oil objectives.

Image systems including various commercially available digital cameras and computer software packages.

3 Methods

3.1 Chromatin Fiber Preparation

As stated earlier, chromatin fiber-FISH is more effective to study larger areas of the genome than DNA fiber. For example, when an individual chromosomal locus displays high levels of gene amplification, it is better to use chromatin fiber. Furthermore, it is necessary to use chromatin fiber if the goal is to study DNA/chromatin protein interactions at the chromatin level.

3.1.1 Releasing Chromatin Fibers with Alkaline Buffer

The harvested cells are resuspended in an alkaline or borate buffer at room temperature for 2–10 min. Since different types of cells responded differently to this alkaline-releasing procedure, it is necessary to adjust the time of incubation and KCl concentration accordingly (*see* **Note 1**).

1. Harvest cells using a trypsin treatment (avoid prolonged trypsinization). Divide suspended cells into 5 × 0.2–0.4 mL aliquots (~10^4 cells) in 15-mL culture tubes.
2. Add 2 mL alkaline buffer to each tube, mix contents gently by tapping the tube, and incubate at room temperature for 2, 4, 6, 8, and 10 min, respectively.
3. Add 3 mL of fixative to each tube to stop alkaline treatment immediately. Mix well.
4. Centrifuge at 200 × *g* for 7 min to collect chromatin fibers.
5. Resuspend the pellet in 4 mL of fresh fixative and fix at room temperature for 10 min. Centrifuge again at 200 × *g* for 7 min.
6. Resuspend the pellet in 0.2 mL of fixative and mix by gently tapping the tube. Drop the suspension on a prechilled slide. Air dry.
7. Examine the slide with a phase-contrast microscope to check the quality of preparation and identify the optimal duration of alkaline treatment. Alternatively, stain the slide with 4 % Giemsa stain before the quality check.
8. Prepare additional slides according to the optimized condition tested from **step 2**. Dry the good quality slides at room temperature for 1 day for FISH detection. Slides can be stored up to several weeks at −20 °C in a slide box sealed with Parafilm.

3.1.2 Inducing Chromatin Fibers from Cultured Lymphocytes by Drug Treatment

For liquid cancer samples, the induction of chromatin fiber can be achieved by various drug treatments, including ethidium bromide, BrdU, or m-AMSA. These drugs are thought to interfere with chromosome condensation, but the mechanism is not fully understood. Compared to chromatin fibers prepared by alkaline or detergent treatments, this protocol seems to produce more consistent results in lymphocytes, and the morphology of free chromatin appears to be more homogeneous.

1. Isolate the lymphocytes from 3 to 5 mL of fresh peripheral blood by low-speed centrifugation at 10 × *g* for 5 min or unit-gravity sedimentation. Collect buffy coat including lymphocytes using a transfer pipette, with a gentle aspiration.
2. Transfer 0.5–0.8 mL of isolated cells to 20 mL of RPMI-1640 medium with serum in a 25-cm^2 tissue culture flask (or 0.2 mL of isolated lymphocyte in 5 mL of medium using a 15-mL culture tube, if blood amount is limited). Culture in CO_2 incubator at 37 °C for 48 h.
3. Add 40 μL of 5 mg/mL m-AMSA or 20 μL of 10 mg/mL ethidium bromide (10 μg/mL final concentration of either drug). Culture in CO_2 incubator at 37 °C for 2 h (*see* **Note 2**).
4. Transfer 4 mL of culture to a 15-mL polypropylene tube and harvest drug-treated cells by centrifuging at 200 × *g* for 7 min

at room temperature. The culture should contain ~10^4 cells/mL. Do not use >4 mL of culture as an overcrowded chromatin fiber suspension is not ideal for subsequent FISH analyses.

5. Resuspend the cell pellet in 0.3 mL of RPMI-1640 medium. Add 5 mL of 0.4% KCl solution and mix well. Incubate at 37 °C for 15 min (*see* **Note 3**).
6. Add 0.1–0.2 mL of freshly prepared fixative. Mix gently by tapping and inverting the tube. Centrifuge at 200 × *g* for 7 min.
7. Discard the supernatant. Add a few drops of fresh fixative and tap bottom of tube gently to loosen pellet. Add 5 mL of fixative to resuspend the cells, and incubate at room temperature for 20 min.
8. Centrifuge at 200 × *g* for 7 min. Discard the supernatant and resuspend the pellet in 0.5 mL of fresh fixative. Place two drops of free chromatin suspension on a prechilled slide. Air dry the slide.
9. Examine the slide with a phase-contrast microscope or stain the slide with Giemsa to check the quality of fibers.
10. Prepare more fiber slides using the optimal tested conditions in **step 3**. The slides can be used for FISH detection following a few hours baking on slide warmer or store up to several months at −20 °C in slide box sealed with Parafilm (*see* **Note 4**).

3.2 DNA Fiber Preparation

The main difference between protocols generating chromatin or DNA fiber is the releasing power. In general, a harsher treatment (e.g., hypotonic treatment, alkaline treatment, use of detergents, extracting protein, etc.) favors the generation of DNA fibers. Among published protocols, many steps can be interchanged or modified to achieve better results (*see* **Note 5**).

3.2.1 Preparing DNA Fibers Using Alkaline Treatment Followed by Mechanical Stretching

1. Transfer the cultured cancer cells into a 15-mL centrifuge tube and centrifuge at 200 × *g* for 7 min to collect the cells.
2. Discard the supernatant and resuspend the cell pellet in 0.3 mL of RPMI-1640 medium, and add 4 mL of 0.4% KCl. Incubate at 37 °C for 10 min.
3. Centrifuge at 200 × *g* for 7 min.
4. Discard the supernatant. Add 5 mL of fixative and mix well.
5. Repeat **steps 3** and **4** for an additional 20 min fixation. Centrifuge, discard the supernatant, and resuspend the pellet in 0.5 mL of fresh fixative. Drop the fixed nuclear materials (two drops) onto a slide. Quickly air-dry the slide for 1 min.
6. The slide is then soaked in 1× PBS at room temperature for 1 min (the slide must not be allowed to dry out), then add 200 μL of alkaline solution onto the slide (*see* **Note 6**).

7. The coverslip lands on its edge at one end of the slide and then the coverslip is pulled along the slide from one end to the other.
8. Cover the slide with 400 μL of fixative for a 2–5 min followed by air-drying. Ready for FISH or stored at −20 °C in a sealed box.

3.2.2 Releasing DNA Fibers Using Chemical Lysis and Gravity

1. Harvest the cultured cancer cells and resuspend in 1× PBS to give a concentration of 100–5000 cells in 2 μL (5×10^4–2.5×10^6 cells/mL).
2. Place 2 μL of cell suspension at one end of a glass slide and air dry.
3. Apply 5–8 μL of lysis buffer to cells on the slide and incubate in a moist chamber at room temperature for 5 min.
4. Gently tilt the slide to vertical position with cells at the top end. Allow DNA to stream toward the bottom end of slide, then air dry almost completely.
5. Cover the slide with 400 μL of fixative at or shortly before the time that the DNA stream dries. Wait for 3 min.
6. Tilt the slide to let excess fixative drain off. Then air dry the slide. Mark the area around the DNA stream with an etching pen to help identify the area of interest.
7. Slides can be used for FISH or stored at −20 °C.

3.2.3 Preparing DNA Fiber from Halo Preparation

1. Harvest the cells from the culture.
2. Wash the cells twice with 1× PBS, and resuspend the cells in 10 mL of isotonic CSK buffer (keep the tube in ice) for 10 min.
3. Apply 40 μL of suspended cells onto the slide and centrifuge at 65 × *g* for 5 min in a cytocentrifuge. For optimal halo preparations, the cells should be at the density of 10–15/mm^2. The amount of cells for each slide can be adjusted.
4. Rinse twice with 1× PBS for 2 min each (keep the Coplin jar in ice from **steps 4** to 7).
5. Extraction in 35 mL of 2 M NaCl buffer for 4 min.
6. Rinse through a series of PBS buffer; 10×, 5×, and 2× for 1 min each, and then 1× PBS for 2 min.
7. Pass the slide in a series of ethanol; 10, 30, 70, and 95 % for 1 min each. Air dry slides at room temperature for 30 min. Bake the slides at 70 °C for 2 h using a slide warmer.
8. Slides are ready for FISH (*see* **Note** 7).

3.3 FISH Signal Detection

The challenge for fiber-FISH is the fiber preparation and image interpretation. There are no special requirements for the standard FISH protocol. Different investigators might choose their own favored protocol of FISH detection; nevertheless, 2 or 3-color FISH is required when there is more than one probe involved.

3.3.1 DNA Probe Preparation

1. To label 1 μg of probe DNA, mix 4 μL of Biotin-Nick Translation Mix (or Dig-Nick Translation Mix) and bring the total reaction volume to 20 μL with distilled water, then gently mix them (*see* **Note 8**).
2. Perform the labeling at 15 °C for 1 h for small size probes or 2 h for large size probes (BAC/PAC/YAC). Stop the reaction by adding 1 μL of stop buffer and put on ice.
3. Use the Nick column to separate the unincorporated nucleotides from the labeled probe. Load the labeled products on an equilibrated column. Add 400 μL of equilibration buffer and let it enter into the gel bed. Elute the purified sample with 400 μL of equilibration buffer. (The separation of incorporated nucleotides using nick-column is an optional step.)
4. Add 6 μL of sonicated salmon sperm DNA (60 μg) to the eluted probe solution along with 40 μL of 3 M sodium acetate.
5. Add 880 μL of cold ethanol to precipitate the probe.
6. Wash the pellet with 70% ethanol and air dry.
7. Resuspend the pellet in 20 μL of 10 mM TE buffer (pH 7.5). Probes can be stored at −20 °C for at least 1 year.

3.3.2 Probe/Slide Denaturation, Hybridization and Post-Washing

1. For cosmid-size or smaller probes: Mix 20 ng of each labeled probe with 10 μg of sonicated genomic DNA or Cot-1 DNA in 30 μL of hybridization buffer in a 1.5-mL microcentrifuge tube. For large size probes (e.g., BACs): increase the DNA of probe up to 200 ng.
2. Denature probes at 75 °C for 5 min, place the tube in a 37 °C water bath for 10 min for pre-hybridization. For probes of repetitive sequences, the pre-hybridization step should not be used. The denatured probes should be place in ice immediately.
3. Apply 50 μL of 100 μg/mL RNase to area on glass slide containing streams of stretched chromatin or DNA fibers. Cover with 22 mm × 40 mm coverslip. Incubate at 37 °C in a moist chamber for 1 h.
4. Heat jars with formamide/SSC to 75 °C in a water bath. Chill a jar with 70% ethanol on ice or use ethanol from a −20 °C freezer. Prepare two jars of 90% and 100% ethanol at room temperature.
5. Gently lift the coverslip off slide, and immerse the slide in 70% formamide/2× SSC Coplin jar at 75 °C for 2 min. Agitate the slide slightly with forceps.
6. Quickly transfer the slide to Coplin jar containing ice-cold 70% ethanol and dehydrate for 2 min, agitating slide slightly. Continue the dehydration process sequentially at room temperature in 90 and 100% ethanol for 2 min each. Air dry the slide.

7. Load the denatured probe solution to the area of the chromatin or DNA fiber and then cover with a 22 mm × 40 mm coverslip. Gently press on coverslip with forceps to force air bubbles out and seal edges with rubber cement. Incubate at 37 °C for overnight (~18 h) in a moist chamber.
8. On the next day, set up two Coplin jars with 40 mL wash solution A and two Coplin jars containing 40 mL of 2× SSC. Keep in 45 °C water bath.
9. Remove slides from moist chamber. Peel off rubber cement and carefully lift off coverslip with forceps. Immerse slide in Coplin jars of formamide/2× SSC solution for 3 min each and subsequent in Coplin jars of 2× SSC solution for 2 min each. For repetitive DNA probes, use wash solution B at 43 °C and 2× SSC at 37 °C.
10. Remove slides and drain off washing solution without letting target area dry out. Do not allow slide to dry out at any point during the following detection procedure.

3.3.3 Detection and Amplification of Fluorescence Signal (See Note 9)

1. Load 50 μL of preavidin block solution to slide. Cover with a 22 mm × 40 mm plastic coverslip. Incubate at room temperature for 10 min in a moist chamber.
2. Remove coverslip. Apply 40 μL of 5 μg/mL fluorescein-avidin DN solution to slide and cover with a plastic coverslip. Incubate at 37 °C for 20 min in a moist chamber.
3. Remove coverslip. Immerse slide sequentially in Coplin jars with 4× SSC, 4× SSC/0.1% Triton X-100, 4× SSC, and PN buffer at room temperature for 2 min each.
4. Immerse slides in 0.2 μg/mL DAPI/2× SSC at room temperature for 5 min. Rinse slides in 2× SSC, three times for 1 min each.
5. Load 10 μL of antifade solution and cover with 22 mm × 44 mm coverslip. Gently press the coverslip to exclude excessive liquid. The slides are ready for examination.
6. For signal amplification (*see* **Note 10**), add 50 μL of NGS/PN solution to the slide and cover with plastic coverslip. Incubate at room temperature for 10 min in a moist chamber.
7. Remove plastic coverslip. Apply 40 μL of 5 μg/mL biotinylated anti-avidin D antibody to area containing hybridized DNA and cover with coverslip. Incubate at 37 °C for 20 min in a moist chamber.
8. Repeat washes as described in **step 3**.
9. Repeat blocking with preavidin block solution as described in **step 1**.
10. Repeat application of fluorescein-avidin as described in **step 2**. The one color amplification is now completed, proceed to **step 11** for counterstaining. However, if two-color detection is required, skip **step 11** and proceed directly to **step 12**.

11. Repeat **steps 3–5** (for one color only). The slides are now ready for examination.
12. For the second color detection (*see* **Note 11**), wash the slide from **step 10**. Immerse slide sequentially in Coplin jars with 4× SSC, 4× SSC/0.1% Triton X-100, 4× SSC, and PN buffer at room temperature for 2 min each. (A newly prepared washing solution set is recommended for the second color detection).
13. Add 50 μL of NGS/PN solution to the slide and cover with a plastic coverslip. Incubate at room temperature for 10 min in a moist chamber.
14. Remove the coverslip. Tilt the slide to let the NGS/PN solution drain off. Apply 40 μL of 10 μg/mL mouse anti-digoxigenin antibody to the slide and cover with a coverslip. Incubate at 37 °C for 20 min in a moist chamber.
15. Repeat washes as described in **step 12**.
16. To amplify the signals, repeat **step 13**.
17. Remove the coverslip. Apply 40 μL of 10 μg/mL digoxigenin-labeled anti-mouse Ig $F(ab')_2$ fragment to the slide and cover with a coverslip. Incubate at 37 °C for 20 min in a moist chamber.
18. Repeat washes as described in **step 12**.
19. Repeat blocking with NGS/PN solution as described in **step 13**.
20. Remove the coverslip. Apply 40 μL of 10 μg/mL rhodamine-conjugated anti-digoxigenin Fab fragment to the slide and cover with a coverslip. Incubate the slide at room temperature for 20 min in a moist chamber.
21. Repeat washes as described in **step 12**.
22. Apply **steps 4** and **5**.

3.3.4 Image and Analyses

Due to the issues of fiber folding, hybridization efficiency, and background noises, quantitative analysis is of importance during fiber-FISH data interpretation. There are a few rudimentary considerations. When measuring the insert size or the physical distance between genetic markers, it is essential to include nearby markers with known genomic size. The size of the known probe can serve as a ruler for measurement. Comparative analyses using data generated from chromatin fiber, DNA fiber, and metaphase/interphase FISH are often helpful as well. One specific concern for cancer cytogenetic/cytogenomic analysis is the issue of chromosomal/genome heterogeneity. The measurements of copy number variations, the levels of gene amplification, chromosomal region amplification, and chromosomal translocations can be altered drastically among different cells/loci. It is thus important to report such heterogeneity. Knowing that genome chaos, including chromothripsis and chromoplexy, is a common phenomenon in cancer cells, and that fuzzy inheritance is a key feature in cancer evolution, fiber-FISH analysis should play an increasingly significant role.

4 Notes

1. A few factors to be considered: (a) KCl concentration and working solution pH can also be adjusted to optimal levels. Both lower pH and higher concentration (up to 2% of KCl) can reduce the releasing power. (b) Released chromatin fibers tend to stick together when present in high density, which can be avoided by reducing cell numbers or the duration of treatment. (c) A good preparation would be at the density of 2–10 chromatin fibers per 100× field. To ensure optimal density of chromatin fibers on the slide, cell concentration or duration of alkaline treatment should be adjusted. (d) Two criteria are used to judge the quality of chromatin fiber preparations: good morphology of chromatin fiber (which should be in the shape of an elongated spindle or strand-like structure with smooth edges), and minimal aggregation (i.e., contact between chromatin bundles and neighboring structures).
2. Even though the recommended drug concentration of 10 μg/mL works well for most blood samples, optimal concentrations may vary for different samples. If necessary, concentrations of 5, 10, and 20 μg/mL may be tested with small portions of the culture at ~48 h incubation. The entire process of testing (from **steps 3** to **9**) can be finished in 3–4 h. The drug concentration yielding the chromatin fibers of the most satisfactory result will then be applied for the remaining culture at ~52 h incubation.
3. Over-hypotonic treatment also promotes the release of free chromatin; duration of this step may be extended to 20–30 min if the yield of chromatin fiber is too low.
4. Metaphase FISH is often performed prior to fiber FISH analyses. This is important as the general information (including the probe quality, the number of loci, the distribution pattern cross the entire genome, and the level of noise) is essential for suitable hybridization/washing conditions as well as correct analyses of fiber FISH data. One approach is to load metaphase chromosome and chromatin/DNA fibers onto the same slide. One drop of chromatin fiber suspension and one drop of chromosome suspension should fit on the same slide longitudinally. The two preparations may be made at different times; either suspension can be kept at 4 °C before the second sample is ready.
5. Different protocols have been developed to release DNA fiber, including nuclei lysis and DNA release in a gel block and

fiber-linearization by a mechanical or an electronic pulling force. Particularly, as DNA fibers can be stretched on any hydrophobic surface with variable efficiency, the alignment of DNA molecules has been achieved using molecular combing [14]. A combing device has since been developed by the Pasteur Institute in France. Interestingly, for further improvement, salinization has been used to ensure irreversible fixation and alignment of DNA fibers onto a surface [46]. While molecular combing methods can generate more homogenous DNA fibers, the methods we discussed in this chapter are easier to follow. Again, it should be noted that, when studying the genome structure, the combination of DNA/chromatin fibers is of importance.

6. The duration of alkaline solution treatment can be adjusted. If a greater amount of release from the nuclei is needed, a longer treatment should be used. This protocol can also be used to generate chromatin fiber by adjusting the releasing conditions.
7. The duration of **steps 2** and **5** can be modified to control the degrees of fiber release. When preparing halo fiber, if a cytocentrifuge is not available, the cells can be directly cultured on slides, then simply follow **steps 2**, and **4–7**.
8. DNA probes can be labeled by different methods (nick translation vs. random primers; direct labeling with fluorescent dyes vs. indirectly labeling with biotin, digoxigenin, then detected by avidin or anti-Dig antibody conjugated with fluorescent dyes). There are many commercial labeling kits available. Supplier's instructions should be followed when the commercial kits are used.
9. Without signal amplification, signals may appear faint. With improved direct labeling, sensitive image capture systems, and software enhancement, the amplification step could be potentially eliminated.
10. When detecting small size probes, signal amplification is often required. In this case, upon finishing **step 3**, one should avoid **steps 4** and **5**, and directly proceed to **step 6**. If a large-sized probe's signal is too weak upon examination, the amplification step can be added on. To do so, just carefully remove the coverslip, and briefly wash the slides in 2× SSC, before proceeding to **steps 6–11**.
11. For multiple color FISH detection without amplification, anti-digoxigenin-rhodomin fragments and FITC-avidin can be detected simultaneously within the same step. If signal amplification is required, sequential detection/amplification of each probe is preferred to avoid higher background.

References

1. Heng H, Chen WY (1985) The study of the chromatin and the structure for Bufo gargarizans by the light microscope. J Sichuan Union Univ Nat Sci 2:105–109
2. Heng HH, Shi XM (1997) From free chromatin analysis to high resolution fiber FISH. Cell Res 7:119–124
3. Heng HH, Tsui LC (1998) High resolution free chromatin/DNA fiber fluorescent in situ hybridization. J Chromatogr A 806:219–229
4. Heng HH, Spyropoulos B, Moens P (1997) Fish technology in chromosome and genome research. BioEssays 10:75–84
5. Heng HH, Liu G, Stevens JB et al (2013) Karyotype heterogeneity and unclassified chromosomal abnormalities. Cytogenet Genome Res 139:144–157
6. Heng HH, Squire J, Tsui LC (1991) Chromatin mapping - a strategy for physical characterization of the human genome by hybridization in situ. Proc 8th Int Cong Hum Gen Am J Hum Genet 49:368
7. Heng HH, Squire J, Tsui LC (1992) High resolution mapping of mammalian genes by in situ hybridization to free chromatin. Proc Natl Acad Sci U S A 89:9509–9513
8. Wiegant J, Kalle W, Mullenders L et al (1992) High resolution in situ hybridization using DNA halo preparation. Hum Mol Genet 1:587–592
9. Parra I, Windle B (1993) High resolution visual mapping of stretched DNA by fluorescent hybridization. Nat Genet 5:17–21
10. Houseal TW, Dackowski WR, Landes GM et al (1994) High resolution mapping of overlappingcosmids by fluorescence in situ hybridization. Cytometry 15:193–198
11. Fidlerova H, Senger G, Kost M et al (1994) Two simple procedures for releasing chromatin from routinely fixed cells for fluorescence in situ hybridization. Cytogenet Cell Genet 65:203–205
12. Haaf T, Ward DC (1994) High resolution ordering of YAC contigs using extended chromatin and chromosomes. Hum Mol Genet 3:629–633
13. Heiskanen M, Karhu R, Hellsten E et al (1994) High resolution mapping using fluorescence in situ hybridization to extended DNA fibers prepared from agarose embedded cells. Bio Techniques 17:928–933
14. Bensimon A, Simon A, Chiffaudel A et al (1994) Alignment and sensitive detection of DNA by a moving interface. Science 265:2096–2098
15. Heng HH (2002) High resolution FISH mapping using chromatin and DNA fiber. In: Beatty B, Mai S, Squire J (eds) FISH: a practical approach. Oxford University Press, Oxford, pp 77–92
16. Heng HH, Windle B, Tsui LC (2005) High -resolution FISH analysis. In: Dracopoli NC, Haines JL, Korf BR (eds) Current protocols in human genetics. John Wiley & Sons, New York, Volume 23 (Suppl 44) 4.5.1–4.5.23
17. Fransz PF, Alonso-Blanco CM, Liharska TB et al (1996) High-resolution physical mapping in Arabidopsis thaliana and tomato by fluorescence in situ hybridization to extended DNA fibres. Plant J 9:421–430
18. Jackson SA, Wang ML, Goodman HM et al (1998) Application of fiber-FISH in physical mapping of Arabidopsis thaliana. Genome 41:566–572
19. Tsuchiya D, Taga M (2001) Application of fibre-FISH (fluorescence in situ hybridization) to filamentous fungi: visualization of the rRNA gene cluster of the ascomycete Cochliobolus heterostrophus. Microbiology 147:1183–1187
20. Pauciullo A, Fleck K, Lühken G et al (2013) Dual-color high-resolution fiber-FISH analysis on lethal white syndrome carriers in sheep. Cytogenet Genome Res 140:46–54
21. Wang K, Zhang W, Jiang Y et al (2013) Systematic application of DNA fiber-FISH technique in cotton. PLoS One 8, e75674
22. Iafrate AJ, Feuk L, Rivera MN et al (2004) Detection of large-scale variation in the human genome. Nat Genet 36:949–951
23. Horelli-Kuitunen N, Aaltonen J, Yaspo ML et al (1999) Mapping ESTs by fiber-FISH. Genome Res 9:62–71
24. Lestou VS, Strehl S, Lion T et al (1996) High-resolution FISH of the entire integrated Epstein-Barr virus genome on extended human DNA. Cytogenet Cell Genet 74:211–217
25. Gervasini C, Bentivegna A, Venturin M et al (2002) Tandem duplication of the NF1 gene detected by high-resolution FISH in the 17q11.2 region. Hum Genet 111:465–467
26. Vesa J, Hellsten E, Verkruyse LA et al (1995) Mutations in the palmitoyl protein thioesterase gene causing infantile neuronal ceroid lipofuscinosis. Nature 376:584–587
27. Trower MK, Orton SM, Purvis IJ et al (1996) Conservation of synteny between the genome of the pufferfish (Fugu rubripes) and the region on human chromosome 14 (14q24.3) associated with familial Alzheimer

disease (AD3 locus). Proc Natl Acad Sci U S A 93:1366–1369

28. Gusso Goll L, Matiello RR, Artoni RF et al (2015) High-resolution physical chromosome mapping of multigene families in Lagria villosa (Tenebrionidae): occurrence of interspersed ribosomal genes in coleoptera. Cytogenet Genome Res 146:64–70
29. Rottger S, Yen PH, Schempp W (2002) A fiber-FISH contig spanning the non-recombining region of the human Y chromosome. Chromosome Res 10:621–635
30. Heng HH, Chamberlain JW, Shi XM et al (1996) Regulation of meiotic chromatin loop size by chromosomal position. Proc Natl Acad Sci U S A 93:2795–2800
31. Heng HH, Krawetz SK, Lu W et al (2001) Re-defining the chromatin loop domain. Cytogent Cell Genet 93:155–161
32. Heng HH, Goetze S, Ye CJ et al (2004) Chromatin loops are selectively anchored using scaffold/matrix attachment regions. J Cell Sci 117:999–1008
33. Haaf T (1996) High-resolution analysis of DNA replication in released chromatin fibers containing 5-bromodeoxyuridine. Biotechniques 21:1050–1054
34. Florijn RJ, Bonden LA, Vrolijk H et al (1995) High-resolution DNA Fiber-FISH for genomic DNA mapping and colour bar-coding of large genes. Hum Mol Genet 4:831–836
35. Riemersma SA, Jordanova ES, Schop RF et al (2000) Extensive genetic alterations of the HLA region, including homozygous deletions of HLA class II genes in B-cell lymphomas arising in immune-privileged sites. Blood 96:3569–3577
36. Inoue K, Osaka H, Imaizumi K et al (1999) Proteolipid protein gene duplications causing Pelizaeus-Merzbacher Disease: molecular mechanism and phenotypic manifestations. Ann Neurol 45:624–632
37. Jiang F, Lin F, Price R et al (2002) Rapid detection of IgH/BCL2 rearrangement in follicular lymphoma by interphase fluorescence in situ hybridization with bacterial artificial chromosome probes. J Mol Diagn 4:144–149
38. Poulsen TS, Silahtaroglu AN, Gisselo CG et al (2001) Detection of illegitimate rearrangement within the immunoglobulin locus on 14q32.3 in B-cell malignancies using end-sequenced probes. Genes Chromosomes Cancer 32:265–274
39. Heng HH (2009) The genome-centric concept: resynthesis of evolutionary theory. Bioessays 31:512–525
40. Heng HH, Liu G, Stevens JB et al (2011) Decoding the genome beyond sequencing: the new phase of genomic research. Genomics 98:242–252
41. Heng HH (2016) Debating cancer: the paradox of cancer research. World Scientific, Hackensack, NJ
42. Stevens JB, Abdallah BY, Horne SD et al (2013) Genetic and epigenetic heterogeneity in cancer. eLs – Wiley Online Library. doi:10.1002/9780470015902.a0023592
43. Liu G, Stevens JB, Horne SD et al (2014) Genome chaos: survival strategy during crisis. Cell Cycle 13:528–537
44. Heng HH, Regan SM, Liu G et al (2016) Why it is crucial to analyze non clonal chromosome aberrations or NCCAs? Mol Cytogenet 9:e15
45. Heng HH, Bremer SW, Stevens JB et al (2013) Chromosomal instability (CIN): what it is and why it is crucial to cancer evolution. Cancer Metastasis Rev 32:325–340
46. Labit H, Goldar A, Guilbaud G et al (2008) A simple and optimized method of producing silanized surfaces for FISH and replication mapping on combed DNA fibers. BioTechniques 45:649–658

Chapter 15

Array-Based Comparative Genomic Hybridization (aCGH)

Chengsheng Zhang, Eliza Cerveira, Mallory Romanovitch, and Qihui Zhu

Abstract

Copy number variations (CNVs) in the genomes have been suggested to play important roles in human evolution, genetic diversity, and disease susceptibility. A number of assays have been developed for the detection of CNVs, including fluorescent in situ hybridization (FISH), array-based comparative genomic hybridization (aCGH), PCR-based assays, and next-generation sequencing (NGS). In this chapter, we describe a microarray method that has been used for the detection of genome-wide CNVs, loss of heterozygosity (LOH), and uniparental disomy (UPD) associated with constitutional and neoplastic disorders.

Key words Microarray, Array-based comparative genomic hybridization (aCGH), Copy number variation (CNV), Single nucleotide polymorphism (SNP), Loss of heterozygosity (LOH), Uniparental disomy (UPD)

1 Introduction

Structural variations (SVs) in the human genome are present in many forms, including single nucleotide polymorphisms (SNPs), small insertion/deletions (Indels), inversions, translocations, repetitive sequences, and copy number variations (CNVs) [1–3]. CNVs, which encompass more total nucleotides than SNPs in the human genomes, have been suggested to play important roles in human evolution, genetic diversity, and disease susceptibility [4–12]. In addition, CNVs have been shown to be associated with a variety of constitutional and neoplastic disorders. For instance, a number of microdeletion/microduplication syndromes (e.g., Williams-Beuren syndrome, Angelman Syndrome, DiGeorge syndrome, Pallister Killian syndrome, and Potocki-Lupski syndrome) result from copy number gain or loss in the genome [13]. Cancer is a genetic disease, which is driven by genetic changes in the oncogenes, tumor suppressor genes, and DNA repair genes, as well as the chromosomal instability [14]. Numerous studies from the Cancer Genome Atlas (TCGA) Consortium and other research groups have indicated that CNVs may also play significant roles in the process of tumorigenesis [15–17].

Thomas S.K. Wan (ed.), *Cancer Cytogenetics: Methods and Protocols*, Methods in Molecular Biology, vol. 1541,
DOI 10.1007/978-1-4939-6703-2_15,

A number of assays have been developed for detection of CNVs in the human genomes, including fluorescence in situ hybridization (FISH), array-based comparative genomic hybridization (aCGH), PCR-based assays, and next-generation sequencing [1–3, 13]. The aCGH has many advantages over the conventional cytogenetic techniques, such as genome-wide coverage, high resolution, and amenable to automation. However, it also has a number of limitations. For instance, it is unable to detect the balanced chromosomal rearrangements (e.g., inversions and translocations). In early CGH experiments, the DNA targets were analyzed with the metaphase chromosome spreads [18–20]. This technology later evolved so that the DNA targets are hybridized to immobile cDNA fragments or bacterial artificial chromosomes (BACs) on a microarray surface [21–25]. The current advanced technology measures copy number differences using oligonucleotide microarrays from Agilent, Affymetrix, and Illumina [26–28]. Some of the aCGH arrays label the test and normal reference DNA samples with different fluorescent dyes (e.g., Cy5 and Cy3) respectively, and co-hybridized to the microarray [28]. The fluorescence intensity ratio of the two labeled dyes at each DNA fragment reflects the copy number ratio of that DNA sequence in the test DNA compared to the reference DNA [28]. Others are not required to be hybridized simultaneously with the test DNA sample [29]. The test sample data is compared to the data of normal reference samples in the database developed by the manufacturers through bioinformatics analysis. Regions of DNA that have been deleted or amplified are seen as changes in the ratio of test data against the normal control data along the target chromosomes. The SNP arrays are able to detect CNVs, loss of heterozygosity (LOH), and uniparental disomy (UPD) [29].

In this chapter, we describe an aCGH assay using the CytoScan HD platform from Affymetrix [29]. This array contains roughly 2.7 million probes throughout the human genome and offers the highest resolution coverage for constitutional and cancer genes. It covers all 36,000 RefSeq genes including 12,000 OMIM, all ISCA constitutional regions, and Sanger cancer genes. The effective resolution is 12 kilobase pairs (kb) on OMIM genes, 22 kb on other RefSeq genes, 10 kb on ISCA and cancer genes, and 50 kb on the backbone. It provides a genome-wide approach for detection of CNVs (gains or losses), LOH, regions identical-by-descent, and UPD on a single array. This array platform has been widely used in research and clinical laboratories for studies of constitutional and neoplastic disorders [30–38]. In 2010, the American College of Medical Genetics and Genomics (ACMGG) recommended employing chromosomal microarray as a first-tier test for patients with unexplained developmental or intellectual disability, autism spectrum disorders, and congenital anomalies [39]. In 2014, Affymetrix received the clearance from the U.S. Food and Drug

Administration (FDA) to market its CytoScan Dx assay for pediatric patients with developmental delay and/or intellectual disability [40]. However, for DNA samples extracted from the formalin-fixed, paraffin-embedded (FFPE) tissue specimens, we are using the Affymetrix OncoScan CNV FFPE array platform, which has been developed and optimized specifically for FFPE DNA samples [41–43].

2 Materials

2.1 Equipment and Software

1. Gene Chip® Hybridization Oven 645 (Affymetrix).
2. GeneChip® Fluidics Station 450 (Affymetrix).
3. GeneChip® 3000 Scanner (Affymetrix).
4. Nanodrop™ 2000 (ThermoFisher Scientific).
5. GeneChip® Command Console (Affymetrix).
6. Chromosome Analysis Suite (Affymetrix).
7. DynaMag-2™ Magnet (ThermoFisher Scientific).
8. Microtube foam adapter for vortexer.
9. GeneAmp® PCR System 9700, 96-Well Gold-Plated (ThermoFisher Scientific). Program the thermal cycler with the programs listed below (**Items 10–15**).
10. DIGEST thermal cycler program: 37 °C for 2 h, 65 °C for 20 min, hold at 4 °C.
11. LIGATION thermal cycler program: 16 °C for 3 h, 70 °C for 20 min, hold at 4 °C.
12. PCR thermal cycler program: 1 cycle of 94 °C for 3 min; 30 cycles of 94 °C for 30 s, 60 °C for 45 s and 68 °C for 15 s; 1 cycle of 68 °C for 7 min; hold at 4 °C.
13. FRAGMENTATION thermal cycler program: 37 °C for 35 min, 95 °C for 15 min, hold at 4 °C.
14. LABELING thermal cycler program: 37 °C for 4 h, 95 °C for 15 min, hold at 4 °C.
15. HYBRIDIZATION thermal cycler program: 95 °C for 10 min, hold at 49 °C.

2.2 Reagents and Consumables

It is critical that the reagents from Affymetrix and Clontech are stored at −20 °C, unless otherwise noted. Arrays should be stored at 4 °C until use.

1. 96-well un-skirted PCR plate.
2. Adhesive film for 96-well PCR plate.
3. Tough Spots, 1/2″ and 3/8″ (ThermoFisher Scientific).
4. 50–2000 base pairs (bp) DNA marker.

5. 25 bp DNA Marker.
6. CytoScan® HD Array and Reagent kit (Affymetrix). For purification wash buffer, add 45 mL of 100% ethanol to bottle before use. Make Master Mixes immediately before use [8–13] and prepare on ice.
7. Titanium® DNA Amplification kit (Clontech). Make Master Mix immediately before use and prepare on ice.
8. Digestion Master Mix: Add 2.0 μL of 10× NspI buffer, 0.2 μL of 100× BSA, 1.0 μL of NspI; total per reaction 3.2 μL.
9. Ligation Master Mix: Add 2.50 μL of 10× T4 DNA Ligase buffer, 0.75 μL of 50 μM Adaptor (NspI), 2 μL of T4 DNA Ligase; total per reaction 5.25 μL.
10. PCR Master Mix: Add 39.5 μL of Nuclease-Free water, 10.0 μL of 10× TITANIUM™ Taq PCR buffer, 20 μL of GC-Melt Reagent, 14 μL of dNTP Mixture (2.5 mM each), 4.5 μL PCR Primer (002), 2 μL of 50× TITANIUM™ Taq DNA Polymerase; total per reaction 90.0 μL.
11. Fragmentation Master Mix: Add 90.4 μL of Nuclease-Free water, 114.6 μL of 10× Fragmentation buffer, 3.3 μL of 2.5 U/μL Fragmentation reagent; total per reaction 208.3 μL.
12. Labeling Master Mix: Add 14.0 μL of 5× TdT buffer, 2 μL of 30 mM DNA Labeling reagent, 3.5 μL of TdT; total per reaction 19.5 μL.
13. Hybridization Master Mix: Add 165.0 μL of Hyb buffer Part 1, 15.0 μL of Hyb buffer Part 2, 7 μL of Hyb buffer Part 3, 1 μL of Hyb buffer Part 4, 2 μL of Oligo control reagent 0100; total per reaction 190 μL.

3 Methods

Listed below are the laboratory methods for the CytoScan® HD Assay. The assay can be completed in 3 or 4 days depending on the timing of each step (*see* **Note 1**). In order to assure the quality of performance, reactions should be set up in designated Pre-PCR or Post-PCR areas to decrease the likelihood of amplicon contamination (*see* **Note 2**). For quality control and troubleshooting purposes, a positive and a negative control may be run alongside of the test samples (*see* **Note 3**). Perform all steps on ice unless otherwise specified.

3.1 Sample Preparation

1. Good quality double-stranded DNA must be used for this protocol (*see* **Note 4**).
2. Add 250 ng of DNA to nuclease-free water in a 96-well plate. The final dilution volume is 16.6 μL.
3. Seal, vortex, and spin down the plate (*see* **Notes 5** and **6**).

3.2 Restriction Enzyme Digestion

1. Thaw reagents (*see* **Note 7**). Prepare the Digestion Master Mix (*see* **Note 8**). Briefly vortex master mix and spin down. Add 3.2 μL of Digestion Master Mix to each sample well in the plate (*see* **Note 9**). Seal, vortex, and spin down the plate.
2. Load the plate onto the thermal cycler (*see* **Note 10**) and run the DIGEST program.
3. When the program is complete, spin plate (*see* **Note 11**). Proceed to Ligation or store plate at −20 °C (*see* **Note 12**).

3.3 Ligation

1. Prepare the Ligation Master Mix. Briefly vortex master mix and spin down. Add 5.25 μL of Ligation Master Mix to each sample well in the plate. Seal, vortex, and spin down the plate.
2. Load the plate onto the thermal cycler and run the LIGATION program.
3. When the program is complete, spin plate. Proceed to PCR or store the *Ligation* plate at −20 °C.

3.4 PCR

1. Dilute the ligated samples by adding 75 μL of chilled nuclease-free water. Seal, vortex, and spin down the plate.
2. Transfer 10 μL of the diluted sample to each of the corresponding four wells of a new 96-well plate to be used for PCR. For example, the sample in A1 in the *Ligation* plate will be transferred to wells A1, B1, C1, and D1 of the *new PCR* plate, respectively (*see* **Note 13**). Store the *Ligation* plate at −20 °C (*see* **Note 14**). Proceed to PCR setup or store the *PCR* plate at −20 °C.
3. Prepare the PCR Master Mix (*see* **Note 15**). Briefly vortex master mix and spin down. Add 90 μL of PCR Master Mix to each sample well in the plate (*see* **Note 16**). Seal, vortex, repeat vortex, and spin down the plate.
4. Load the plate onto the thermal cycler in the Post-PCR area and run the PCR program.

3.5 Gel QC and PCR Product Purification

1. After the PCR program is complete, remove plate from thermal cycler and spin down.
2. Use 3 μL of PCR product from the first row of samples and run a 2% gel. Use a 50–2000 bp marker for determining the size distribution. The PCR was successful if the majority of the product distribution is between 150 and 2000 bp (*see* **Note 14**).
3. Pool the four wells of each sample from the *PCR* plate into a new 1.5-mL tube (A total of 400 μL will be pooled for each sample). Add 720 μL of Purification Beads to each pooled sample (*see* **Note 17**). Mix sample tubes well by inverting ten times. Incubate at room temperature for 10 min. Centrifuge tubes at 16,000 × *g* for 3 min (*see* **Note 18**).

4. Place tubes on magnetic stand to separate the beads from the supernatant (*see* **Note 19**). Pipette supernatant and discard. Add 1 mL of the Purification Wash Buffer to each tube on the stand. Cap tubes and load onto the foam adapter. Vortex tubes at maximum speed for 2 min and then centrifuge at 16,000 × *g* for 3 min.
5. Place tubes on magnetic stand to separate the beads from the supernatant. Pipette supernatant and discard. Spin tubes at 16,000 × *g* for 30 s. Place tubes on magnetic stand to separate the beads from the supernatant. Pipette and discard any residual Purification Wash Buffer. Remove tubes from magnetic stand, leave caps open, and allow remaining Purification Wash Buffer to evaporate for 10 min.
6. Add 52 μL of Elution Buffer to each tube, dispensing directly on the beads. Cap the tubes and vortex in the foam adaptor for 10 min (*see* **Note 20**). Centrifuge at 16,000 × *g* for 3 min. Place tubes on magnetic stand for 10 min to separate the beads from the supernatant.
7. Transfer 47 μL of eluted sample to a new 96-well plate for Fragmentation. Seal and spin the plate. Proceed to Quantification or store the *Fragmentation* plate at −20 °C.

3.6 Quantification of the Purified PCR Product

1. Aliquot 2 μL of each purified sample from the *Fragmentation* plate to 18 μL of nuclease-free water, for a 1:10 dilution. Vortex and spin.
2. Measure the concentration by Nanodrop. Calculate the undiluted concentration for each sample in μg/μL (*see* **Note 21**). Samples pass the quality control check if they are ≥2.5 μg/μL (*see* **Note 14**).

3.7 Fragmentation and Gel QC

1. Set plate centrifuge to 4 °C (*see* **Note 22**).
2. Prepare the Fragmentation Master Mix (*see* **Note 23**). Briefly vortex master mix and spin down. Add 10 μL of Fragmentation Master Mix to each sample well in the plate. Seal, vortex, and spin down the plate.
3. Load plate onto the thermal cycler and run the FRAGMENTATION program (*see* **Note 24**).
4. After the FRAGMENTATION program is complete spin plate. Prepare sample for gel QC by aliquoting 4 μL of Fragmentation product to 28 μL of nuclease-free water for a 1:8 dilution. Seal Fragmentation plate and proceed to Labeling on the same day (*see* **Note 25**).
5. Use 8 μL of diluted Fragmentation product to run a 4% gel. Use a 25 bp marker for determining the size distribution. The Fragmentation is successful if the majority of the product distribution is between 25 and 125 bp (*see* **Note 14**).

3.8 Labeling

1. Prepare the Labeling Master Mix. Briefly vortex master mix and spin down. Add 19.5 µL of Labeling Master Mix to each sample well in the plate. Seal, vortex, and spin down the plate.
2. Load the plate onto thermal cycler and run the LABELING program.
3. When the program is complete, spin plate. Proceed to Hybridization or store plate at −20 °C.

3.9 Hybridization

1. Unpack arrays and allow them to equilibrate at room temperature. Preheat the hybridization oven for at least 1 h at 50 °C with rotation at 60 rpm.
2. If using Affymetrix GeneChip® Command Console® (AGCC) software, generate and enter information into a sample batch registration file. Open the "AGCC Scan Control" application from the "Affymetrix Launcher." Download a batch file from the program and fill out the user fields. Scan the array barcodes and verify that the correct array type was assigned as "CytoScan HD." Once the file is complete, upload the sample and array information to AGCC.
3. Place the arrays on a clean bench top area designated for hybridization. Insert a 200 µL pipette tip into the upper right septum of each array. Paste two 1/2″ Tough-Spots® on the top edge of the array for later use.
4. Prepare the Hybridization Master Mix. Briefly vortex master mix and spin down. Add 190 µL of Hybridization Master Mix to each sample well in the plate (*see* **Note 26**). Seal, vortex, repeat vortex, and spin down the plate. Load the plate onto thermal cycler and run the HYBRIDIZATION program.
5. When the HYBRIDIZATION program is complete, ensure that samples incubate at 49 °C for at least 1 min. Keeping the plate on the thermal cycler at 49 °C, remove the seal and pipette 200 µL of the sample and immediately inject it into the lower left septum of the array (*see* **Note 27**). Cover both septa on the array with the 1/2" Tough-Spots®, leaving a small overhang for easy removal. When six to eight arrays are loaded and the septa are covered, balance in bins and place in preheated oven. Allow the arrays to rotate at 50 °C, 60 rpm for 16–18 h.

3.10 Washing, Staining, and Scanning Arrays

1. Aliquot the following reagents into separate 1.5-mL microfuge tubes for each array:
   (a) 500 µL of Stain Buffer 1 into amber tubes.
   (b) 500 µL of Stain Buffer 2 into clear tubes.
   (c) 800 µL of Array Holding Buffer into blue tubes.

2. Prime the Fluidics Stations with Wash A, Wash B and distilled water by selecting "Prime450" as the method in the Fluidics Control section of the AGCC (*see* **Note 28**).
3. Select the "CytoScan_Array_450" program on the Fluidics Control, and follow the prompts to load the stain solutions. After the 16–18 h incubation, remove the arrays from the hybridization oven. Remove the Tough-Spots® from each array and follow the prompts to load onto the Fluidics Stations and run the program.
4. Once the washing and staining protocol is complete, examine the arrays and ensure there are no visible bubbles. Debubble by inserting the array back into the fluidics station if necessary (*see* **Note 29**).
5. Turn on scanner and allow it to warm up for at least 10 min prior to use. Cover the array septa with 3/8″ Tough-Spots®, clean the array window with a lint-free tissue.
6. Open the Scan Control from the AGCC. Load the arrays into the autoloader of the scanner. Once all the arrays are loaded, click the "Start" icon to initiate the scan. Select the check box "arrays in carousel positions 1–4 at room temperature." If the arrays are not at room temperature, do not select this option. The scanner will wait 10 min before scanning begins to allow the arrays to reach room temperature.
7. The scanner generates images of the array and converts the data into a .cel file. Analysis of the data files for structural variation, including CNVs, SNPs, and LOH, is completed by uploading the .cel file to the Affymetrix Chromosome Analysis Suite (ChAS). Please refer to the Affymetrix user manual to set up appropriate parameters determined by experiment setup and sample type. *See* Fig. 1 for examples of the different types of chromosomal aberrations that can be detected by this assay.

4 Notes

1. A 4- or 3-day protocol works well for this assay.
   (a) CytoScan® HD 4-day protocol.
   - Day 1: Digestion, Ligation (stay on thermal cycler overnight).
   - Day 2: PCR, PCR Gel QC, Purification, Quantification (store samples at −20 °C overnight).
   - Day 3: Fragmentation, Fragmentation Gel QC, Labeling, Hybridization (overnight).
   - Day 4: Wash, Stain, and Scan.

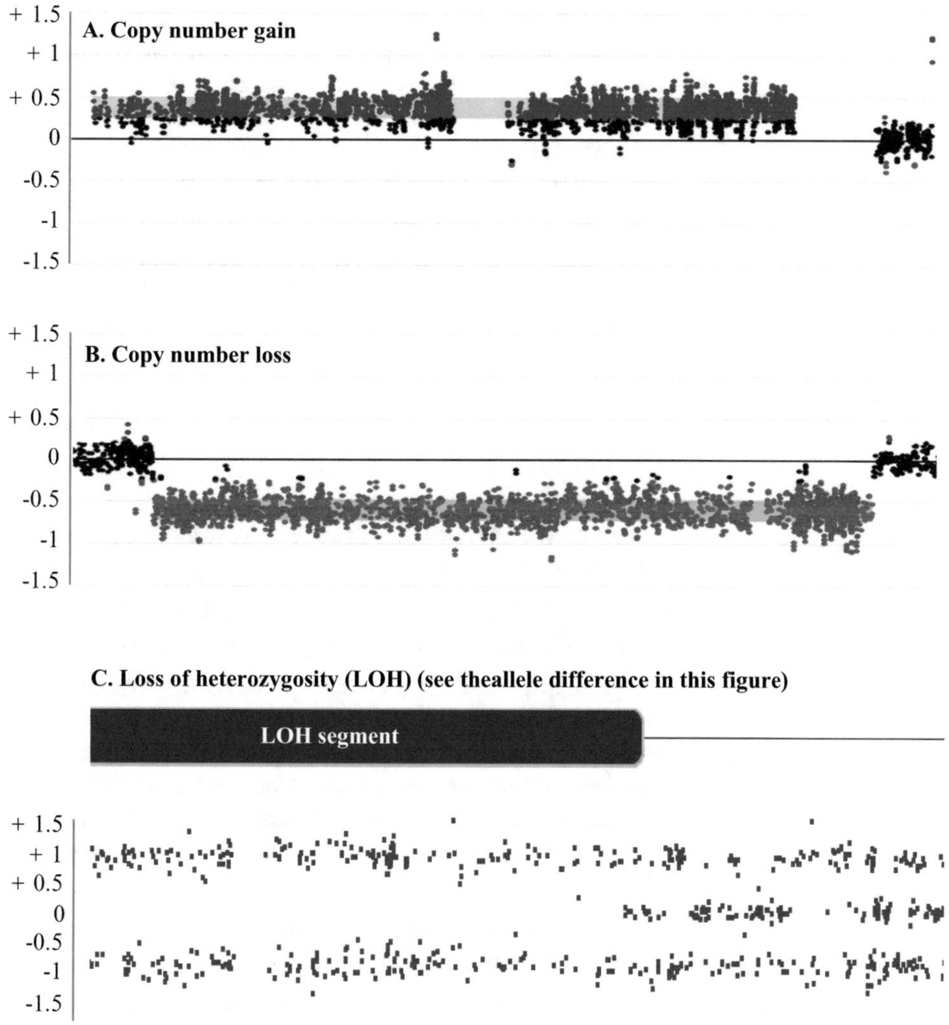

Fig. 1 Chromosomal aberrations detected by aCGH using Affymetrix CytoScan® HD platform. (**a**) Copy number gain, (**b**) Copy number loss, (**c**) Loss of heterozygosity (LOH) (see the allele difference in this figure)

(b) CytoScan® HD 3-day protocol.

- Day 1: Digestion, Ligation, PCR (stay on thermal cycler overnight).
- Day 2: PCR Gel QC, Purification, Quantification, Fragmentation, Fragmentation Gel QC, Labeling, Hybridization (overnight).
- Day 3: Wash, Stain, and Scan.

2. The following steps should be performed in the Pre-PCR area: Sample Prep, Digestion, Ligation, and the setup for PCR. The remaining steps are to be performed in the Post-PCR area.
3. The CytoScan® HD kit comes with a positive control that meets the DNA requirements. It is helpful to run this control

when familiarizing oneself with the protocol and for troubleshooting purposes. A negative control can also be run by loading nuclease-free water to the reaction instead of template DNA. The negative control is helpful for determining if contamination is an issue, which is seen in the QC steps. The negative control should not be hybridized to an array.

4. Genomic DNA must be of high quality as the PCR amplification requires fragments between 150 and 2000 bp in size. The sample must be double-stranded, free of PCR inhibitors, not contaminated with other sources, and not degraded. The Qiagen Gentra Purgene kit has provided high-quality DNA for this method. DNA concentration is recommended to be >50 ng/μL.
5. Always use a new seal and ensure it is tight before vortexing. For all plate vortexing, use the **5-sector method**: vortex each corner of the plate for 1 s and then an additional 1 s vortex at the center of the plate.
6. For all centrifugations, use a plate centrifuge and spin for 1 min at 800 × *g* at room temperature, unless otherwise noted.
7. For all steps, thaw reagents except enzymes at room temperature. Briefly vortex reagents three times, one second each and quickly spin down. Place reagents on ice and ensure they are cool before use. Enzymes should be kept at −20 °C until use. Quickly vortex for one second and spin briefly. Always keep enzymes on a cooling chamber and return immediately to −20 °C after use.
8. When preparing master mixes for all steps, always make 20% extra to account for dead volume and pipetting error.
9. When working with more than a few samples, it can be helpful to aliquot the master mix into a strip tube and then use a multichannel pipette to dispense the master mix to the reaction plate.
10. For all programs, preheat the lid of the thermal cycler before loading the plate. The block can be left at room temperature.
11. At the end of all thermal cycling programs, ensure seal is sufficiently tight on the plate before removing from the thermal cycler. This will reduce the likelihood of contamination between wells.
12. The reaction plate can sit on the thermal cycler overnight for all programs except Cytoscan FRAGMENTATION, as the Fragmentation step is extremely sensitive. In addition, the samples can also be stored at −20 °C for up to a week after each step, except Fragmentation.
13. Four PCR reactions per sample will be run to increase total yield for further processing.

14. The remaining volume of the *Ligation* plate is 60 μL. If a processing error occurs at any point, including failed QC steps, the assay can be repeated starting from the PCR step using the remaining Ligation product.
15. It is important to remember that there are four PCR reactions per sample when preparing the master mix. Prepare enough master mix for the total number of samples multiplied by 4, plus 20% dead volume.
16. For the PCR Master Mix, it is sometimes easier to pour it into a trough on ice and use a multichannel pipette to dispense into the plate.
17. It is crucial to mix the Purification Beads thoroughly before addition to the samples; invert several times or quickly vortex and ensure mixture is homogeneous. In addition, take the Purification Beads out of the refrigerator and allow them to warm to room temperature for at least 15 min before use. Pipette the beads slowly as they are viscous.
18. When centrifuging tubes, always have tube hinges facing out, away from the rotor.
19. When allowing the beads to separate from the supernatant, ensure the solution is clear before removing supernatant. This typically takes around 5 min. Be careful to not disturb the bead pellet when removing the supernatant.
20. After 10 min vortex, gently flick the tubes to ensure pellet has been dislodged. If not, vortex for an additional 2 min. Repeat the vortex again if necessary.
21. Calculate the concentration for each sample in μg/μL as follows: Undiluted concentration in μg/μL = (Nanodrop Concentration in ng/μL × 10) ÷ (1000).
22. The Fragmentation step is very temperature sensitive. Spin the plate in a cold (4 °C) centrifuge, keep all reagents cold, and move quickly. Over or under fragmentation can yield poor QC results.
23. The Fragmentation master mix recipe provided is the minimum amount to make per experiment due to pipetting accuracy of the enzyme. This recipe can be multiplied if more than eight samples are processed.
24. It is critical at this stage to ensure that both the lid and the block of thermal cycler are preheated for the Fragmentation step.
25. Always proceed immediately to labeling on the same day. Do NOT store the fragmented samples overnight as they are very unstable.
26. For the Hybridization Master Mix, it is sometimes easier to pour it into a trough on ice and use a multichannel pipette to dispense into the plate.

27. If hybridizing more than eight samples at one time, only remove the seal from six to eight samples at a time only using a razor blade. Leave the remaining wells covered to help prevent cross-contamination and evaporation.
28. It is good practice to prime all modules on the fluidics station to reduce the chance that an array would be loaded on an unprimed module. The fluidics system will prompt the user to raise/lower tips and eject wash block.
29. If the debubbling does not work, manually fill the array with Array Holding Buffer. Stick a p200 pipette tip into the top septa of the array. Remove about half of the Array Holding Buffer from the lower septa. Add fresh Array Holding Buffer to the array through the lower septa until it is full. If the fluidics stations are not removing the bubbles from the array, it is likely that the system is due for maintenance.

Acknowledgment

We would like to thank Dr. Charles Lee and other colleagues for their kind help and support.

References

1. The 1000 Genomes Project Consortium (2012) An integrated map of genetic variation from 1092 human genomes. Nature 491:56–65
2. 1000 Genomes Project Consortium (2015) A global reference for human genetic variation. Nature 256:68–74
3. Sudmant PH, Rausch T, Gardner EJ et al (2015) An integrated map of structural variation in 2,504 human genomes. Nature 526:75–81
4. Iafrate AJ, Feuk L, Rivera MN et al (2004) Detection of large-scale variation in the human genome. Nat Genet 36:949–951
5. Sebat J, Lakshmi B, Troge J et al (2004) Large-scale copy number polymorphism in the human genome. Science 305:525–528
6. Freeman JL, Perry GH, Feuk L et al (2006) Copy number variation: new insights in genome diversity. Genome Res 16:949–961
7. Redon R, Ishikawa S, Fitch KR et al (2006) Global variation in copy number in the human genome. Nature 444:444–454
8. McCarroll SA, Kuruvilla FG, Korn JM et al (2008) Integrated detection and population-genetic analysis of SNPs and copy number variation. Nat Genet 40:1166–1174
9. Korn JM, Kuruvilla FG, McCarroll SA et al (2008) Integrated genotype calling and association analysis of SNPs, common copy number polymorphisms and rare CNVs. Nat Genet 40:1253–1260
10. Conrad DF, Pinto D, Redon R et al (2010) Origins and functional impact of copy number variation in the human genome. Nature 464:704–712
11. McCarroll SA (2010) Copy number variation and human genome maps. Nat Genet 42:365–366
12. Park H, Kim JI, Ju YS et al (2010) Discovery of common Asian copy number variants using integrated high-resolution array CGH and massively parallel DNA sequencing. Nat Genet 42:400–405
13. Gersen SL, Keagle MB (2013) The principle of clinical cytogenetics, 3rd edn. Springer Science + Business Media, New York
14. Hanahan D, Weinberg RA (2011) Hallmarks of cancer: the next generation. Cell 144:646–674
15. The Cancer Genome Atlas Research Network (2011) Integrated genomic analyses of ovarian carcinoma. Nature 474:609–615
16. The Cancer Genome Atlas Research Network (2012) Comprehensive molecular portraits of human breast tumours. Nature 490:61–70

17. Yang L, Luquette LJ, Gehlenborg N et al (2013) Diverse mechanisms of somatic structural variations in human cancer genomes. Cell 153:919–929
18. Kallioniemi A, Kallioniemi OP, Sudar D et al (1992) Comparative genomic hybridization for molecular cytogenetic analysis of solid tumors. Science 258:818–821
19. Pinkel D, Segraves R, Sudar D et al (1998) High resolution analysis of DNA copy number variation using comparative genomic hybridization to microarrays. Nat Genet 20:207–211
20. Roylance R (2001) Comparative genomic hybridization. Methods Mol Med 57:223–240
21. Cai WW, Mao JH, Chow CW et al (2002) Genome-wide detection of chromosomal imbalances in tumors using BAC microarrays. Nat Biotechnol 20:393–396
22. Cowell JK, Matsui S, Wang YD et al (2004) Application of bacterial artificial chromosome array-based comparative genomic hybridization and spectral karyotyping to the analysis of glioblastoma multiforme. Cancer Genet Cytogenet 151:36–51
23. Shaffer LG, Bejjani BA (2004) A cytogeneticist's perspective on genomic microarrays. Hum Reprod Update 10:221–226
24. Tchinda J, Lee C (2006) Detecting copy number variation in the human genome using comparative genomic hybridization. BioTechniques 41:385–392
25. Carter NP (2007) Methods and strategies for analyzing copy number variation using DNA microarrays. Nat Genet 39:S16–S2
26. Hester SD, Reid L, Nowak N et al (2009) Comparison of comparative genomic hybridization technologies across microarray platforms. J Biomol Tech 20:135–151
27. Holcomb IN, Trask BJ (2011) Comparative genomic hybridization to detect variation in the copy number of large DNA segments. Cold Spring Harb Protoc 2011:1323–1333
28. Pinto D, Darvishi K, Shi X et al (2011) Comprehensive assessment of array-based platforms and calling algorithms for detection of copy number variants. Nat Biotechnol 29:512–520
29. UserGuide: Cytoscan® Assay [PDF] (2011–2012) Santa Clara CA: Affymetrix Inc
30. Shaw-Smith C, Redon R, Rickman L et al (2004) Microarray based comparative genomic hybridisation (array-CGH) detects submicroscopic chromosomal deletions and duplications in patients with learning disability/mental retardation and dysmorphic features. J Med Genet 41:241–248
31. Rickman L, Fiegler H, Shaw-Smith C et al (2005) Prenatal detection of unbalanced chromosomal rearrangements by array CGH. J Med Genet 43:353–361
32. Pfeifer D, Pantic M, Skatulla I et al (2006) Genome-wide analysis of DNA copy number changes and LOH in CLL using high-density SNP arrays. Blood 109:1202–1210
33. Jacobs S, Thompson ER, Nannya Y et al (2007) Genome-wide, high-resolution detection of copy number, loss of heterozygosity, and genotypes from formalin-fixed, paraffin-embedded tumor tissue using microarrays. Cancer Res 67:2544–2551
34. Bowden W, Skorupski J, Kovanci E et al (2009) Detection of novel copy number variants in uterine leiomyomas using high-resolution SNP arrays. Mol Hum Reprod 15:563–568
35. Scott SA, Cohen N, Brandt T et al (2009) Detection of low-level mosaicism and placental mosaicism by oligonucleotide array comparative genomic hybridization. Genet Med 12:85–92
36. Heim S, Mitelman F (eds) (2015) Cancer cytogenetics: chromosomal and molecular genetic abberations of tumor cells. Wiley-Blackwell, New York
37. Heim S, Mitelman F (2009) Cancer cytogenetics. Wiley-Blackwell, Hoboken, NJ
38. Beroukhim R, Mermel CH, Porter D et al (2010) The landscape of somatic copy-number alteration across human cancers. Nature 463:899–905
39. Conlin LK, Thiel BD, Bonnemann CG et al (2010) Mechanisms of mosaicism, chimerism and uniparental disomy identified by single nucleotide polymorphism array analysis. Hum Mol Genet 19:1263–1275
40. Miller DT, Adam MP, Aradhya S et al (2010) Consensus statement: chromosomal microarray is a first-tier clinical diagnostic test for individuals with developmental disabilities or congenital anomalies. Am J Hum Genet 86:749–764
41. FDA News Release (2014) FDA allows marketing for first of-its-kind post-natal test to help diagnose developmental delays and intellectual disabilities in children. http://www.fda.gov/NewsEvents/Newsroom/PressAnnouncements/ucm382179.htm
42. Affymetrix UserGuide (2015) UserGuide: OncoScan® CNV FFPE Assay Kit [PDF]. Affymetrix Inc, Santa Clara, CA
43. Foster JM, Oumie A, Togneri FS et al (2015) Cross-laboratory validation of the OncoScan® FFPE Assay, a multiplex tool for whole genome tumour profiling. BMC Med Genomics 8:5

Chapter 16

Multicolor Karyotyping and Fluorescence In Situ Hybridization-Banding (MCB/mBAND)

Thomas Liehr, Moneeb A.K. Othman, and Katharina Rittscher

Abstract

Multicolor fluorescence in situ hybridization (mFISH) approaches are routine applications in tumor as well as clinical cytogenetics nowadays. The first approach when thinking about mFISH is multicolor karyotyping using human whole chromosome paints as probes; this can be achieved by narrow-band filter-based multiplex-FISH (M-FISH) or interferometer/spectroscopy-based spectral karyotyping (SKY). Besides, various FISH-based banding approaches were reported in the literature, including multicolor banding (MCB/mBAND) the latter being evaluated by narrow-band filters, and using specific software. Here, we describe the combined application of multicolor karyotyping and MCB/mBAND for the characterization of simple and complex acquired chromosomal changes in cancer cytogenetics.

Key words Multicolor karyotyping, Multicolor fluorescence in situ hybridization (mFISH), Multiplex-FISH (M-FISH), Spectral karyotyping (SKY), Multicolor banding (MCB/mBAND)

1 Introduction

In cancer, more specifically in leukemia and lymphoma diagnostics, karyotyping is still one of the most crucial approaches to be done for correct disease assessment, treatment decisions, and follow-up [1]. However, as chromosome morphology and black and white banding pattern are the only two evaluated parameters in banding cytogenetics [2], origin of additional material in a structurally altered acquired tumor-chromosome often remained unresolved. This kind of limitations was overcome in major parts by the introduction of fluorescence in situ hybridization (FISH) approaches in the 1980s [3] and more recently by multicolor FISH (mFISH) techniques. mFISH is "the simultaneous use of at least three different ligands or fluorochromes for the specific labeling of DNA, excluding the counterstain" [4]. Following this definition first successful mFISH experiments were done not before the end of the 1990s [5] and first mFISH probe sets were established by the mid-1990s [6, 7] enabling multicolor karyotyping. The latter describes

Thomas S.K. Wan (ed.), *Cancer Cytogenetics: Methods and Protocols*, Methods in Molecular Biology, vol. 1541,
DOI 10.1007/978-1-4939-6703-2_16,

the simultaneous staining of each of the 24 human chromosomes in different colors using whole chromosome painting (wcp) probes (Fig. 1A-1). Interestingly, multicolor karyotyping was reported at least eight times in the literature as M-FISH (=multiplex-FISH) [6], SKY (=spectral karyotyping) [7], multicolor FISH [8, 9], COBRA-FISH (=COmbined Binary RAtio labeling FISH) [10], 24-color FISH [11], as well as IPM-FISH (=IRS-PCR multiplex FISH) [12]. While SKY and COBRA-FISH are interferometer/ spectroscopy-based, all other approaches have evaluation systems that are narrow-band filter-based. All mentioned multicolor karyotyping possibilities are based on four to seven different

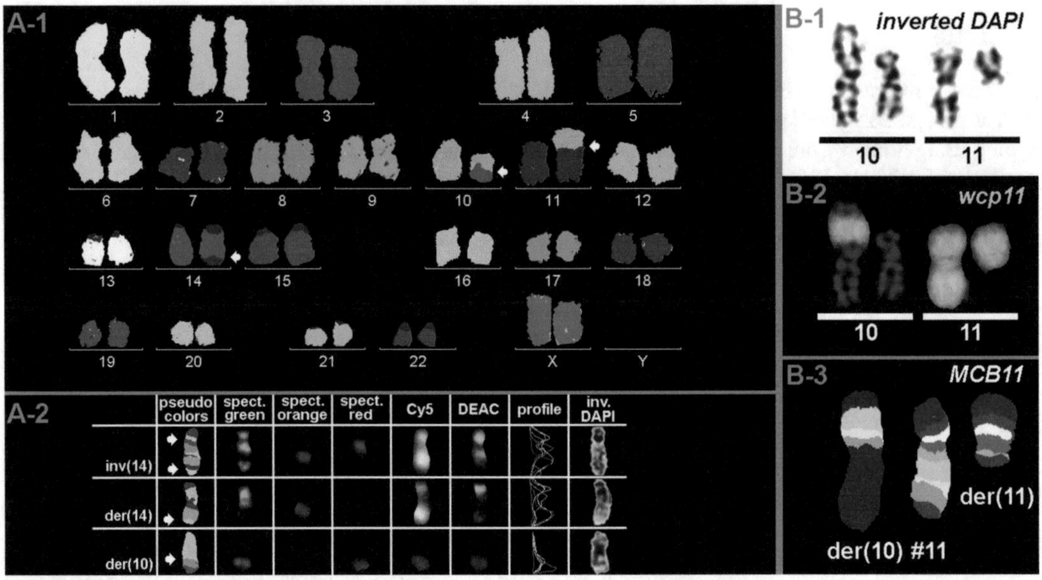

Fig. 1 Examples for multicolor karyotyping and FISH-banding (MCB/mBAND) (**A**) In case of an acute lymphatic leukemia [1] a complex karyotype was found in GTG-banding (result not shown). M-FISH showed that indeed the three following chromosomes were involved in the rearrangement: 10, 11, and 14 (*arrows* in A-1). The rearrangements of all chromosomes were further characterized by chromosome-specific homemade MCB probes. In A-2 only the result for chromosome 14 is depicted. MCB revealed that indeed no normal chromosome 14 was present; one chromosome 14 had a paracentric inversion, the second was involved in a translocation with chromosome 11, and a derivative der(10)t(10;14) was also stained by MCB-14-probe set. Overall, a final karyotype was determined as: 46,XX,der(10)(10pter->10p12.31::11q23.3->11q23.3::10p12.31->10q11.23::14q24.2->14qter),der(11)(10qter->10q11.23::11p15.3->11q23.3::10p12.31->10p12.31::11q23.3->11qter),der(14)t(11;14)(q15.3;q24.2),inv(14)(q11q23) using additional probes and approaches (see also [1]). [Abbreviations: *Cy5* cyanine 5, *DAPI* 4,6-diamidino-2-phenylindole.2HCl, *DEAC* diethylaminocoumarine, *inv.* inverted, *spect.* spectrum] (**B**) A simple insertion translocation between chromosomes 10 and 11 was suggested in this acute myeloid leukemia case according to banding cytogenetics (result not shown). No M-FISH was done, but first a whole chromosome paint (wcp) probe for chromosome 11 was used together with inverted DAPI banding (B-1) to characterize the breakpoint in chromosome 10 to subband p12.31 (B-2). In B-3 the result of MCB probe set for chromosome 11 is shown, characterizing the breakpoints in 11q13.1 and 11q23.3. This part is inserted directly in the derivative chromosome 10. The rearrangement after MCB could be reported as ins(10;11)(p12.31;q13.1q23.3)

fluorescence dyes. However, those that are routinely used by the majority of laboratories are M-FISH and SKY, which work with five fluorochromes used for combinatorial labeling and one counterstain (DAPI = 4,6-diamidino-2-phenylindole·2HCl) [13].

As multicolor karyotyping reaches its limits when an exact localization of a chromosomal breakpoint is required, or when intrachromosomal aberrations need to characterized, different so-called FISH banding approaches were developed to overcome this kind of limitations. As defined in 2002, FISH-banding methods are any kind of FISH technique, which provide the possibility of characterizing simultaneously several chromosomal subregions smaller than a chromosome arm (excluding the short arms of the acrocentric chromosomes). FISH banding methods fitting that definition may have quite different characteristics, but share the ability to produce a DNA-specific chromosomal banding [14]. For humans the following FISH banding probe sets were established yet: IPM-FISH [12], cross-species color banding (Rx-FISH) [15], locus-specific probe-based [16–19] and somatic cell hybrid-based chromosome bar coding [20], multicolor banding (MCB) [21–23], multitude multicolor banding (mMCB) [24], spectral color banding (SCAN) [25, 26], and M-FISH using chromosome-region-specific probes (CRP) [27]. To the best of our knowledge, the only commercially available FISH-banding probe set is MCB/mBAND.

The applications of M-FISH and SKY or MCB/mBAND cover the whole spectrum of human cytogenetics including tumor cytogenetics; while in leukemia and lymphoma these probe sets may be used in routine diagnostics, solid tumors (including cell lines) are most often studied by these approaches mainly under research aspects [13].

The protocol how to do M-FISH for characterization of chromosomes involved in a complex rearrangement and MCB/mBAND to resolve the breakpoints in more detail are provided here. In case of more simple rearrangements those may be resolved by directly starting with chromosome-specific MCB/mBAND probe sets. Examples for a complex rearrangement resolved by both M-FISH and MCB and only by MCB are given in Fig. 1. For research-associated screening of cancer cytogenetic cases appearing unaltered according to banding cytogenetics it might be better first to do M-FISH or SKY followed by mMCB [1]. Also, it is necessary to keep in mind that M-FISH and MCB/mBAND have resolution limitations of 3–10 megabase pairs; thus in cases higher resolution of breakpoints needs to be achieved locus-specific probes and/or MLPA and array-comparative genomic hybridization need to be applied (the latter two approaches for sure can only resolve unbalanced rearrangements) [1].

2 Materials

To perform M-FISH and/or MCB/mBAND a fully equipped molecular cytogenetic laboratory is the prerequisite.

2.1 Chemicals and Solutions

1. 20 × Saline-sodium citrate (SSC) buffer.
2. DAPI (4,6-diamidino-2-phenylindol·2HCl) stock solution.
3. DAPI solution: Dissolve 1.5 μl of 1 M DAPI stock solution in 1 ml of antifade mounting medium, make fresh as required.
4. Denaturation buffer: 70% deionized formamide, 20% double distilled water, 10% 20 × SSC, make fresh as required.
5. Ethanol (100, 90, 70%).
6. Probe solution – here we describe the application of molecular karyotyping "Xcyte Human Multicolor FISH Probe Kit" and for MCB/mBAND "XCyte mBAND Human mBAND Probe Kit" (*see* Subheading 2.2).
7. Rubber cement.
8. Tween 20.
9. Vectashield antifade.
10. Washing buffer 1: 4 × SSC, 0.05% Tween 20.
11. Washing buffer 2: 1 × SSC.

2.2 Probe Sets

Probe sets suited for multicolor karyotyping are commercially available by providers like MetaSystems and ASI. mBAND probes are commercially exclusively available at MetaSystems. M-FISH, MCB, and other probe sets can also be obtained in frame of cooperation from the corresponding author of this chapter.

2.3 Image Acquisition and Evaluation Software

In standard mFISH 5 fluorochromes and one counterstain are routinely used; thus at least a fluorescence microscope equipped with six filter sets is necessary. A charge-coupled device (CCD) camera attached to computer-based image acquisition and evaluation software is also required. For M-FISH in combination with MCB/mBAND there is only one provider available on the market, i.e., MetaSystems (Altlussheim, Germany) (*see* **Note 1**). However, mFISH results principally can also be analyzed by other supplier's software.

3 Methods

Here, we describe how to do FISH when using commercial M-FISH or mBAND kit and how to evaluate the results using the corresponding software (ISIS, MetaSystems).

3.1 Fluorescence In Situ Hybridization (FISH) Procedure

1. Per slide with metaphases to be hybridized, add 100 μl of denaturation buffer and cover with a 24 mm × 60 mm coverslip.
2. Incubate slides on a heating plate at 75 °C for ~3 min (*see* **Note 2**).
3. Let swim off the coverslip by placing slides in a Coplin jar with 70% ethanol at −20 °C for 3 min.
4. Dehydration of slides in 90 and 100% ethanol series at room temperature for 3 min each and let air-dry.
5. Add 10 μl of denatured (at 95 °C for 2–3 min) and prehybridized (at 37 °C for 15–20 min) probe solution onto each denatured slide, put a 24 mm × 24 mm coverslip on the region of interest, and seal with rubber cement (*see* **Note 3**).
6. Incubate slides at 37 °C for 16–60 h in a humid chamber (*see* **Note 4**).
7. Remove the rubber cement and coverslips, e.g., by letting them swim off in washing buffer 1 in 100 ml Coplin jar at room temperature.
8. Post-wash the slides in washing buffer at 62–64 °C for 23 min with gentle agitation.
9. Transfer slides in 100 ml of washing buffer 1 at room temperature for 5 min on a shaker.
10. Dehydrate slides in 70, 90, 100%, ethanolseries for 3 min each and air-dry.
11. Counterstain the slides with 20 μl of DAPI solution (antifade already included), cover with a coverslip 24 mm × 60 mm, and look at the results under a fluorescence microscope.

3.2 Evaluation

For evaluation, the above-mentioned (*see* Subheading 2.3) hard and software are necessary. Software program most suited for MCB/mBAND evaluation is ISIS (MetaSystems). Here, we cannot discuss details of evaluation, as this is mostly software dependent. Only the following general statements can be made:

1. In cancer cytogenetics, it is essential to evaluate as many metaphases as possible (at least 20 per case and hybridization) not to miss small acquired cell clones and/or subclones reflecting karyotypic evolution.
2. Metaphase quality is often limited in cancer cytogenetics. While reliable MCB/mBAND results may also be obtained even from clumpy metaphase spreads, such metaphases should not be evaluated in case of molecular karyotyping. In molecular karyotyping this attempt may lead to wrong separated chromosomes and misclassified rearrangements.

3. Evaluation should be done using the six different fluorochrome channels and pseudocolor depictions for M-FISH and MCB/mBAND to come to correct conclusions (*see* **Note 5**).

4 Notes

1. SKY-results could only be obtained and evaluated by a microscope equipped with a SpectraCube provided exclusively by Spectral Imaging Systems (ASI, Inc., Vista, CA, USA) and the fitting 2 filter sets. However, fluorochromes need to be inside the frame covered by the SKY-1 filter (~450–850 nm).
2. Here the supplier recommends basic solution denaturation; it may be possible to do but as we use heat denaturation routinely this was never tested in our laboratory.
3. As all mFISH probe sets are expensive one may save probe using following tricks: use smaller coverslips with less probe solution and/or dilute probe solution; also prolonged hybridization time [instead of up to 16 or 60 h (*see* **Note 4**), >72 h can also be used] can reduce necessary probe amount drastically.
4. Hybridization time should be for M-FISH at least 60 h, while for MCB/mBAND probes 16 h is normally sufficient.
5. Reliable pseudocolor depictions like those shown in Fig. 1 cannot always be achieved in mFISH. In case of poor hybridization quality several candidate chromosomes may by suggested to be involved in a certain rearrangement after molecular karyotyping. This can be helpful to continue with only two or three specific whole chromosome painting probes to verify the M-FISH results. Also features provided by the software should be used to establish experiment-specific pseudocolors. For MCB/mBAND also the possibility of creating fluorochrome profiles along the analyzed chromosomes (Fig. 1A-2) should be used besides the multicolor-banding feature.

Acknowledgments

Supported in parts by the Wilhelm Sander Stiftung (2013.032.1) and German academic exchange service (DAAD).

References

1. Othman MA, Melo JB, Carreira IM et al (2015) High rates of submicroscopic aberrations in karyotypically normal acute lymphoblastic leukemia. Mol Cytogenet 8:45
2. Claussen U, Michel S, Mühlig P et al (2002) Demystifying chromosome preparation and the implications for the concept of chromosome condensation during mitosis. Cytogenet Genome Res 98:136–146

3. Chang SS, Mark HF (1997) Emerging molecular cytogenetic technologies. Cytobios 90:7–22
4. Liehr T, Starke H, Weise A et al (2004) Multicolor FISH probe sets and their applications. Histol Histopathol 19:229–237
5. Nederlof PM, Robinson D, Abuknesha R et al (1989) Three-color fluorescence in situ hybridization for the simultaneous detection of multiple nucleic acid sequences. Cytometry 10:20–27
6. Speicher MR, Gwyn Ballard S, Ward DC (1996) Karyotyping human chromosomes by combinatorial multi-fluor FISH. Nat Genet 12:368–375
7. Schröck E, du Manoir S, Veldman T et al (1996) Multicolor spectral karyotyping of human chromosomes. Science 273:494–497
8. Tanke HJ, De Haas RR, Sagner G et al (1998) Use of platinum coproporphyrin and delayed luminescence imaging to extend the number of targets FISH karyotyping. Cytometry 33:453–459
9. Senger G, Chudoba I, Plesch A (1998) Multicolor-FISH – the identification of chromosome aberrations by 24 colors. BIOforum 9:499–503
10. Tanke HJ, Wiegant J, van Gijlswijk RP et al (1999) New strategy for multi-colour fluorescence in situ hybridisation: COBRA: COmbined Binary RAtio labelling. Eur J Hum Genet 7:2–11
11. Azofeifa J, Fauth C, Kraus J et al (2000) An optimized probe set for the detection of small interchromosomal aberrations by use of 24-color FISH. Am J Hum Genet 66:1684–1688
12. Aurich-Costa J, Vannier A, Gregoire E et al (2001) IPM-FISH, a new M-FISH approach using IRS-PCR painting probes: application to the analysis of seven human prostate cell lines. Genes Chromosomes Cancer 30:143–160
13. Liehr T (2016) Basics and literature on multicolor fluorescence in situ hybridization application. http://fish-tl.com/mfish.html. Accessed 15 September 2016
14. Liehr T, Heller A, Starke H et al (2002) FISH banding methods: applications in research and diagnostics. Expert Rev Mol Diagn 2:217–225
15. Müller S, O'Brien PC, Ferguson-Smith MA et al (1998) Cross-species colour segmenting: a novel tool in human karyotype analysis. Cytometry 33:445–452
16. Lichter P, Tang CJ, Call K et al (1990) High-resolution mapping of human chromosome 11 by in situ hybridization with cosmid clones. Science 247:64–69
17. Lengauer C, Green ED, Cremer T (1992) Fluorescence in situ hybridization of YAC clones after Alu-PCR amplification. Genomics 13:826–828
18. Liehr T, Weise A, Heller A et al (2002) Multicolor chromosome banding (MCB) with YAC/BAC-based probes and region-specific microdissection DNA libraries. Cytogenet Genome Res 97:43–50
19. Hamid AB, Kreskowski K, Weise A et al (2012) How to narrow down chromosomal breakpoints in small and large derivative chromosomes--a new probe set. J Appl Genet 53:259–269
20. Müller S, Rocchi M, Ferguson-Smith MA et al (1997) Toward a multicolor chromosome bar code for the entire human karyotype by fluorescence in situ hybridization. Hum Genet 100:271–278
21. Chudoba I, Plesch A, Lörch T et al (1999) High resolution multicolorbanding: a new technique for refined FISH analysis of human chromosomes. Cytogenet Cell Genet 84:156–160
22. Liehr T, Heller A, Starke H et al (2002) Microdissection based high resolution multicolor banding for all 24 human chromosomes. Int J Mol Med 9:335–339
23. Weise A, Mrasek K, Fickelscher I et al (2008) Molecular definition of high-resolution multicolor banding probes: first within the human DNA sequence anchored FISH banding probe set. J Histochem Cytochem 56:487–493
24. Weise A, Heller A, Starke H et al (2003) Multitude multicolor chromosome banding (mMCB)—a comprehensive one-step multicolor FISH banding method. Cytogenet Genome Res 103:34–39
25. Kakazu N, Ashihara E, Hada S et al (2001) Development of spectral colour banding in cytogenetic analysis. Lancet 357:529–530
26. Kakazu N, Bar-Am I, Hada S et al (2003) A new chromosome banding technique, spectral color banding (SCAN), for full characterization of chromosomal abnormalities. Genes Chromosomes Cancer 37:412–416
27. Tjia WM, Sham JS, Hu L et al (2005) Characterization of 3p, 5p, and 3q in two nasopharyngeal carcinoma cell lines, using region-specific multiplex fluorescence in situ hybridization probes. Cancer Genet Cytogenet 158:61–66

Chapter 17

Cytogenetics for Biological Dosimetry

Michelle Ricoul, Tamizh Gnana-Sekaran, Laure Piqueret-Stephan, and Laure Sabatier

Abstract

Cytogenetics is the gold-standard in biological dosimetry for assessing a received dose of ionizing radiation. More modern techniques have recently emerged, but none are as specific as cytogenetic approaches, particularly the dicentric assay. Here, we will focus on the principal cytogenetic techniques used for biological dosimetry: the dicentric assay in metaphase cells, the micronuclei assay in binucleated cells, and the premature condensed chromosome (PCC) assay in interphase cells. New fluorescence in situ hybridization (FISH) techniques (such as telomere–centromere hybridization) have facilitated the analysis of the dicentric assay and have permitted to assess the dose a long time after irradiation by translocation analysis (such as by Tri-color FISH or Multiplex-FISH). Telomere centromere staining of PCCs will make it possible to perform dose assessment within 24 h of exposure in the near future.

Key words Chromosomal aberrations, Radiation effects, Biological dosimetry, Telomere, Centromere

1 Introduction

Biological dosimetry is routinely performed for the estimation of the absorbed dose in the individuals exposed to radiation. Radiation is a form of energy that comes from naturally occurring radionuclides or man-made sources. One of the earliest and most direct methods of dose determination following radiation exposure is the recording of daily counts of various cell types circulating in the peripheral blood; the extent and duration of the decline and subsequent recovery of specific cell-types correlate well with the received dose [1] despite poor sensitivity. Biological samples are used to quantify radiation damage, hence the term biological dosimetry. There are many biological indicators of radiation exposure such as mutations [2–4], gene expression [5], cytogenetics [6], proteins such as γ-H2AX [7], metabolic intermediates [8], and proteomics [9]. Cytogenetic biomarkers are considered to be the most sensitive and reliable of the various biological indicators reported to quantify the absorbed dose of radiation. The radiation absorbed by

Thomas S.K. Wan (ed.), *Cancer Cytogenetics: Methods and Protocols*, Methods in Molecular Biology, vol. 1541,
DOI 10.1007/978-1-4939-6703-2_17,

exposed cells can induce DNA strand breaks on the chromosomes, which are subsequently repaired by the DNA repair machinery of the cell. Misrepaired breaks can result in abnormal chromosome structures. Various types of abnormal chromosomes can be identified and counted, of which the number is related to the dose, providing a reliable dose-effect relationship.

The most common aberration is the dicentric chromosome (DC). It is an aberrant chromosome with two centromeres which is formed when two chromosome segments, each with a centromere, fuse end to end, with rejoining or not of their acentric fragments. DCs are unstable, highly specific to ionizing radiation, and can be used to estimate the unknown absorbed dose during a radiation emergency by counting their frequency [6]. Biodosimetry based on DC counts can also discriminate between whole and partial body exposures as DC formation is not influenced by any other factors. The background frequency is very low (0.001/cell) and the sensitivity of the DC assay is 0.1 Gray (Gy), hence it is the "gold standard" for biodosimetry applications [6]. The assay has been used in many accidental incidents in Chernobyl [10], Istanbul [6], Goiania [11], and Bangkok [12]. However, it is time consuming, laborious, and requires skilled and highly trained personnel to score the chromosomal aberrations. The other principal cytogenetic marker is micronuclei (MN). These are formed from lagging chromosomal fragments or whole chromosomes at anaphase which are not included in the nuclei of daughter cells. They are seen as distinct, separate, and small spherical objects in the cytoplasm of the daughter cells with the same morphology and staining properties as nuclei [13]. MN reflect chromosomal damage and are a useful index for monitoring environmental effects on genetic material in human cells [14]. This assay has been shown to be a promising and potential tool for triage in the medical management of a nuclear emergency due to its simplicity and the rapidity of scoring. However, its sensitivity is only 0.25 Gy due to a spontaneous MN frequency of 0.002–0.036/cell [6]. This assay was used in the Chernobyl [14] and Istanbul [15] radiation accidents. The abovementioned techniques require an incompressible culture time and the report can only be generated after a minimum of 72 h. During a mass radiation exposure event, the potentially exposed individuals cannot wait for 72 hr to start treatment. Thus, a technique was introduced by Johnson and Rao [16] in which the mitotic cells of Chinese hamster ovary (CHO) cells induce the condensation of chromosomes in interphase cells of lymphocytes following fusion using polyethylene glycol or Sendai virus [16]. This technique allows the study of radiation-induced damage without stimulating the cells and the aberrations can be assessed within 2 h of exposure [17]; thus, the chances of losing information due to interphase cell death are reduced. Another advantage of this assay is that it can be used for high dose (>5 Gy) estimations because conventional cytogenetic dosimetry based on the frequency of chromosomal aberrations becomes difficult due to mitotic delay and the disappearance of lymphocytes in peripheral blood circulation [18, 19]. The minimum dose detection limit of this technique is 0.05 Gy [6]. The premature condensed chromosome (PCC) assay using peripheral blood lymphocytes (PBLs) is recommended as a rapid method for biodosimetry [20]. This technique was also performed on three seriously exposed victims of the Tokaimura criticality accident in Japan [21].

Potential scenarios of radiation exposure resulting in mass casualties require individual, early, and definitive radiation dose assessment to provide medical aid within days of the occurrence of a disaster. The preliminary dose estimation and segregation of exposed and nonexposed individuals are the main steps in triage medical management. Biological dosimetry in "triage" mode must provide an answer as quickly as possible. A rough estimate of the dose is sufficient as long as it permits the classification of the victims into three categories that will guide medical follow up (<1 Gy, 1–2 Gy, and >2 Gy). Alternative strategies are being developed to meet the demands of triage. These include the use of automated scoring, as manual scoring of classical cytogenetic methods (DC, MN, and PCC) is time consuming.

The quantification of DC is not reliable for retrospective dosimetry (>1 year after exposure), as they decrease by 50% with each cell division. Stable chromosome rearrangements, such as translocations, are mostly scored using Tri-color FISH. Multiplex-FISH (M-FISH) can permit the detection of translocations involving any chromosome but it is time consuming and expensive. Some approaches are focused on the detection of radiation-induced inversions, the most stable chromosomal aberrations, using cross-species FISH (RxFISH) or directional genomic hybridization [22].

Sharing of the workload among expert groups (i.e., the European RENEB (Realizing the European Network of Biodosimetry) network [23], the IAEA RANET (International Atomic Energy Agency Response and Assistance Network), REMPAN (Radiation Emergency Medical Preparedness and Assistance Network), and WHO BioDoseNet (World Health Organization biodosimetry network) is necessary, especially for triage. It also permits expert training, protocol harmonization, and dissemination of up-to-date developments, such as the automation of analytical methods and the use of early markers of ionizing radiation that are among the most recent advances in biodosimetry. In this chapter, we will focus on the principal techniques used for biological dosimetry in cytogenetics consisting of the dicentric assay and translocation assays in metaphase cells, the micronuclei assay in bi-nucleate cells, and the premature condensed chromosome (PCC) assay in interphase cells.

2 Materials

2.1 Blood Culture and Spreading

2.1.1 Chromosomal Aberrations

1. T25 culture flask.
2. 37 °C, 5 % CO_2 incubator.
3. Growth medium: Add 2 mL of penicillin-streptomycin antibiotics and 55 mL of fetal calf serum (FCS) to 500 mL of RPMI 1640 medium, mix well and store at 4 °C.
4. Bromodeoxyuridine (BrdU): use at a final concentration of 10 μg/mL.
5. Phytohemagglutinin-M (PHA): use at a final concentration of 1.5 %.
6. Colcemid: use at a final concentration of 0.1 μg/mL.
7. 0.075 M KCl: Dissolve 2.795 g of KCl in 500 mL of sterile water. Warm to 37 °C before use.
8. Carnoy's II fixative: add three volumes of ethanol to one volume of acetic acid (*see* **Note 1**).
9. Microscopic slides: Wash three times with deionized water and keep cool in a beaker filled with deionized water on ice until use. Keep the beaker on ice during spreading.
10. Phase-contrast microscope.
11. Water bath.

2.1.2 Cytokinesis Blocked Micronucleus (CBMN) Assay

1. T25 culture flask.
2. 37 °C, 5 % CO_2 incubator.
3. Growth medium: Add 2 mL of penicillin-streptomycin antibiotics and 55 mL of FCS to 500 mL of RPMI 1640 medium, mix well and store at 4 °C.
4. Cytochalasin-B (Cyto-B):

   Dissolve 5 mg of Cyto-B in 5 mL of dimethyl sulfoxide (DMSO) and filter through a 0.2 μ syringe filter. Store at −20 °C in the dark and labeled as *stock solution*. For *working solution* (100 μg/mL): Dissolve 1 mL of the stock solution in 9 mL of RPMI 1640 medium. Then add 600 μL of working solution to the 10 mL of culture to obtain a final concentration of 6 μg/mL.
5. PHA: use at a final concentration of 2 %.
6. 0.075 M KCl: Dissolve 2.795 g of KCl in 500 mL of sterile water. Cool to 4 °C before use.
7. Modified Carnoy's fixative: Add five volumes of ethanol to one volume of acetic acid (*see* **Note 1**).

8. Microscopic slides: Wash three times with deionized water and keep cool in a beaker filled with deionized water on ice until use. Keep the beaker on ice during spreading.
9. Phase-contrast microscope.

2.1.3 Premature Condensed Chromosome (PCC) Assay

1. T25 culture flask.
2. 37 °C, 5% CO_2 incubator.
3. Ficoll density gradient media.
4. Growth medium: Add 2 mL of penicillin-streptomycin antibiotics and 55 mL of FCS to 500 mL of RPMI 1640 (with HEPES) medium, mix well and store at 4 °C.
5. Growth Medium for Hamster cells: DMEM/F12 medium with 10% FCS.
6. Colcemid: use at a final concentration of 0.1 μg/mL.
7. PHA: use at a final concentration of 2%.
8. 50% Polyethylene glycol (PEG) (w/v): Dissolve 50 g of PEG in 100 mL of 1× PBS and heat in microwave oven at 600 W for 20 s.
9. 0.075 M KCl: Add 2.795 g of KCl in 500 mL of sterile water. Warm to 37 °C before use.
10. Carnoy's II fixative: Add three volumes of ethanol to one volume of acetic acid (*see* **Note 1**).
11. Microscopic slides: Wash three times with deionized water and keep cool in a beaker filled with deionized water on ice until use. Keep the beaker on ice during spreading.
12. Phase-contrast microscope.
13. Water bath.

2.2 Staining

2.2.1 Giemsa Staining

1. Giemsa stock solution: Mix 2.5 g of Giemsa powder with 135 mL of glycerol in a 500-mL conical flask and dissolve completely at 60 °C for 3 h. Allow it to cool to room temperature and add 210 mL of methanol. Mix thoroughly overnight, filter using Whatmann paper, and store at 4–8 °C.
2. Giemsa working solution: Add 4 mL of Giemsa stock solution, 4 mL of sodium hydrogen phosphate, and 4 mL of sodium dihydrogen phosphate buffers to 38 mL of distilled water. Mix well to obtain a final volume of 50 mL 8% Giemsa working stain.

2.2.2 Telomere–Centromere Hybridization

1. Pepsin: Prepare 0.1 M HCl (pH 2.0) by mixing 90 mL of sterile water and 10 mL of 1 M HCl. Add pepsin to obtain a final concentration of 0.2 mg/mL.
2. 1× Phosphate buffered saline (PBS).
3. 4% Formaldehyde: Add 11 mL of 36% formaldehyde to 89 mL of 1x PBS (*see* **Note 2**).

4. Ethanol series: 50, 70, and 100% ethanol. Keep on ice.
5. Probe solution: 50 μL of telomere [$(CCCTAA)_3$ labeled with cyanine 3 (Cy3)] and centromere-specific sequence [labeled with fluorescein isothiocyanate (FITC)] peptide nucleic acid (PNA) probes at 0.3 μg/mL each.
6. Wash I: Add 140 mL of formamide and 2 mL of 1 M Tris–HCl (pH 7.2) to 58 mL of distilled water (*see* **Note 2**).
7. Wash II: Add 15 mL of 1 M Tris–HCl (pH 7.2), 9 mL of 5 M NaCl, and 150 μL of Tween 20 to 276 mL of distilled water in a bottle and mix (*see* **Note 3**).
8. DAPI: 1 μg/mL 4′,6-diamidino-2-phenylindole.
9. PPD: Add 100 mg of p-phenylenediamine to 10 mL of 1× PBS and 90 mL of glycerol (*see* **Note 4**).
10. Hotplate.
11. Water bath.

2.2.3 Tri-Color FISH

1. 2× SSC (pH 6.3): Keep 100 mL on ice and 100 mL in 37 °C water bath (*see* **Note 5**).
2. 4% Formaldehyde: Add 11 mL of 36% formaldehyde to 89 mL of 1× PBS (*see* **Note 2**).
3. 1× PBS.
4. Ethanol series: 50, 70, and 100% ethanol for dehydration. Keep on ice.
5. 70% Formamide/2× SSC (pH 5.6): Add 70 mL of formamide and 10 mL of 20× SSC (pH 5.6) to 20 mL of distilled water. Warm the solution to 70 °C in water bath (*see* **Note 2**).
6. FISH probes: MetaSystems chromosome painting probes for chromosomes 1 (TexasRed, TR), 4 (mix of TR and FITC probes), and 11 (FITC) (*see* **Note 6**).
7. 1× SSC (pH 6.3): Warm 100 mL in 75 °C water bath (*see* **Notes 5** and **7**).
8. 2× SSC (pH6.3)/0.05% Tween 20: Add 100 mL of 2× SSC (pH 6.3) with 50 μL of Tween 20 (*see* **Notes 3**, **5**, and **7**).
9. DAPI: use at final concentration 1 μg/mL.
10. PPD: Add 100 mg of p-phenylenediamine to 10 mL of 1× PBS and 90 mL of glycerol (*see* **Note 4**).
11. Hotplate.
12. Water bath.

2.2.4 M-FISH

1. 1× PBS.
2. 0.07 N NaOH: Add 700 μL of 10 N NaOH to 100 mL of water.

3. FISH probes: M-FISH probes (MetaSystems, Germany), ready to use.
4. 0.1× SSC (pH 6.3): Keep 100 mL on ice and 100 mL at room temperature (*see* **Note 5**).
5. 2× SSC (pH 6.3): Keep 100 mL on ice and 100 mL at 70 °C in a water bath (*see* **Note 5**).
6. Ethanol series: 30, 50, 70, and 100% ethanol for dehydration; keep on ice.
7. 0.4× SSC (pH 6.3): Prepare 200 mL of 0.4x SSC (pH 6.3) in distilled water and warm it to 72 °C in a water bath (*see* **Notes 5** and 7).
8. 2× SSC (pH6.3) 0.05% Tween 20: Prepare 100 mL of 2X SSC pH 6.3 in distilled water in a bottle and add 50 μL of Tween 20 (*see* **Notes 3**, **5**, and 7).
9. 1 μg/mL DAPI.
10. PPD: Add 100 mg of p-phenylenediamine to 10 mL of 1x PBS and 90 mL of glycerol (*see* **Note 4**).
11. Water bath.

2.3 Image Capture and Analysis

1. Metaphases, micronuclei, and PCC images are captured using MetaSystems software on a Zeiss axioplan II microscope coupled to a CCD camera.
2. Images are analyzed using ISIS software (MetaSystems) for Tri-color FISH, M-FISH, Telomere–Centromere hybridization, and Giemsa staining. Telomere–Centromere hybridization images can also be analyzed using TC-Score [24] or PCC-TC-Score [20].

2.4 Dose Reference Curve

To assess the dose according to the number of scored chromosomal aberrations, CABAS (http://www.ujk.edu.pl/ibiol/cabas/) [25] software and/or dose estimate [26] are used according to the calibration curve of the laboratory.

3 Methods

3.1 Blood Culture and Spreading

3.1.1 Chromosomal Aberrations

1. Add 0.5 mL of lithium heparinized-blood to10 mL of growth medium in T25 culture flask. Then, add 100 μL of BrdU and 150 μL of PHA to stimulate the T lymphocytes and incubate in a 37 °C, 5% CO_2 incubator for 46 h.
2. Add 100 μL of colcemid to the culture to block the mitotic cells and incubate in a 37 °C, 5% CO_2 incubator for 2 h.
3. Transfer the cells with the medium into a 15-mL tube and centrifuge at 328*g* for 7 min.

4. Discard the supernatant, add 10 mL pre-warmed hypotonic KCl solution (*see* **Note 8**) and incubate in a 37 °C water bath for 15 min.
5. Add 2–3 drops of Carnoy's fixative for pre-fixation (*see* **Note 9**) and centrifuge at 328 × *g* for 7 min.
6. Discard the supernatant, add 10 mL of Carnoy's fixative (*see* **Note 8**), and centrifuge at 328 × *g* for 7 min.
7. Repeat **step 6** and fix the cells at 4 °C overnight.
8. On the next day, repeat **step 6**.
9. Discard the supernatant and adjust the remaining volume of the supernatant to twice that of the cell pellet. Resuspend the cells well (*see* **Note 10**).
10. Spread 15 μL of the suspension on cold, wet slides (*see* **Notes 11** and **12**). Keep the slide at −20 °C until staining.

3.1.2 Cytokinesis Blocked Micronucleus (CBMN) Assay

1. Add 1 mL of blood and 200 μL of PHA to 10 mL of growth medium in T25 culture flask and incubate in a 37 °C, 5 % CO_2 incubator for 44 h.
2. Add Cyto-B aseptically and further incubate in a 37 °C, 5 % CO_2 incubator for 28 h.
3. Transfer the culture into a 15-mL centrifuge tube and centrifuge at 328 × *g* for 7 min.
4. Discard the supernatant, add 10 mL of prechilled hypotonic KCl solution (*see* **Notes 8**, **13** and **14**) and immediately centrifuge at 328 × *g* for 7 min.
5. Discard the supernatant, add 10 mL of Carnoy's fixative (*see* **Notes 8** and **15**), and centrifuge at 328 × *g* for 7 min.
6. Repeat **step 5** and fix the cells at 4 °C overnight.
7. On the next day, repeat **step 5**. Discard the supernatant until the remaining volume is twice that of the cell pellet. Resuspend the cells well (*see* **Note 10**).
8. Spread 15 μL of the suspension on cold, wet slides (*see* **Notes 11**, **12**, **16** and **17**). Keep the slides at −20 °C until staining (Fig. 1).

3.1.3 Premature Condensed Chromosomes (PCC)

1. *To isolate lymphocytes*, dilute whole blood with RPMI 1640 medium (1:1) and layer it onto 2 mL of Ficoll density gradient medium.
2. Centrifuge the tube at 543 × *g* for 20 min at 20 °C.
3. Remove the mononuclear cell layer and transfer to a 15-mL centrifuge tube containing 5 mL growth medium.
4. Centrifuge at 377 × *g* for 10 min at 4 °C.

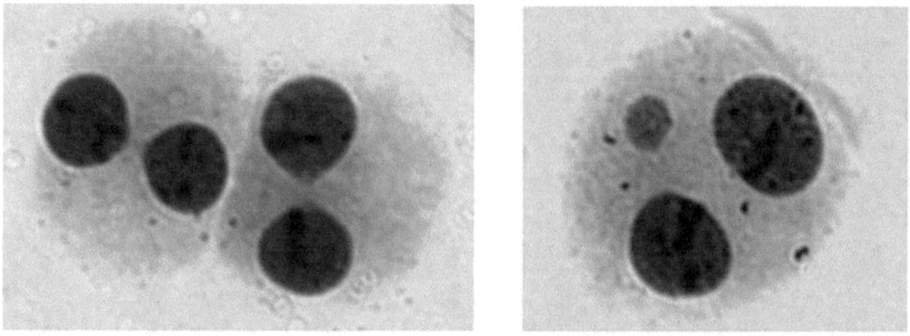

Fig. 1 Binucleate cells with or without micronuclei obtained from human peripheral blood

5. Discard the supernatant and resuspend the pellet with 3 mL growth medium and keep on ice until use.
6. *To collect of mitotic CHO cells*, add colcemid (with a final concentration of 0.1 μg/mL) to the CHO cells and keep at 37 °C for 4 h.
7. Discard the medium and tap the flask to obtain the mitotic cells.
8. Add 8 mL of DMEM/F12 medium and 80 μL of colcemid and transfer the contents to a 15-mL centrifuge tube, rinse the flask with DMEM/F12 medium containing colcemid, transfer the rinse to the same tube, and centrifuge at 377 × *g* for 10 min at 20 °C.
9. Discard the supernatant, tap the pellet, and add 3 mL of DMEM/F12 medium containing colcemid. Keep in ice until use.
10. *To induce of fusion*, transfer the collected mitotic CHO cells to round-bottom culture tubes containing the lymphocyte suspension and centrifuge at 377 × *g* for 10 min at 20 °C.
11. Discard the supernatant, add 150 μL of 50% PEG followed by 1.5 mL of RPMI 1640 with colcemid, and centrifuge at 377 × *g* for 10 min at 20 °C.
12. Discard the supernatant, add 0.7 mL of growth medium with colcemid and 2% PHA, and incubate at 37 °C for 90 min.
13. Add 6 mL of pre-warmed 0.075 M KCl and incubate at 37 °C for 5 min.
14. Centrifuge at 328 × *g* for 7 min and discard the supernatant.
15. Add 7 mL of Carnoy's fixative (*see* **Note 18**) and keep at 4 °C overnight.
16. On the next day, wash the fixed cells twice with Carnoy's fixative and drop 15 μL onto clean glass slides (*see* **Notes 10–12** and **16**). Keep the slides at −20 °C until staining (Fig. 2).

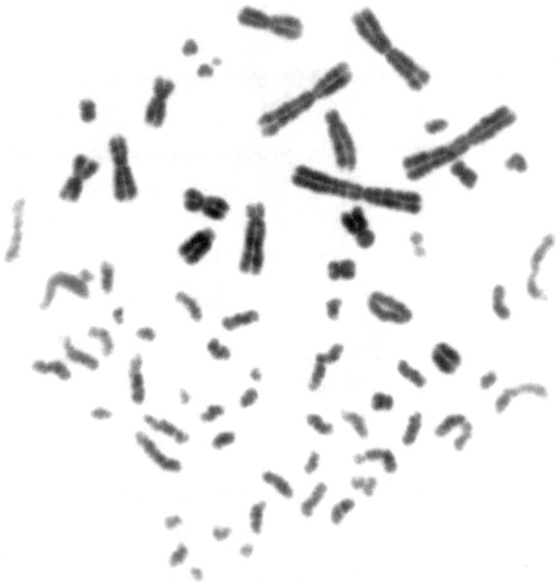

Fig. 2 Premature chromosome condensation obtained from the fusion of human peripheral blood and CHO cells

3.2 Staining

3.2.1 Giemsa Staining

1. Remove the slides from the freezer and allow them to come to room temperature.
2. Immerse dried slides in Coplin jar containing Giemsa stain for 20 min.
3. Transfer the slides to Coplin jar containing distilled water, to remove excess stain, for a few seconds.
4. Air dry and visualize under the microscope for scoring (*see* **Note 19**).

3.2.2 Telomere–Centromere Hybridization

1. Remove the slides from the freezer the day before the experiment and allow them to come to room temperature overnight (*see* **Note 20**).
2. Wash the slides in PBS for 5 min and fix with 4% formaldehyde for 2 min.
3. Wash the slides three times in PBS for 5 min each, and digest in pre-warmed pepsin solution in Coplin jar for 7 min in 37 °C water bath.
4. Wash the slides in PBS for a few seconds, fix with 4% formaldehyde for 2 min.
5. Wash the slides three times in PBS for 5 min each.
6. Dehydrate with 50, 70, and 100% ethanol series for 5 min each and air dry at room temperature for 1 h.

7. Add 50 μL of probe per slide and cover with a plastic coverslip, then denature for 3 min at 80 °C on a hotplate.
8. Keep the slides in a moist chamber at room temperature for 90 min for hybridization.
9. Wash the slides in Wash I twice at room temperature for 15 min each.
10. Wash the slides with Wash II three times at 37 °C for 5 min each (*see* **Note 3**).
11. Wash the slides with PBS at room temperature for 5 min, counter stain with DAPI for 5 min, and mount with one or two drops of antifade mounting medium such as PPD (Figs. 3 and 4). Keep the slides at 4 °C in the dark or at −20 °C if the slides cannot be captured within a few days.

3.2.3 Tri-Color FISH

1. Remove the slides from the freezer the day before the experiment and allow them to come to room temperature overnight (*see* **Note 20**).
2. Wash the slides in 2× SSC at 37 °C in a water bath for 30 min.
3. Fix the cells with 4% formaldehyde for 2 min at room temperature.
4. Wash the slides three times in PBS at room temperature for 5 min each.

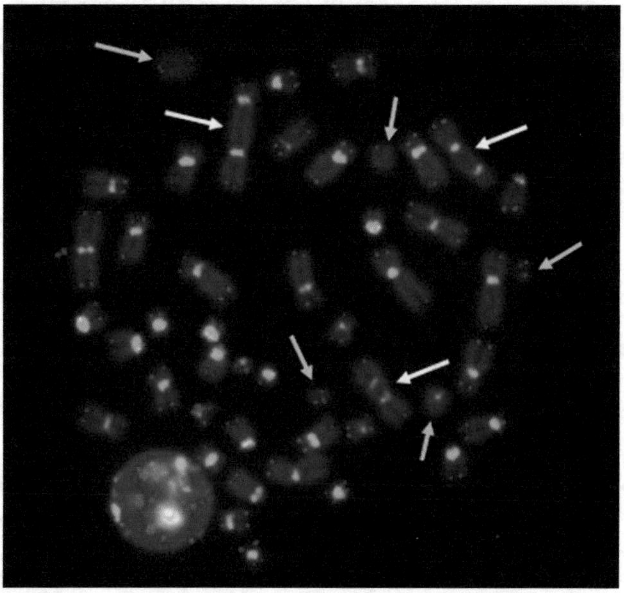

Fig. 3 Telomere–Centromere hybridization of a metaphase spread (cell irradiated at 4 Gy). Dicentrics are indicated by the *white arrows*, rings by the *green arrow*, and acentrics by the *yellow arrows*

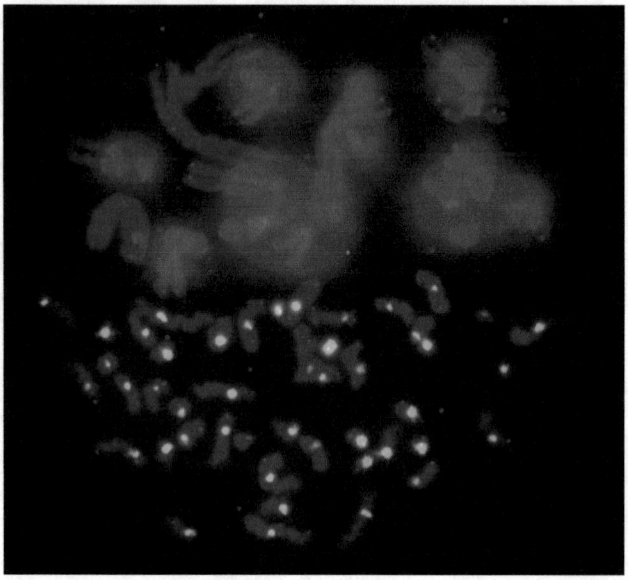

Fig. 4 Premature chromosome condensation obtained from human peripheral blood stained with PNA probes

5. Dehydrate with 50, 70, and 100% ethanol series for 5 min each and air dry at room temperature for 20 min.
6. Denature the slides with 70% formamide/2× SSC (pH 5.6) in Coplin jar at 70 °C in a water bath for 2 min.
7. Rinse rapidly with 2× SSC at 4 °C to stop the denaturation.
8. Dehydrate in 50, 70, and 100% ethanol series for 5 min each on ice and air dry for 20–30 min.
9. Denature the 3 FISH probes at 75 °C in water bath for 5 min (*see* **Note 21**) and pre-hybridize the centromeric and homologous regions at 37 °C for 45 min (*see* **Note 22**).
10. Drop 7–10 μL of the mixed probes onto each slide, cover with a plastic coverslip, and hybridize in a moist chamber containing 50% formamide, for better hybridization of the DNA probes, in a 37 °C incubator overnight.
11. On the next day, remove the plastic cover slip and rinse with 1× SSC at 75 °C for 3–4 min, then with 2× SSC/0.05% Tween 20 at room temperature for 5 min.
12. Wash the slides with PBS at room temperature for 5 min, counter stain with DAPI for 5 min, and mount with one or two drops of antifade mounting medium such as PPD (Fig. 5). Keep the slides at 4 °C in the dark or at −20 °C if the images cannot be captured within a few days.

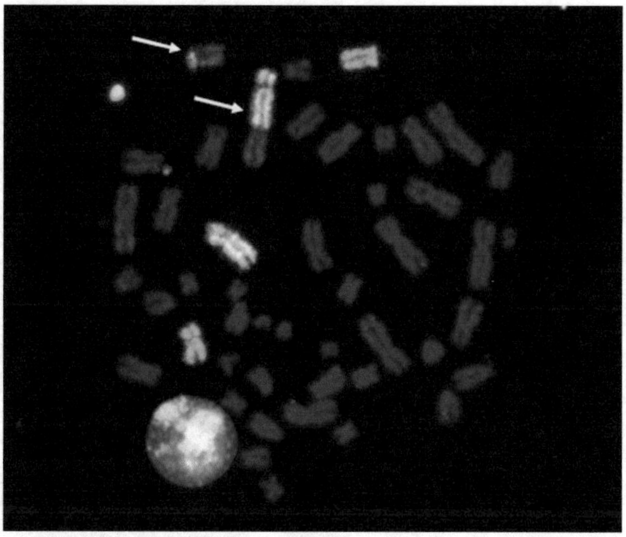

Fig. 5 Tri-color FISH on the same metaphase as shown in Fig. 3 (cell irradiated at 4 Gy). Chromosomes 1 in TR, 11 in FITC, and 4 in TR plus FITC. Translocations are indicated by the *white arrows*

3.2.4 M-FISH

1. Remove the slides from the freezer the day before the experiment and allow them to come to room temperature overnight (*see* **Note 20**).
2. Wash the slides with 0.1× SSC (pH 6.3) for 1 min and then 2× SSC (pH 6.3) in Coplin jar in 70 °C water bath for 30 min. Remove the Coplin jar from water bath and let it cool to 37 °C. Then, wash the slides in 0.1× SSC (pH 6.3) for 1 min.
3. Denature the slides with 0.07 N NaOH at room temperature for 1 min and stop the denaturation with 0.1× SSC (pH 6.3) on ice for 1 min, then 2× SSC (pH 6.3) on ice for 1 min.
4. Dehydrate the slides with 30, 50, 70, and 100% ethanol series for 1 min each and air dry at room temperature for 20 min.
5. Denature the probe cocktail at 75 °C in a water bath for 5 min (*see* **Note 21**) and pre-hybridize the centromeric and homologous regions at 37 °C for 30 min.
6. Add 10–15 μL of probe cocktail per slide, cover with a plastic coverslip, and hybridize in a moist chamber containing 50% formamide, for better hybridization of the DNA probes, in a 37 °C incubator for 3–4 days.
7. Remove the plastic coverslip and wash the slides in 0.4× SSC (pH 6.3) at 72 °C in a water bath for 2 min and then 2× SSC (pH6.3)/0.05% Tween 20 at room temperature for 30 s.
8. Wash the slides with PBS for 5 min, counter stain with DAPI for 5 min, and mount with one or two drops of antifade mounting medium such as PPD (Fig. 6). Keep the slides at 4 °C in the dark or at −20 °C if the images cannot be captured within a few days.

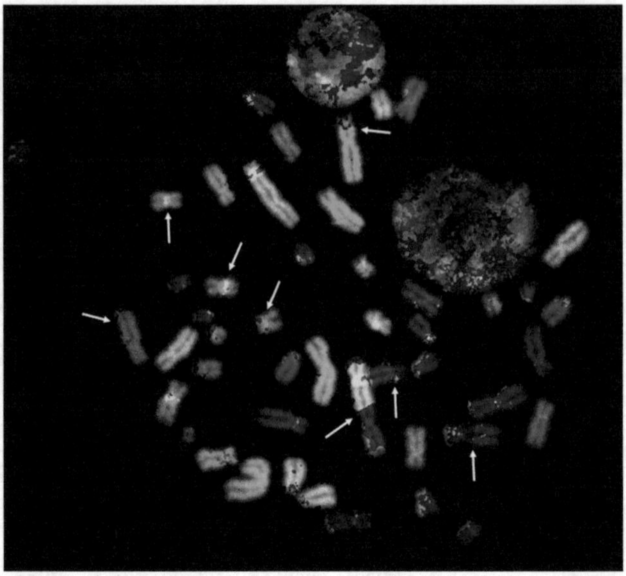

Fig. 6 M-FISH of metaphase spread (cell irradiated at 4 Gy). Translocations are indicated by the *white arrows*

3.3 Image Capture and Analysis for Chromosomal Aberrations

For biological dosimetry dedicated to triage, 50 metaphases are scored for the dicentric assay or other chromosomal aberration assays. For a precise dose estimate, 200–500 metaphases are scored. Up to 1000 metaphases can be analyzed when the dose appears to be low (<1 Gy).

3.3.1 Image Capture

1. *Giemsa stained*: Metaphase images are captured using an integration time of 0.093 s.
2. *Telomere–Centromere hybridization*: Metaphase images are captured using AutoCapt Metafer (Metasystems) with integration times of 0.485 s for Cy3 (telomeres) and in automatic mode with a maximum integration time of 0.04 and 4.2 s for DAPI and FITC (centromeres), respectively.
3. *Tri-color FISH*: Metaphase images are captured in automatic mode with a maximum integration time of 1.48 s for the 3-colors (DAPI, FITC, and TR).
4. *M-FISH*: Metaphase images are captured in automatic mode with a maximum integration time of 1.04, 3.04, 3.52, 3.52, 8.68, and 2.08 s for DAPI, FITC, SpO, TR, near infrared (NIR), and AQUA, respectively.

3.3.2 Analysis

For the analysis of the dicentric assay, first generation metaphases are analyzed only (*see* **Note 23**).

1. *Giemsa stain*: Chromosomal aberrations are difficult to analyze and require a high level cytogenetics experience. The misrepaired or unrepaired DNA double stranded breaks (DSBs) can be estimated from the number and types of chromosomal aberrations (CAs) (i.e., DC and rings) and excess acentric fragments. A DC or a centric ring associated with an acentric fragment is counted as two DSBs. A tricentric chromosome with two associated acentric fragments is counted as four DSBs. DC Score (Dicentric scoring, Metasystems) software can be used for automatic DC scoring alone, but the number of counted DCs is lower than that obtained by manual scoring.
2. *Telomere–Centromere hybridization*: Chromosomal aberrations are easily detected due to labeling of the centromeres, telomeres, and chromatin. A DC or a centric ring associated with an acentric fragment with four telomeres is counted as two DSBs. A tricentric chromosome associated with two acentric fragments, with four telomeres each, is counted as four DSBs. Excess acentric fragments with two telomeres are counted as one DSB (this is a terminal deletion), and those with no telomere are counted as two DSBs (this is an interstitial deletion). DC Score FL (Dicentric scoring fluorescence PNA-FISH telomeres-centromeres, Metasystems) can be used for automatic DC scoring alone, but the number of counted DCs is lower than that obtained by manual scoring. Quantification of the total breaks is explained in Fig. 7a.

A

Metaphases

Dics	Trics	Rings	Total Dics + rings	Total breaks Dics + rings	Frags 4 Telo	Frags 3 Telo	Frags 2 Telo	Frags 1 Telo	Total breaks frags Telo	Frags 0 Telo	Total breaks issues frags 0 Telo	Total breaks
number	number	number	number		number	number	number	number		number		
1 dic	(=2 dic)	(=1 r)			w	y	a	b	Z = 2(w+y)+a+b	H		if and only if (Z-2X) >0
2 DSB	4 DSB	2 DSB	X	2X	2 DSB	2 DSB	1 DSB	1 DSB	Z	2 DSB	2H	Total breaks = 2X +(Z-2X) + 2H

B

PCC

Dics	Trics	Rings	Total Dics + rings	Total breaks Dics + rings	Frags 2 Telo	Frags 1 Telo	Total breaks frags Telo	Frags 0 Telo	Total breaks issues frags 0 Telo	Total breaks
number	number	number	number		number	number		number		
1 dic	(=2 dic)	(=1 r)			w	y	Z = 2w+y	H		if and only if (Z-2X) >0
2 DSB	4 DSB	2 DSB	X	2X	2 DSB	1 DSB	Z	2 DSB	2H	Total breaks = 2X +(Z-2X) + 2H

Fig. 7 Scoring sheet for dicentric assay (**a**) and PCC assay (**b**)

3. *Tri-Color FISH*: The total number of translocations is counted on the three chromosomes and can be converted to genomic frequencies (FG) according to the proposed model of Lucas et al. [27, 28]. According to their formula, for the analysis of chromosomes 1, 4, and 11, approximately 19% of the genome is painted (that is fraction painted (fp) = 0.0828, 0.0639, and 0.0454, respectively).
4. *M-FISH*: DCs or translocations involving two chromosomes are generally counted as two DSBs, whereas more complex rearrangements involving three or more chromosomes can be counted and then converted into DSBs [28].

3.4 Image Capture and Analysis for Cytokinesis Blocked Micronucleus (CBMN) Assay

For biological dosimetry, 1000 binucleate cells with or without micronuclei (Fig. 1) are scored.

3.4.1 Image Capture

For Giemsa, binucleate cell images are captured using an integration time of 0.093 s with AutoCapt Metafer (Metasystems).

3.4.2 Analysis

1. The frequency and the distribution of the number of micronuclei per binucleate cell are counted.
2. Binucleate cells must fulfill several criteria such as (a) intact membranes for both nuclei located in the same cytoplasmic boundary, (b) similar size and staining pattern and intensity for both nuclei, (c) the two nuclei are not attached and do not overlap, (d) intact cytoplasmic membranes are distinguishable from other adjacent cytoplasmic boundaries.
3. Micronuclei must also fulfill several criteria such as (a) no connection to the main nuclei, (b) a diameter between 1/16 and 1/3 that of the mean diameter of the main nuclei, (c) no overlap with other micronuclei and must be distinguishable from the nuclear boundary, (d) staining of similar or superior intensity to that of the main nuclei.
4. CBMN Score (Metasystems) software can be used for automatic scoring.

3.5 Image Capture and Analysis for Premature Condensed Chromosomes (PCC)

For biological dosimetry, at least 20 PCC spreads may be sufficient for triage.

3.5.1 Image Capture

1. *Giemsa*: PCC images are captured using an integration time of 0.093 s.
2. *Telomere–Centromere hybridization*: Metaphase images are captured using AutoCapt Metafer (Metasystems) with integration times of 0.76 s for Cy3 (Telomeres) and FITC (human Centromeres), and in automatic mode with a maximum integration time of 0.12 s for DAPI.

3.5.2 Analysis

1. *Giemsa*: Excess fragments are counted.
2. *Telomere–Centromere hybridization*: DC or centric ring associated with an acentric fragment with two telomeres is counted as two DSBs. A tricentric chromosome associated with two acentric fragments with two telomeres each is counted as four DSBs. Excess acentric fragments with one telomere are counted as one DSB (this is a terminal deletion), and those with no telomere are counted as two DSBs (this is an interstitial deletion). Quantification of the total breaks is explained in Fig. 7b.

3.6 Dose Reference Curve

The number of chromosomal aberrations is plotted on a dose reference curve, established using data from at least five different donors with eight different doses. The IAEA has published a dose reference curve for Giemsa analysis of dicentric assays, but it is preferable that every laboratory establish their own. The curve is generally linear quadratic (aberration/cell = $aD^2 + bD + c$, where D is the dose). The mean score for chromosomal aberrations for all cells analyzed is plotted and the dose estimated. An example of a dose reference curve is shown in Fig. 8 for Telomere–Centromere analysis.

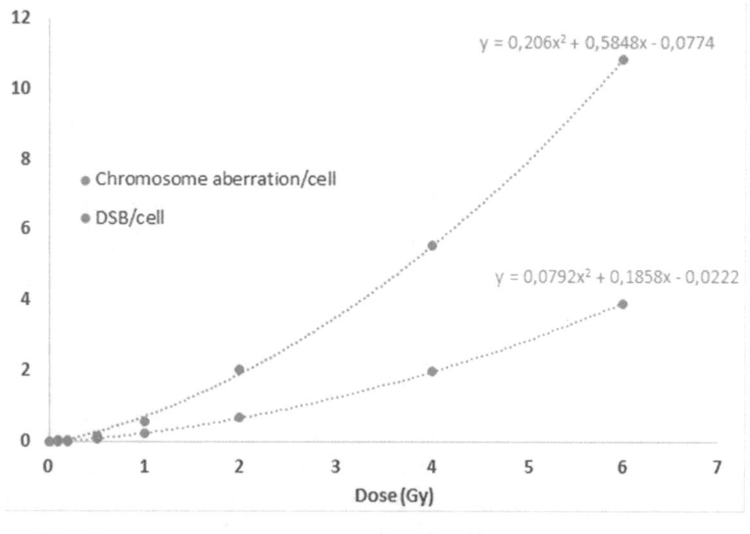

Fig. 8 Dose reference curves for chromosomal aberrations (CAs) per cell (*blue*) and per number of DSBs (DSB is defined as misrepaired or unrepaired DNA DSBs generating CAs) per cell (*orange*) after telomere–centromere hybridization for a dose rate of 0.5 Gy/min with γ-rays (^{137}Cs)

4 Notes

1. Carnoy's II fixative should be freshly prepared before use. Carnoy's fixative is normally composed of methanol but it can be replaced by ethanol to reduce toxicity.
2. Use formaldehyde and formamide under the hood.
3. The washing solutions can be pre-warmed to 37 °C before use to improve washing.
4. During and after the preparation of the PPD, keep it away from light with aluminum foil at −20 °C.
5. A stock solution of 20× SSC can be prepared with 175.2 g of NaCl and 88.2 g of Tris sodium citrate diluted in sterile water in a final volume of 1 L. The pH is adjusted with HCl or NaOH depending on the initial pH measured.
6. Other combinations of chromosomes are possible.
7. Solution to be prepared on day 2 of the experiment.
8. When removing the supernatant, always leave a small amount of medium above the cell pellet because the mitotic cells are on the top of the cell pellet. Discard supernatant by aspiration. To resuspend the cell pellet, first add 2 mL of the solution, vortex, and then add the rest of the solution. Eliminate the clumps if necessary by pipetting up and down with a Pasteur pipette [29].
9. Mix the tube well by inversion before and after adding the pre-fixative.
10. Use a P200 pipette with a tip with no filter.
11. Depending on the ambient humidity, it may be preferable to spread as a smear or as a drop.
12. Check the concentration of the cells using an inverted light microscope. If the density of the suspension is too high, add several drops of Carnoy's fixative, and if it is too low, centrifuge at 328 × *g* for 7 min and remove some of the fixative.
13. Gentle handling is required for the CBMN and PCC assays.
14. During hypotonic treatment in the CBMN assay, add potassium chloride, and process one tube at a time to obtain intact cytoplasm.
15. Gentle tapping is required. Modified Carnoy's fixative is at 5:1 instead of 3:1 to conserve the cytoplasm.
16. Cast the slides by dropping the fixed cells from a low height, so as to preserve the cytoplasm for the CBMN assay. It also helps to prevent over spreading of chromosomes for PCC.
17. To detect the effect of clastogens and anugens, Telomere–Centromere hybridization can be performed on CBMN to identify the type of fragments or whole chromosomes included in the micronuclei.

18. Add the fixative dropwise and do not vortex.
19. It is possible to add a coverslip to the slide and affix it with permanent glue, but further experiments on the same slide will be difficult. In any case, coverslips can be removed using xylene in a 37 °C incubator in a ventilated room until removal (may take a few days).
20. If the slides are not coming directly from the freezer and have already been hybridized, put the slide in PBS at 37 °C in a water bath until removal of the coverslip.
21. Rapidly stop the denaturation of the probes by placing on ice for a few seconds.
22. Denature each probe separately and mix them after prehybridization to avoid cross-hybridization.
23. To analyze first generation metaphases only, two techniques are possible: (a) 24 h incubation in colcemid during culture or (b) adding BrdU at the beginning of the culture.

Acknowledgements

This work is supported by the European Commission (FP7, Fission-2011-295513 (RENEB) and NRBC-C2. TGS is a post-doctoral fellow from EUROTALENTS CEA-EC Cofund program. We acknowledge Dr. P. Venkatachalam, SRU, Chennai, and Dr. N.K. Chaudhury, INMAS, Delhi, for their input to improve the CBMN assay.

References

1. Vorobiev AI (1997) Acute radiation disease and biological dosimetry in 1993. Stem Cells 15:269–274
2. Leonhardt EA, Trinh M, Forrester HB et al (1997) Comparisons of the frequencies and molecular spectra of HPRT mutants when human cancer cells were X-irradiated during G1 or S phase. Radiat Res 148:548–560
3. Lin J, Weiss A (2001) T cell receptor signalling. J Cell Sci 114:243–244
4. Langlois RG, Akiyama M, Kusunoki Y et al (1993) Analysis of somatic mutations at the glycophorinA locus in atomic bomb survivors: a comparative study of assay methods. Radiat Res 136:111–117
5. Paul S, Amundson SA (2008) Development of gene expression signatures for practical radiation biodosimetry. Int J Radiat Oncol Biol Phys 71:1236–1244
6. IAEA (International Atomic Energy Agency) (2011) applications in preparedness for and response to radiation emergencies, IAEA, Vienna
7. Viau M, Testard I, Shim G et al (2015) Global quantification of γH2AX as a triage tool for the rapid estimation of received dose in the event of accidental radiation exposure. Mutat Res Genet Toxicol Environ Mutagen 793:123–131
8. Li H, Eichler GS, Krausz KW et al (2008) UPLC-ESI-TOFMS based metabolomics and gene expression dynamics inspector self-organizing metabolomic maps as tools for understanding the cellular response to ionizing radiation. Anal Chem 80:665–674
9. Matsuoka S, Ballif BA, Smogorzewska A et al (2007) ATM and ATR substrate analysis reveals extensive protein networks responsive to DNA damage. Science 316:1160–1166
10. Sevankaev AV (2000) Results of cytogenetic studies of the consequences of the Chernobyl accident. Radiats Biol Radioecol 40:589–595

11. Ramalho AT, Nascimento AC (1991) The fate of chromosomal aberrations in ^{137}Cs-exposed individuals in the Goiânia radiation accident. Health Phys 60:67–70
12. Jinaratana V (2002) The radiological accident in Thailand. The medical basis for radiation accident preparedness. The Parthenon, New York, pp 283–301
13. Fenech M, Morley A (1985) Solutions to the kinetic problem in the micronucleus assay. Cytobios 43:233–246
14. Mikhalevich LS, De Zwart FA, Perepetskaya GA et al (2000) Radiation effects in lymphocytes of children living in a Chernobyl contaminated region of Belarus. Int J Radiat Biol 76:1377–1385
15. IAEA (International Atomic Energy Agency) (2001) Cytogenetic analysis for radiation dose assessment – A manual. 405:71-87
16. Johnson RT, Rao PN (1970) Mammalian cell fusion: induction of premature chromosome condensation in interphase nuclei. Nature 226:717–722
17. Pantelias GE, Maillie HD (1984) The use of peripheral blood mononuclear cell prematurely condensed chromosomes for biological dosimetry. Radiat Res 99:140–150
18. Sreedevi B, Shirsath K, Bhat N et al (2010) Biodosimetry for high dose accidental exposures by drug induced premature chromosome condensation assay. Mutat Res 699:11–16
19. Lamadrid AI, Garcia O, Delbos M et al (2007) PCC-ring induction human lymphocytes exposed to gamma and neutron irradiation. J Radiat Res 48:1–6
20. M'kacher R, El Maalouf E, Terzoudi G et al (2015) Detection and automated scoring of Dicentric chromosomes in nonstimulated lymphocyte prematurely condensed chromosomes after telomere and centromere staining. Int J Radiat Oncol Biol Phys 91:640–649
21. Hayata I, Kanda R, Minamihisamatsu M et al (2001) Cytogenetical dose estimation for 3 severely exposed patients in the JCO criticality accident in Tokaimura. J Radiat Res 42:149–155
22. Ray FA, Robinson E, McKenna M et al (2014) Directional genomic hybridization: inversions as a potential biodosimeter for retrospective radiation exposure. Radiat Environ Biophys 53:255–263
23. Kulka U, Ainsbury L, Atkinson M et al (2012) Realising the European Network of Biodosimetry (RENEB). Radiat Prot Dosimetry 151:621–625
24. M'kacher R, Maalouf EE, Ricoul M et al (2014) New tool for biological dosimetry: reevaluation and automation of the gold standard method following telomere and centromere staining. Mutat Res 770:45–53
25. Deperas J, Szluinska M, Deperas-Kaminska M et al (2007) CABAS: a freely available PC program for fitting calibration curves in chromosome aberration dosimetry. Radiat Prot Dosimetry 124:115–123
26. Ainsbury EA, Lloyd DC (2010) Dose estimation software for radiation biodosimetry. Health Phys 98:290–295
27. Lucas JN, Awa A, Straume T et al (1992) Rapid translocation frequency analysis in humans decades after exposure to ionizing radiation. Int J Radiat Biol 62:53–63
28. Lucas JN, Deng W (2000) Views on issues in radiation biodosimetry based on chromosome translocations measured by FISH. Radiat Protect Dosim 88:77–86
29. Dutrillaux B, Couturier J (1981) La pratique de l'analyse chromosomique. Eds Masson

Chapter 18

Recurrent Cytogenetic Abnormalities in Myelodysplastic Syndromes

Meaghan Wall

Abstract

Cytogenetic analysis has an essential role in diagnosis, classification, and prognosis of myelodysplastic syndromes (MDS). Some cytogenetic abnormalities are sufficiently characteristic of MDS to be considered MDS defining in the appropriate clinical context. MDS with isolated del(5q) is the only molecularly defined MDS subtype. The genes responsible for many aspects of 5q- syndrome, the distinct clinical phenotype associated with this condition, have now been identified. Cytogenetics forms the cornerstone of the most widely adopted prognostic scoring systems in MDS, the international prognostic scoring system (IPSS) and the revised international prognostic scoring system (IPPS-R). Cytogenetic parameters also have utility in chronic myelomonocytic leukemia (CMML) and have been incorporated into specific prognostic scoring systems for this condition. More recently, it has been appreciated that submicroscopic copy number changes and gene mutations play a significant part in MDS pathogenesis. Integration of molecular genetics and cytogenetics holds much promise for improving clinical care and outcomes for patients with MDS.

Key words Myelodysplasia, Karyotype, Cytogenetics, Chronic myelomonocytic leukemia, Therapy-related myeloid neoplasms, IPSS-R, Diagnosis, Prognosis, SNP-A, Mutations

1 Introduction

Myelodysplastic syndromes (MDS) are a heterogeneous group of disorders characterized by clonal and ineffective hematopoiesis. Ineffective blood production manifests morphologically as dysplasia and leads to one or more cytopenias. The blast count may be normal or elevated but is less than 20% in the bone marrow and peripheral blood. There is a heightened risk of progression to acute leukemia. Therapy-related cases are set apart from de novo MDS by a history of exposure to DNA-damaging agents. Chronic myelomonocytic leukemia (CMML) shares the dysplastic morphologic changes and leukemia risk found in MDS. However, it is distinguished by evidence of myeloproliferation in the form of a peripheral blood monocytosis, which may be accompanied by leucocytosis and neutrophilia, and it is therefore categorized as a myelodysplastic/myeloproliferative syndrome.

Thomas S.K. Wan (ed.), *Cancer Cytogenetics: Methods and Protocols*, Methods in Molecular Biology, vol. 1541,
DOI 10.1007/978-1-4939-6703-2_18, © Springer Science+Business Media LLC 2017

MDS and CMML are predominantly disorders of aging with a median age at diagnosis of 73–77 years [1, 2]. X chromosome inactivation studies [3], and more recent studies using massively parallel sequencing techniques, have shown that a significant proportion of older people have evidence of clonal hematopoiesis without compromise of blood production sufficient for diagnosis of a myeloid malignancy [4, 5]. This condition has been labeled clonal hematopoiesis of indeterminate potential (CHIP) [6]. CHIP carries a risk of approximately 1% per year of developing a hematological malignancy, analogous to the risk of plasma cell myeloma in monoclonal gammopathy of uncertain significance.

Metaphase cytogenetics identifies abnormalities in approximately 50% of MDS cases and 30% of CMML cases. Cytogenetic abnormalities have broad-ranging clinical utility with implications for diagnosis and prognosis. MDS with isolated del(5q) is known to be a lenalidomide-responsive condition with a clearly elucidated molecular mechanism. Integration of additional genomic information, provided by DNA microarrays and sequencing, holds great promise in further refining the classification and management of these disorders.

2 Diagnosis and Classification of MDS and CMML

Cytogenetic abnormalities are present in 35–50% of de novo MDS cases [2, 7–9]. The World Health Organization (WHO) classification of tumors of hematopoietic tumors and lymphoid tissue recognizes six categories of MDS: refractory cytopenia with unilineage dysplasia (RCUD), refractory anemia with ring sideroblasts (RARS), refractory cytopenia with multilineage dysplasia (RCMD), refractory anemia with excess blasts (RAEB), MDS with isolated deletion of 5q and MDS unclassifiable (MDS-U) [10]. MDS with unilineage dysplasia (RCUD and RARS subtypes) tend have more favorable outcomes than RCMD and then RAEB in turn, and cytogenetic abnormality rates vary accordingly. Abnormalities are identified by metaphase cytogenetics in approximately 11–34, 32–43, 46, and 50–59% cases of RARS, RCUD, RCMD, and RAEB, respectively [7, 8].

By definition, according to the 2008 version of the WHO classification, del(5q) is present as a sole abnormality in all cases of MDS with isolated deletion of 5q and so the abnormality rate is 100% in this subtype. In recent years, data have emerged indicating that del(5q) cases with one additional abnormality, other than −7 or del(7q), have equivalent clinical outcomes to cases where del(5q) is present as the sole abnormality [9, 11, 12]. Therefore, the 2016 revision of the WHO classification will allow cases with del(5q) plus one other abnormality to be categorized as MDS with isolated del(5q), providing the second abnormality is not del(7q) or −7 [13]. MDS with isolated del(5q) is the only molecularly defined MDS category and 5q- syndrome is the best understood contiguous gene syndrome in MDS. It has been shown that macrocytic anemia is the result of haploinsufficiency for the *RPS14* gene at 5q33 [14] and deletion of nearby microRNA clusters are responsible for the hypolobated megakaryocyte phenotype [15]. Haploinsufficiency of a third gene, *CSNK1A1* is required for lenalidomide sensitivity [16].

In contrast to acute myeloid leukemia (AML) where balanced abnormalities predominate, unbalanced abnormalities are more common in MDS. Overall, the most frequent abnormalities are loss of the Y chromosome (-Y), del(5q), +8, del(20q), and −7 [2, 7–9]. Assessment of morphologic dysplasia in cases of possible MDS can be challenging and is subject to significant interobserver variability [17]. In the setting of persistent cytopenia where morphologic criteria for a diagnosis of MDS have not been met, the WHO classification considers some cytogenetic abnormalities sufficiently characteristic of this condition to be MDS defining [10]. Cases that qualify for an MDS diagnosis by virtue of a characteristic cytogenetic abnormality fall into the MDS-U category. Unbalanced abnormalities considered presumptive evidence of MDS include −5, del(5q), −7, del(7q), del(9q), del(11q), del(12p) or translocations involving 12p, −13 or del(13q), i(17q) or translocations involving 17p, and the isodicentric Xq (Fig. 1). These abnormalities occur in MDS with estimated frequencies between 1 and 10%. Balanced abnormalities are more unusual in MDS. None occur with a frequency of more than 1%. However, the t(1;3)(p36.1:q26), t(2;11)(p21;q23), t(6;9)(p22;q34), and inv(3)(q21q26) recur with sufficient frequency to be considered MDS defining. Notably,

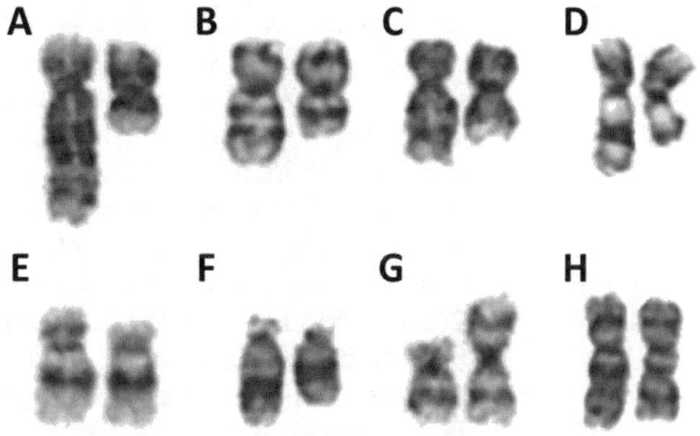

Fig. 1 Partial G-banded karyotypes of unbalanced, structural abnormalities considered presumptive evidence of MDS. In each panel the abnormal chromosome is shown on the *right* with the normal chromosome on the *left* for comparison. (**a**) del(5)(q12q34), (**b**) del(7)(q22q36), (**c**) del(9)(q22q33), (**d**) del(11)(q14q23), (**e**) del(12)(p12p13), (**f**) del(13)(q12q14), (**g**) i(17)(q10), (**h**) idic(X)(q13)

detection of MDS-defining abnormalities by fluorescence in situ hybridization (FISH) or other molecular techniques is not considered presumptive evidence of MDS. To be MDS defining, abnormalities must be identified by conventional karyotyping [13]. Loss of the Y chromosome, although common in men with MDS, may be observed as an age-related phenomenon in the absence of a hematological disorder and so cannot be considered presumptive evidence of MDS. Trisomy 8 and del(20q) are also common in MDS, but are not sufficiently specific to this disorder. Consequently, they are also excluded from the list of MDS-defining cytogenetic abnormalities.

Cytogenetic abnormalities are more frequent in therapy-related MDS (t-MDS) than de novo MDS, being reported in 70–90% cases [18, 19]. Presentations in t-MDS vary according to the regimen used to treat the primary malignancy. Patients with a history of exposure to alkylating agents most often present after 5–10 years with a t-MDS phenotype and unbalanced chromosomal abnormalities. Abnormalities of chromosomes 5, 7, and 17 that lead to loss of 5q, −7 or loss of 7q and loss of 17p are particularly common. These abnormalities often occur in the context of a complex karyotype in which three or more abnormalities are present. In contrast, those patients with a history of prior exposure to topoisomerase II inhibitors have a shorter latency, presenting within 1–5 years of cytotoxic therapy. Balanced translocations are characteristic of this group and include rearrangements involving the *KMT2A* gene (formerly known as *MLL*) or *RUNX1*. The balanced translocation, topoisomerase II inhibitor-provoked group of therapy-related myeloid neoplasms are more likely to present with therapy-related AML (t-AML) than t-MDS, or to progress rapidly to t-AML when fewer than 20% blasts are present at diagnosis [10].

The spectrum of cytogenetic abnormalities in CMML is similar to MDS, although overall abnormality rates are lower and del(5q) is rare [7, 8, 20, 21]. Reported abnormality rates range from 27 to 37%. The most common abnormalities are +8, loss of Y, −7, del(7q), and del(20q) [20, 21]. A CMML diagnosis requires exclusion of *BCR-ABL1* fusion gene formation. In cases where eosinophilia is present, abnormalities of *PDGFRA*, *PDGFRB*, and *FGFR1* should also be excluded. Myeloid/lymphoid neoplasm with *PCM1-JAK2* will be introduced a provisional entity in the 2016 revision of the WHO classification [13]. Therefore, the t(8;9)(p22;p24) involving *PCM1* and *JAK2* should also be excluded. In practice, in the setting of presentation with a CMML-like phenotype and eosinophilia, the most common translocation detected is the t(5;12)(q33;p13) involving the *PDGFRB* and *ETV6* genes. This translocation may be subtle, and FISH testing with a *PDGRFB* break-apart probe should be considered in cases where the pretest probability of the t(5;12) is high and chromosome morphology is suboptimal.

3 Prognosis of MDS and CMML

In 1997, the International MDS Risk Analysis Workshop generated a landmark, consensus prognostic scoring system for MDS known as the IPSS [22]. The statistical power gained by integrating data from a number of databases allowed the IPSS to define cytogenetic groups with superior prognostic accuracy to smaller, previous studies. The IPSS good cytogenetic risk group included normal karyotype as well as -Y, del(5q) and del(20q) as sole abnormalities. Complex karyotypes (containing ≥3 abnormalities) and abnormalities of chromosome 7 were defined as poor cytogenetic risk abnormalities. All other changes were classified as intermediate cytogenetic risk. As the survival benefit of azacitidine was demonstrated for patients in the IPSS intermediate 2 and high-risk groups [23], many regulatory agencies still use the IPSS score for drug approval purposes.

Following widespread acceptance and uptake of the IPSS, it became apparent that counting guidelines to reproducibly enumerate the number of abnormalities in a karyotype were required to apply the IPSS in a consistent fashion. To this end, the International Working Group on MDS Cytogenetics (IWGMC) published standardized guidelines for counting aberrations in MDS karyotypes in 2010 [24]. The key recommendation of this group was to count each item between commas in the International System for Human Cytogenomic Nomenclature (ISCN) string as one abnormality. More specifically this means: (1) each balanced translocation, simple structural change to a chromosome and numeric abnormality (including –Y) counts as one abnormality; (2) each complex structural change is counted as one abnormality. Further recommendations to address ambiguity are to (3) count zero for a proven constitutional aberration but count one if the etiology of the aberration is in doubt; (4) add all independent aberrations if multiple clones are present, but where the same abnormality appears in more than one clone, to only count it once; and (5) count tetraploidy as one abnormality. Using the IWGMC guidelines greatly improved consensus among IPSS cytogenetic risk scores assigned to MDS karyotypes by cytogeneticists. However, significant discordance was still observed among hematologists. Accordingly, the IWGMC further recommended that standardized complexity counting be performed by a cytogeneticist and routinely incorporated into the cytogenetics report.

A limitation of the IPSS cytogenetic risk score was that it did not adequately address the cytogenetic heterogeneity of MDS. Less common but recurrent abnormalities, such as deletions of 11q and 12p and trisomies of chromosomes 19 and 21, did not send out a clear prognostic signal in the IPSS. Furthermore, the prognostic significance of pairwise combinations in patients with two abnormalities had not been evaluated. Thus, these abnormalities were essentially ascribed to the IPSS intermediate category by default. In addition, the IPSS abnormal chromosome 7 category included monosomy 7, del(7q) and 7p abnormalities, despite concerns that they may not represent a homogeneous group. To address these concerns Schanz et al. developed a refined cytogenetic risk stratification scheme for MDS in 2012 [9]. Whereas the IPSS was derived from analysis of an 816 patient dataset, Schanz et al. were able to draw on information from 2902 patients. Using this larger dataset, the investigators were able to define 19 cytogenetic categories with predictive prognostic power, distributed across five discrete cytogenetic risk categories.

In an effort to strengthen the predictive power of the IPSS, Greenberg and colleagues studied outcome data from 7012 clinically annotated patients with primary MDS, culminating in the release of the revised IPSS for MDS (IPSS-R) later in 2012 [25]. As in the IPSS, the strongest prognostic factors in the IPPS-R were peripheral blood counts, blast counts, and the karyotype, with karyotyping carrying the most prognostic weight. The cytogenetic risk groups identified by Schanz et al. performed strongly in the extended IPSS-R cohort and were incorporated without change into the IPSS-R. The IPSS-R cytogentic risk groups are as follows:

1. Very good—loss of Y or del(11q) as sole abnormalities.
2. Good—normal karyotype, del(5q), del(12p), del(20q), del(5q) plus one additional abnormality.
3. Intermediate—del(7q), +8, i(17q), +19, +21, other single independent clones, double abnormalities excluding del(5q) and −7/del(7q).
4. Poor—inv(3), t(3q;var), del(3q), −7, any double abnormality including −7/del(7q), complex karyotypes containing three abnormalities.
5. Very poor—complex karyotypes containing >3 abnormalities.

Median overall survival for the very good, good, intermediate, poor, and very poor cytogenetic risk groups were 5.4, 4.8, 2.7, 1.5, and 0.7 years, respectively. Time to AML transformation for 25% patients was not reached for the very good risk group. In remaining four groups it was 9.4, 2.5, 1.7, and 0.7 years in order of increasing risk. It is worth noting that French-American-British (FAB) CMML myelodysplastic syndrome type (CMML-MD) patients (those with a WCC $\leq 12 \times 10^9$/L) but not those with FAB CMML myeloproliferative disorder type (CMML-MP) were included in the IPPS-R cohort, as were patients with FAB RAEB-T (20–30% blasts). Hence, the IPSS-R is applicable to patients with oligoblastic AML and some CMML patients.

There is less data about the prognostic significance of cytogenetic abnormalities in t-MDS cases than in *de novo* MDS. A study of 281 patients treated at the MD Anderson Cancer Center (MDACC) between 1998 and 2007 identified −7 and complex karyotype (≥3 abnormalities) as independent predictors of poor prognosis in t-MDS [19]. As t-MDS cases were not included in the dataset used to construct the IPSS-R it was unclear whether the IPSS-R cytogenetic risk groups retained prognostic power in this setting. A study by the International Working Group for MDS of 1837 t-MDS cases found 2, 36, 17, 15, and 31% cases had very good, good, intermediate, poor, and very poor risk IPSS-R karyotypes, respectively [26]. In comparison, the corresponding figures were 4, 72, 13, 4, and 7% for de novo cases. Thus, although poor risk karyotypes are overrepresented in therapy-related cases relative to de novo MDS, over one-third of therapy-related cases still have favorable risk karyotypes. Overall, the IPSS-R cytogenetic risk schema retained some prognostic power in this therapy-related cohort. However, it did not perform as well in predicting overall survival or AML transformation as it does in de novo MDS.

Cases of CMML-MP were excluded from the dataset used to formulate the IPSS-R. To develop a prognostic scoring system that could be universally applied in CMML, Such et al. used Spanish Registry of MDS data [21]. The investigators defined 3 cytogenetic risk categories: favorable, intermediate, and unfavorable. Normal karyotype and -Y were favorable risk cytogenetic abnormalities. Trisomy 8, chromosome 7 abnormalities, and complex karyotype (≥3 abnormalities) were classified as unfavorable. All other karyotypes were considered intermediate risk. The system retained independent predictive value for survival but not for transformation to AML in multivariable analysis. The CMML-specific cytogenetic risk classification was one of four variables incorporated into the CMML-specific prognostic scoring system (CPSS) published by the same group in 2013 [27].

Subsequently, Tang et al. tested the CPSS in a cohort of CMML patients from the MDACC [20]. Notably, +8 patients had significantly superior overall survival to other patients in the unfavorable cytogenetic risk group. However, leukemia-free survival for +8 patients was equivalent to that of patients with other high-risk cytogenetic abnormalities. Reassignment of +8 cases to the intermediate rather than the high-risk group improved predictive modeling with respect to overall survival and leukemia-free survival. Given the lack of consensus from Spanish Registry data and the MDACC cohort regarding +8 cases, additional studies will be needed to clarify the prognostic significance of this abnormality in CMML. More recently, Padron et al. tested a number of prognostic scoring systems, including the CPSS and the IPSS-R, in a database of 1,832 CMML cases [28]. The CPSS and the IPSS-R performed equally well in predicting survival in this cohort as a whole, despite the fact that the IPPS-R was not designed to predict outcomes in CMML-MP. However, when analysis was confined to CMML-MP cases only, the performance of the IPSS-R was compromised.

As discussed earlier, balanced translocations are rare but recognized in MDS with some considered MDS defining. Yet, with the exception of translocations involving 3q, their prognostic significance is not explicitly addressed in the IPSS-R. A recent study of the Spanish Registry of MDS by Nomdedeu et al. found that a translocation was present in 168 of 1,653 patients with MDS or CMML who had an abnormal karyotype [29]. The presence of a translocation was associated with a poor prognosis in univariable analysis. However, it was not an independent prognostic factor in multivariable analysis, suggesting that any adverse prognostic significance was a function of an association with other poor prognosis variables. Importantly, outcomes were equivalent in those patients with and without a translocation in the intermediate as well as in the poor and very poor IPSS-R cytogenetic risk categories. Thus, this data positively validates assignment of MDS patients with a translocation as a single or double abnormality to the IPPS-R intermediate risk category.

In 2008, Breems et al. demonstrated that a monosomal karyotype (MK) was a superior predictor of poor prognosis in AML [30]. It has since been revealed that there is a strong correlation between MK and mutations in the *TP53* gene, which are also an indicator of poor prognosis in AML [31, 32]. Currently, no clear consensus exists as to whether MK is an independent predictor of poor prognosis in MDS. It may be difficult to separate the impact of complexity from MK in MDS because most MK also meet the criteria for a complex karyotype. Analysis of the Spanish Registry of MDS [33] and the international database of Schanz et al. [34] did not identify MK as an independent prognostic variable. However, in data from the Mayo Clinic database for MDS, MK was an independent predictor of poor prognosis and refined outcome prediction in the IPSS-R poor and very poor cytogenetic risk groups [35, 36]. Furthermore, in a real-world MDS dataset from Australia, MK retained independent predictive value and those patients meeting criteria for complexity plus MK had shorter median survival (6 months) than patients with karyotypic complexity alone (17 months) or MK alone (18 months) [2].

4 Molecular Genetics of MDS and CMML

Molecular karyotyping using comparative genomic hybridization arrays (CGH) and single nucleotide polymorphism arrays (SNP-A) can detect copy number changes in nondividing cells and with higher resolution than metaphase cytogenetics. SNP-A has the added advantage of being able to detect copy-neutral loss of heterozygosity (CN-LOH, also known as acquired uniparental disomy), a manifestation of driver mutations in MDS and CMML. Abnormality rates are generally higher for SNP-A than CGH because CN-LOH events are relatively frequent. In addition to detecting cytogenetically cryptic abnormalities, molecular karyotyping can inform and refine interpretation of structural abnormalities observed by metaphase cytogenetics [37]. However, CGH and SNP-A are not capable of detecting balanced translocations and are limited in their ability to identify low-level mosaicism. Accordingly, CGH and SNP-A play a complementary role to metaphase cytogenetics and increase the detection of abnormalities in MDS and CMML.

Tiu et al. showed that additional abnormalities detected by SNP-A have prognostic significance [38]. The presence of any new abnormality effectively upgraded the IPSS cytogenetic score to the next-highest risk category. Metaphase cytogenetics has a failure rate of 5–15% in MDS and these cases are difficult to stratify because of the absence of an informative karyotype. Arenellas et al. identified copy number abnormalities with prognostic significance in the bone marrow or peripheral blood of 23/62 (37%) patients with a failed cytogenetics result [39]. CN-LOH without copy number change was seen in a further (8/62) 12% cases. These results indicate the molecular karyotyping has clinical utility in this setting.

The advent of massively parallel sequencing has revealed that acquired somatic gene mutations are detected in over 80% MDS patients [40]. Recurrent mutations are observed in genes that play a role in RNA splicing, epigenetic regulation, transcriptional regulation, cell signaling pathways, and the cohesion complex. Mutations in genes involved in RNA splicing and epigenetic regulation are often early or founder mutations in MDS and appear to precede the development of cytogenetics abnormalities in the majority of cases. The mutations observed in MDS show significant overlap with the mutations found in elderly patients with CHIP. Hence, gene mutations cannot be considered diagnostic of MDS at the current time. Bejar et al. found that mutations in *TP53*, *EZH2*, *ETV6*, *RUNX1*, and *ASXL1* were independent prognostic variables in MDS and refined risk stratification [41]. Although validation of these findings in independent MDS cohorts is still ongoing, it is expected that gene mutations will play an important part of MDS prognostication in the near future.

5 Integration of Cytogenetics and Molecular Genetics

Clearly, in MDS, there are nonrandom relationships between copy number changes detected by metaphase cytogenetics or molecular karyotyping and gene mutations and also between CN-LOH and gene mutations. The same genes that are subject to mutation can also be targeted by focal cryptic deletion events that are detected by SNP-A. Mutations in *DNMT3A*, *TET2*, *ETV 6*, and others are known to be recurrent in MDS and deletions in the same genes can also be identified by molecular karyotyping [37, 42]. Known associations between CN-LOH and gene mutations and associations between cytogenetic abnormalities and gene mutations are shown in Table 1.

Table 1
Associations of chromosomal abnormalities with mutations in MDS

Karyotype	Associated mutations (positive correlations)	Associated mutations (negative correlations)	Comments	Reference(s)
Complex karyotype	*TP53* *ASXL1*	*SF3B1*	Poor prognosis.	[40, 43]
Monosomal karyotype	*TP53*		Poor prognosis.	[41]
Loss of Y	*BRCC3*		*BRCC3* mutations have a male predominance.	[44]
CN-LOH 4q	*TET2*			[45, 46]
5q-	*TP53*	*TET2* *SRSF2*	*TP53* mutations confer resistance to lenalidomide and increase the risk of transformation to AML in cases of isolated del(5q).	[40, 47, 48]
CN-LOH 7q	*EZH2*		Poor prognosis.	[49–52]
−7/7q−	*U2AF1* *SETBP1*	*EZH2*	Poor prognosis.	[40, 48, 53–55]
+8	*U2AF1*			[43]
CN-LOH 11q	*CBL*			[56, 57]
CN-LOH17p/17p-	*TP53*		Poor prognosis.	[58, 59]
i(17q)	*SRSF2* *SETBP1* *ASXL1* *NRAS*	*TET2* *TP53*		[53, 55, 60, 61]
20q-	*U2AF1* *SRSF2* *ASXL1*		*ASXL1* mutations associated with a poor prognosis.	[43, 48, 62, 63]

One example in CMML is an association between copy number change or CN-LOH at 4q21 and *TET2* mutations. *TET2* mutations are present in more than 50% CMML cases. They may be heterozygous, compound heterozygous, homozygous with CN-LOH, or hemizygous with deletion of the second copy of *TET2*. Loss of *TET2* may result from interstitial deletion of chromosome 4 or unbalanced translocation (Fig. 2). Thus, cytogenetic changes such as this can signal the presence of clinically relevant gene mutations. Although associations between more common entities are starting to emerge, the heterogeneity of MDS at the cytogenetic and molecular level means larger datasets will be needed to characterize fully cooperating copy number changes and gene mutations.

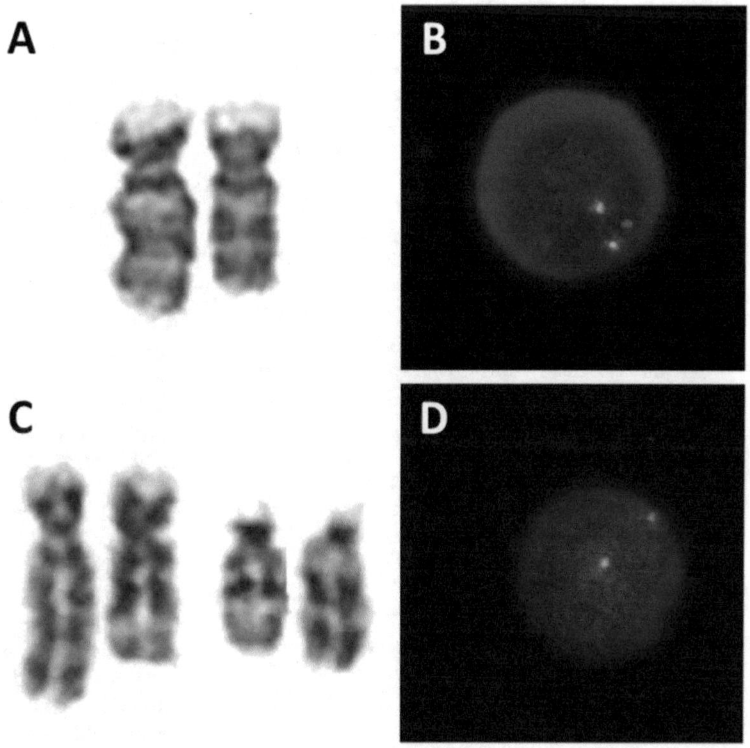

Fig. 2 Loss of *TET2* in CMML in association with an interstitial deletion of 4q and a reciprocal 4;15 translocation. (**a**) Partial G-banded karyotype showing del(4)(q21q24). The abnormal chromosome is shown on the *right* with the normal chromosome 4 on the *left* for comparison. (**b**) FISH using the *SCFD2/TET2* 4q12/4q24 dual color probe (Metasystems) for the case shown in (**a**). The strength of one *TET2* (*red*) signal is greatly diminished. (**c**) Partial G-banded karyotype showing a t(4;15)(q24;q25). The derivative chromosomes in each pair are shown on the *right* with the normal chromosomes on the *left* for comparison. (**d**) FISH in the case shown in (**c**) showed loss of one *TET2* (*red*) signal in keeping with deletion

References

1. Rollison DE, Howlader N, Smith MT et al (2008) Epidemiology of myelodysplastic syndromes and chronic myeloproliferative disorders in the United States, 2001-2004, using data from the NAACCR and SEER programs. Blood 112:45–52. doi:10.1182/blood-2008-01-134858
2. McQuilten ZK, Sundararajan V, Andrianopoulos N et al (2015) Monosomal karyotype predicts inferior survival independently of a complex karyotype in patients with myelodysplastic syndromes. Cancer 121:2892–2899. doi:10.1002/cncr.29396
3. Busque L, Paquette Y, Provost S et al (2009) Skewing of X-inactivation ratios in blood cells of aging women is confirmed by independent methodologies. Blood 113:3472–3474. doi:10.1182/blood-2008-12-195677
4. Genovese G, Kähler AK, Handsaker RE et al (2014) Clonal hematopoiesis and blood-cancer risk inferred from blood DNA sequence. N Engl J Med 371:2477–2487. doi:10.1056/NEJMoa1409405
5. Jaiswal S, Fontanillas P, Flannick J et al (2014) Age-related clonal hematopoiesis associated with adverse outcomes. N Engl J Med 371:2488–2498. doi:10.1056/NEJMoa1408617
6. Steensma DP, Bejar R, Jaiswal S et al (2015) Clonal hematopoiesis of indeterminate potential and its distinction from myelodysplastic syndromes. Blood 126:9–16. doi:10.1182/blood-2015-03-631747
7. Solé F, Luño E, Sanzo C et al (2005) Identification of novel cytogenetic markers with prognostic significance in a series of 968 patients with primary myelodysplastic syndromes. Haematologica 90:1168–1178
8. Haase D, Germing U, Schanz J et al (2007) New insights into the prognostic impact of the karyotype in MDS and correlation with subtypes: evidence from a core dataset of 2124 patients. Blood 110:4385–4395. doi:10.1182/blood-2007-03-082404
9. Schanz J, Tüchler H, Solè F et al (2012) New Comprehensive Cytogenetic Scoring System for Primary Myelodysplastic Syndromes (MDS) and Oligoblastic Acute Myeloid Leukemia After MDS Derived From an International Database Merge. J Clin Oncol 30:820–829. doi:10.1200/JCO.2011.35.6394
10. Swerdlow SH, Campo E, Harris NL et al (eds) (2008) WHO classification of tumours of haematopoietic and lymphoid tissue. IARC, Lyon
11. Germing U, Lauseker M, Hildebrandt B et al (2012) Survival, prognostic factors and rates of leukemic transformation in 381 untreated patients with MDS and del(5q): a multicenter study. Leukemia 26:1286–1292. doi:10.1038/leu.2011.391
12. Mallo M, Cervera J, Schanz J et al (2011) Impact of adjunct cytogenetic abnormalities for prognostic stratification in patients with myelodysplastic syndrome and deletion 5q. Leukemia 25:110–120. doi:10.1038/leu.2010.231
13. Arber DA, Orazi A, Hasserjian R et al (2016) The 2016 revision to the World Health Organization (WHO) classification of myeloid neoplasms and acute leukemia. Blood 127:2391–2405. doi:10.1182/blood-2016-03-643544
14. Ebert BL, Pretz J, Bosco J et al (2008) Identification of RPS14 as a 5q- syndrome gene by RNA interference screen. Nature 451:335–339. doi:10.1038/nature06494
15. Starczynowski DT, Kuchenbauer F, Argiropoulos B et al (2010) Identification of miR-145 and miR-146a as mediators of the 5q- syndrome phenotype. Nat Med 16:49–58. doi:10.1038/nm.2054
16. Krönke J, Fink EC, Hollenbach PW et al (2015) Lenalidomide induces ubiquitination and degradation of CK1α in del(5q) MDS. Nature 523:183–188. doi:10.1038/nature14610
17. Font P, Loscertales J, Benavente C et al (2013) Inter-observer variance with the diagnosis of myelodysplastic syndromes (MDS) following the 2008 WHO classification. Ann Hematol 92:19–24. doi:10.1007/s00277-012-1565-4
18. Smith SM, Le Beau MM, Huo D et al (2003) Clinical-cytogenetic associations in 306 patients with therapy-related myelodysplasia and myeloid leukemia: the University of Chicago series. Blood 102:43–52. doi:10.1182/blood-2002-11-3343
19. Quintás-Cardama A, Daver N, Kim H et al (2014) A prognostic model of therapy-related myelodysplastic syndrome for predicting survival and transformation to acute myeloid leukemia. Clin Lymphoma Myeloma Leuk 14:401–410. doi:10.1016/j.clml.2014.03.001
20. Tang G, Zhang L, Fu B et al (2014) Cytogenetic risk stratification of 417 patients with chronic myelomonocytic leukemia from a single institution. Am J Hematol 89:813–818. doi:10.1002/ajh.23751
21. Such E, Cervera J, Costa D et al (2011) Cytogenetic risk stratification in chronic myelomonocytic leukemia. Haematologica 96:375–383. doi:10.3324/haematol.2010.030957
22. Greenberg P, Cox C, LeBeau MM et al (1997) International scoring system for evaluating prognosis in myelodysplastic syndromes. Blood 89:2079–2088

23. Fenaux P, Mufti GJ, Hellstrom-Lindberg E et al (2009) Efficacy of azacitidine compared with that of conventional care regimens in the treatment of higher-risk myelodysplastic syndromes: a randomised, open-label, phase III study. Lancet Oncol 10:223–232. doi:10.1016/S1470-2045(09)70003-8
24. Chun K, Hagemeijer A, Iqbal A et al (2010) Implementation of standardized international karyotype scoring practices is needed to provide uniform and systematic evaluation for patients with myelodysplastic syndrome using IPSS criteria: An International Working Group on MDS Cytogenetics Study. Leuk Res 34:160–165. doi:10.1016/j.leukres.2009.07.006
25. Greenberg PL, Tuechler H, Schanz J et al (2012) Revised International Prognostic Scoring System (IPSS-R) for myelodysplastic syndromes. Blood 120:2454–2465. doi:10.1182/blood-2012-03-420489
26. Kuendgen A, Tuechler H, Nomdedeu M et al (2015) An analysis of prognostic markers and the performance of scoring systems in 1837 patients with therapy-related myelodysplastic syndrome – a study of the International Working Group (IWG-PM) for Myelodysplastic Syndromes (MDS). Blood 126:609–609
27. Such E, Germing U, Malcovati L et al (2013) Development and validation of a prognostic scoring system for patients with chronic myelomonocytic leukemia. Blood 121:3005–3015. doi:10.1182/blood-2012-08-452938
28. Padron E, Garcia-Manero G, Patnaik MM et al (2015) An international data set for CMML validates prognostic scoring systems and demonstrates a need for novel prognostication strategies. Blood Cancer J 5, e333. doi:10.1038/bcj.2015.53
29. Nomdedeu M, Calvo X, Pereira A et al (2016) Prognostic impact of chromosomal translocations in myelodysplastic syndromes and chronic myelomonocytic leukemia patients. A study by the spanish group of myelodysplastic syndromes. Genes Chromosomes Cancer 55:322–327. doi:10.1002/gcc.22333
30. Breems DA, Van Putten WLJ, De Greef GE et al (2008) Monosomal karyotype in acute myeloid leukemia: a better indicator of poor prognosis than a complex karyotype. J Clin Oncol 26:4791–4797. doi:10.1200/JCO.2008.16.0259
31. Rücker FG, Schlenk RF, Bullinger L et al (2012) TP53 alterations in acute myeloid leukemia with complex karyotype correlate with specific copy number alterations, monosomal karyotype, and dismal outcome. Blood 119:2114–2121. doi:10.1182/blood-2011-08-375758
32. Grossmann V, Schnittger S, Kohlmann A et al (2012) A novel hierarchical prognostic model of AML solely based on molecular mutations. Blood 120:2963–2972. doi:10.1182/blood-2012-03-419622
33. Valcárcel D, Ademà V, Solè F et al (2013) Complex, not monosomal, karyotype is the cytogenetic marker of poorest prognosis in patients with primary myelodysplastic syndrome. J Clin Oncol 31:916–922. doi:10.1200/JCO.2012.41.6073
34. Schanz J, Tüchler H, Solé F et al (2013) Monosomal karyotype in MDS: explaining the poor prognosis? Leukemia 27:1988–1995. doi:10.1038/leu.2013.187
35. Patnaik MM, Hanson CA, Hodnefield JM et al (2011) Monosomal karyotype in myelodysplastic syndromes, with or without monosomy 7 or 5, is prognostically worse than an otherwise complex karyotype. Leukemia 25:266–270. doi:10.1038/leu.2010.258
36. Gangat N, Patnaik MM, Begna K et al (2013) Evaluation of revised IPSS cytogenetic risk stratification and prognostic impact of monosomal karyotype in 783 patients with primary myelodysplastic syndromes. Am J Hematol 88:690–693. doi:10.1002/ajh.23477
37. Kolquist KA, Schultz RA, Furrow A et al (2011) Microarray-based comparative genomic hybridization of cancer targets reveals novel, recurrent genetic aberrations in the myelodysplastic syndromes. Cancer Genet 204:603–628. doi:10.1016/j.cancergen.2011.10.004
38. Tiu RV, Gondek LP, O'keefe CL et al (2011) Prognostic impact of SNP array karyotyping in myelodysplastic syndromes and related myeloid malignancies. Blood 117:4552–4560. doi:10.1182/blood-2010-07-295857
39. Arenillas L, Mallo M, Ramos F et al (2013) Single nucleotide polymorphism array karyotyping: a diagnostic and prognostic tool in myelodysplastic syndromes with unsuccessful conventional cytogenetic testing. Genes Chromosomes Cancer 52:1167–1177. doi:10.1002/gcc.22112
40. Papaemmanuil E, Gerstung M, Malcovati L et al. (2013) Clinical and biological implications of driver mutations in myelodysplastic syndromes. Blood 122:3616-3627– quiz 3699. doi: 10.1182/blood-2013-08-518886
41. Bejar R, Stevenson K, Abdel-Wahab O et al (2011) Clinical effect of point mutations in myelodysplastic syndromes. N Engl J Med 364:2496–2506. doi:10.1056/NEJMoa1013343
42. Haferlach T, Nagata Y, Grossmann V et al (2014) Landscape of genetic lesions in 944 patients with myelodysplastic syndromes.

Leukemia 28:241–247. doi:10.1038/leu.2013.336

43. Wu L, Song L, Xu L et al (2016) Genetic landscape of recurrent ASXL1, U2AF1, SF3B1, SRSF2, and EZH2 mutations in 304 Chinese patients with myelodysplastic syndromes. Tumour Biol 37:4633–4640. doi:10.1007/s13277-015-4305-2
44. Huang D, Nagata Y, Grossmann V et al (2015) BRCC3 mutations in myeloid neoplasms. Haematologica 100:1051–1057. doi:10.3324/haematol.2014.111989
45. Jankowska AM, Szpurka H, Tiu RV et al (2009) Loss of heterozygosity 4q24 and TET2 mutations associated with myelodysplastic/myeloproliferative neoplasms. Blood 113:6403–6410. doi:10.1182/blood-2009-02-205690
46. Langemeijer SMC, Kuiper RP, Berends M et al (2009) Acquired mutations in TET2 are common in myelodysplastic syndromes. Nat Genet 41:838–842. doi:10.1038/ng.391
47. Jädersten M, Saft L, Smith A et al (2011) TP53 mutations in low-risk myelodysplastic syndromes with del(5q) predict disease progression. J Clin Oncol 29:1971–1979. doi:10.1200/JCO.2010.31.8576
48. Pellagatti A, Roy S, Di Genua C et al (2016) Targeted resequencing analysis of 31 genes commonly mutated in myeloid disorders in serial samples from myelodysplastic syndrome patients showing disease progression. Leukemia 30:247–250. doi:10.1038/leu.2015.129
49. Gondek LP, Tiu R, O'keefe CL et al (2008) Chromosomal lesions and uniparental disomy detected by SNP arrays in MDS, MDS/MPD, and MDS-derived AML. Blood 111:1534–1542. doi:10.1182/blood-2007-05-092304
50. Makishima H, Jankowska AM, Tiu RV et al (2010) Novel homo- and hemizygous mutations in EZH2 in myeloid malignancies. Leukemia 24:1799–1804. doi:10.1038/leu.2010.167
51. Nikoloski G, Langemeijer SMC, Kuiper RP et al (2010) Somatic mutations of the histone methyltransferase gene EZH2 in myelodysplastic syndromes. Nat Genet 42:665–667. doi:10.1038/ng.620
52. Ernst T, Chase AJ, Score J et al (2010) Inactivating mutations of the histone methyltransferase gene EZH2 in myeloid disorders. Nat Genet 42:722–726. doi:10.1038/ng.621
53. Hou H-A, Kuo Y-Y, Tang J-L et al (2014) Clinical implications of the SETBP1 mutation in patients with primary myelodysplastic syndrome and its stability during disease progression. Am J Hematol 89:181–186. doi:10.1002/ajh.23611
54. Tiu RV, Visconte V, Traina F et al (2011) Updates in cytogenetics and molecular markers in MDS. Curr Hematol Malig Rep 6:126–135. doi:10.1007/s11899-011-0081-2
55. Fernandez-Mercado M, Pellagatti A, Di Genua C et al (2013) Mutations in SETBP1 are recurrent in myelodysplastic syndromes and often coexist with cytogenetic markers associated with disease progression. Br J Haematol 163:235–239. doi:10.1111/bjh.12491
56. Dunbar AJ, Gondek LP, O'keefe CL et al (2008) 250K single nucleotide polymorphism array karyotyping identifies acquired uniparental disomy and homozygous mutations, including novel missense substitutions of c-Cbl, in myeloid malignancies. Cancer Res 68:10349–10357. doi:10.1158/0008-5472.CAN-08-2754
57. Makishima H, Cazzolli H, Szpurka H et al (2009) Mutations of e3 ubiquitin ligase cbl family members constitute a novel common pathogenic lesion in myeloid malignancies. J Clin Oncol 27:6109–6116. doi:10.1200/JCO.2009.23.7503
58. Jasek M, Gondek LP, Bejanyan N et al (2010) TP53 mutations in myeloid malignancies are either homozygous or hemizygous due to copy number-neutral loss of heterozygosity or deletion of 17p. Leukemia 24:216–219. doi:10.1038/leu.2009.189
59. Svobodova K, Zemanova Z, Lhotska H et al (2016) Copy number neutral loss of heterozygosity at 17p and homozygous mutations of TP53 are associated with complex chromosomal aberrations in patients newly diagnosed with myelodysplastic syndromes. Leuk Res 42:7–12. doi:10.1016/j.leukres.2016.01.009
60. Kanagal-Shamanna R, Luthra R, Yin CC et al (2016) Myeloid neoplasms with isolated isochromosome 17q demonstrate a high frequency of mutations in SETBP1, SRSF2, ASXL1 and NRAS. Oncotarget 7:14251–14258. doi:10.18632/oncotarget.7350
61. Kanagal-Shamanna R, Bueso-Ramos CE, Barkoh B et al (2012) Myeloid neoplasms with isolated isochromosome 17q represent a clinicopathologic entity associated with myelodysplastic/myeloproliferative features, a high risk of leukemic transformation, and wild-type TP53. Cancer 118:2879–2888. doi:10.1002/cncr.26537
62. Graubert TA, Shen D, Ding L et al (2011) Recurrent mutations in the U2AF1 splicing factor in myelodysplastic syndromes. Nat Genet 44:53–57. doi:10.1038/ng.1031
63. Bacher U, Haferlach T, Schnittger S et al (2014) Investigation of 305 patients with myelodysplastic syndromes and 20q deletion for associated cytogenetic and molecular genetic lesions and their prognostic impact. Br J Haematol 164:822–833. doi:10.1111/bjh.12710

Chapter 19

Recurrent Cytogenetic Abnormalities in Acute Myeloid Leukemia

John J. Yang, Tae Sung Park, and Thomas S.K. Wan

Abstract

The spectrum of chromosomal abnormality associated with leukemogenesis of acute myeloid leukemia (AML) is broad and heterogeneous when compared to chronic myeloid leukemia and other myeloid neoplasms. Recurrent chromosomal translocations such as t(8;21), t(15;17), and inv(16) are frequently detected, but hundreds of other uncommon chromosomal aberrations from AML also exist. This chapter discusses 22 chromosomal abnormalities that are common structural, numerical aberrations, and other important but infrequent (less than 1%) translocations emphasized in the WHO classification. Brief morphologic, cytogenetic, and clinical characteristics are summarized, so as to provide a concise reference to cancer cytogenetic laboratories. Morphology based on FAB classification is used together with the current WHO classification due to frequent mentioning in a vast number of reference literatures. Characteristic chromosomal aberrations of other myeloid neoplasms such as myelodysplastic syndrome and myeloproliferative neoplasm will be discussed in separate chapters—except for certain abnormalities such as t(9;22) in de novo AML. Gene mutations detected in normal karyotype AML by cutting edge next generation sequencing technology are also briefly mentioned.

Key words Chromosomal abnormality, Leukemogenesis, Acute myeloid leukemia, WHO classification

1 Major Chromosomal Translocations

1.1 t(8;21)(q22;q22): *RUNX1-RUNX1T1* Rearrangement

The t(8;21)(q22;q22) (Fig. 1) is one of the major recurrent chromosomal translocations, its detection enabling diagnosis of acute myeloid leukemia (AML) regardless of blast count from peripheral blood or bone marrow [1]. It is found in 5–10% of AML, predominantly in young individuals with a median age of 30, and rarely in infants [2, 3]. This translocation correlates with the AML-M2 classification while in some cases of AML-M4 (FAB). Most cases occur as sole chromosomal change but t(8;21) is often found with additional numerical or structural anomalies (e.g., loss of X or Y chromosome, del(9q), +8, del(7q), −7, etc.) [4]. Complex variants involving a third or fourth chromosome are also possible [5].

Thomas S.K. Wan (ed.), *Cancer Cytogenetics: Methods and Protocols*, Methods in Molecular Biology, vol. 1541, DOI 10.1007/978-1-4939-6703-2_19,

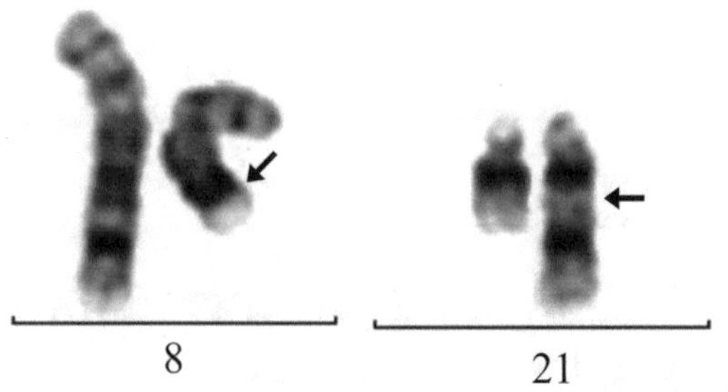

Fig. 1 Partial karyogram showing t(8;21)(q22;q22). *Arrows* indicate the breakpoints

The t(8;21)(q22;q22) involves the *RUNX1* gene (i.e., *AML1* or *CBFA*) located on 21q22 and the *RUNX1T1* gene (i.e., *ETO*, *MTG8*, or *CBFA2T1*) located on 8q22, generating the *RUNX1-RUNX1T1* fusion transcript [6]. It acts through inhibiting apoptosis by up-regulating the expression of anti-apoptotic *BCL2* [7]. However, recent studies indicate that *RUNX1-RUNX1T1* alone is insufficient for leukemogenesis and secondary cooperative mutations are necessary [8]. Such additional mutations found in core-binding factor leukemia include *KRAS*, *NRAS*, *ASXL1*, and *KIT* mutations that are detected in 10–50% of t(8;21) AML patients [9, 10].

Diagnostic strategies include morphology with cytochemical staining, conventional cytogenetics, fluorescent in situ hybridization (FISH) analysis, and reverse transcriptase-polymerase chain reaction (RT-PCR) assays. Target-specific FISH and RT-PCR analyses are especially helpful in variant or cryptic cases [11]. The fusion gene *RUNX1-RUNX1T1* is a target for both diagnosis and minimal residual disease (MRD) monitoring using RT-PCR and real-time (quantitative)-PCR [12].

Prognosis of t(8;21) in AML is considered favorable but leukocytosis, extramedullary leukemia, and *KIT* mutation are the adverse prognostic factors [13]. Most AML with t(8;21) occur de novo and about 5% are therapy-related AML (t-AML) with poor outcome [14]. Recent studies emphasize the importance of cooperative mutations regarding response to treatment and risk of relapse. *ASXL2* mutation is associated with high leukocyte count upon initial presentation and higher risk of relapse [10]. Presence of secondary cytogenetic aberration such as del(9q) and those mentioned above can also influence prognosis. Ethnicity also has impact on prognosis, non-Caucasians are more likely to fail induction chemotherapy [15].

1.2 t(15;17)(q22;q21): PML-RARA Rearrangement

Acute promyelocytic leukemia (APL) is a distinct subtype of AML with predominance of abnormal promyelocytes and numerous Auer rods. Morphologically classified AML-M3 comprises 5–10% of all AML cases, with an occurrence rate similar to t(8;21)(q22;q22) [16]. There are also hypogranular or microgranular variants that classified as M3v (FAB). An important distinctive feature of APL is the frequent association with disseminated

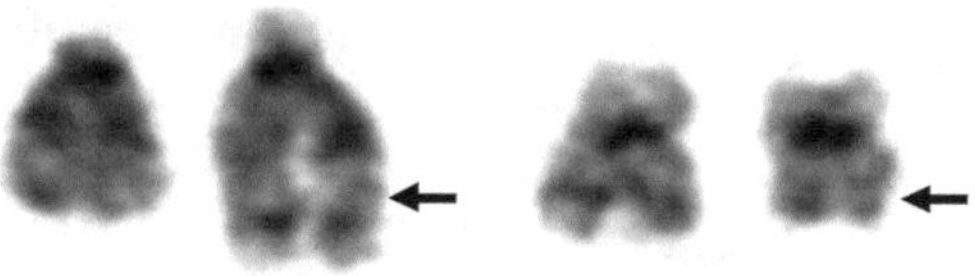

Fig. 2 Partial karyogram showing t(15;17)(q22;q21). *Arrows* indicate the breakpoints

intravascular coagulation (DIC) leading to high mortality and morbidity rate. Leukopenia or pancytopenia with symptoms of weakness, fatigue, and bleeding is common at initial presentation. Hypogranular variants with leukocytosis have higher risk of DIC. Laboratory analysis of d-dimer, fibrinogen, and hemostatic function usually shows abnormal results.

The t(15;17)(q22;q21) (Fig. 2) usually appears as sole chromosomal abnormality but complex translocations involving chromosomes 15 and 17 are also possible. The most common secondary change is +8 which is seen in one third of cases, followed by del(7q), del(9q) and ider(17)(q10)t(15;17) [17].

APL is perhaps the most well-studied hematologic malignancy on account of the discovery of pathogenesis of *PML-RARA*. The t(15;17) generates a fusion transcript between the *PML* gene located on 15q22 and the *RARA* gene located on 17q12-q21. Suspicion of APL based on clinical and morphological evidence warrants an investigation for the *PML-RARA* fusion. There are also cytogenetically cryptic cases, targeted analysis for *PML-RARA* is considered mandatory as those also generate the *PML-RARA* fusion. Among *RARA* rearrangements, APL variants or variant *RARA* translocations can also exist. The *RARA* gene generates fusion transcripts with other partners such as the *ZBT16* [t(11;17)(q23;q21)], *NUMA1* [t(11;17)(q13;q21)], *NPM1* [t(5;17)(q35;q21)], *FIP1L1* [t(4;17)(q12;q21)], *STAT5b* (within 17q21), etc. sharing all the characteristics of APL [18].

While cell morphology is the front line diagnostic method of APL, additional testing strategies are necessary with the advent of advanced technologies nowadays. Besides conventional karyotyping and immunophenotyping, FISH, RT-PCR, and multiplex RT-PCR can also provide additional diagnostic information. FISH analysis is particularly useful for detecting the *PML-RARA* rearrangement [19]. However, existence of FISH-negative cryptic *PML-RARA* rearrangements emphasizes the need of incorporating additional diagnostic methods for the diagnosis of APL such as anti-*PML* immunofluorescence, proximity ligation assay, and genomic breakpoint analysis [20, 21].

APL was considered fatal and malignant since its first description in 1957 [22]. The introduction of differentiation therapy using all-trans retinoic acid (ATRA) and arsenic trioxide (ATO) was a breakthrough in clinical treatment, yielding complete remission (CR) rate over 90% and as high as 5-year disease-free survival rate (>90%). ATRA/ATO therapy that targets on the fusion protein PML-RARA is an excellent model of molecular targeted therapy. The identification of this specific chromosomal abnormality or its fusion transcript has a favorable outcome to APL patients. As a result, initiation of prompt and appropriate treatments is helpful to these patients.

1.3 inv(16)(p13.1q22)/t(16;16)(p13.1;q22): *CBFB-MYH11* Rearrangement

Abnormalities of chromosome 16 are found in about 5–8 % of AML and are one of the three AML defining chromosomal aberrations regardless of blast percentage under the WHO classification [1]. The inv(16)(p13.1q22) or t(16;16)(p13.1;q22) (Fig. 3) associates with morphologic subtypes (FAB) AML-M4 with eosinophilia (AML-M4Eo), M2 and M5 [23, 24]. Leukemic blasts express high CD34 and CD117, and also positive for CD11, CD13, CD14, CD15, CD33, CD36, and HLA-DR. Aberrant co-expression of CD2 is frequently reported [1]. Occurrence is predominant among younger age with median age of 40. It may also present as extramedullary myeloid sarcoma especially during relapse.

The inv(16) is often accompanied by secondary cytogenetic abnormalities (40%). Common additional abnormalities are +22, +8, del(7q), and +21 [15]. Trisomy 22 is a specific change for inv(16)/t(16;16), associating with improved prognosis [25]. Vast majority are found as inv(16) whereas t(16;16) is less common. However, both involve the *CBFB* gene located on 16q22 and the *MYH11* gene located on 16p13.1 leading to the formation of the *CBFB-MYH11* fusion gene [26]. Owing to the variable breakpoints within both genes, more than ten different fusion transcripts are reported [27]. About 85% are type A whereas types D and E each constitute 5–10%. Despite the generally favorable prognosis of inv(16)/t(16;16), each *CBFB-MYH11* fusion can be different. Poor prognostic factors include high WBC count, age >35 years, and *KIT* mutation. Identification of fusion transcript type is important because non-type A fusions and *KIT* mutations are mutually exclusive, and that *KIT* mutation implicates adverse prognosis in type A inv(16)/t(16;16)

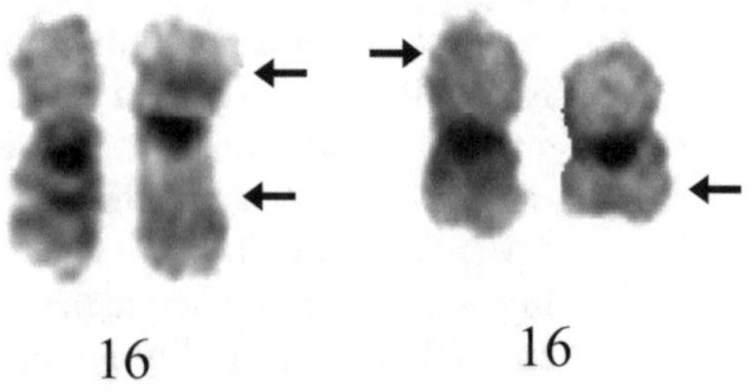

Fig. 3 Partial karyograms showing inv(16)(p13.1q22) (*left panel*) and t(16;16)(p13.1;q22) (*right panel*). *Arrows* indicate the breakpoints

patients [28]. Types also differ in associated secondary chromosomal abnormalities, +8 and +21 are more frequently found in non-type A whereas +22 is exclusive for type A [28].

FISH or RT-PCR are useful methods for confirmation in cases with typical morphologic features and ambiguous cytogenetic result [29]. Utilization of RT-PCR is particularly beneficial and recommendable for MRD monitoring, as RT-PCR negativity is associated with maintenance of complete remission [30]. Favorable prognosis is expected through high dose of cytarabine treatment in consolidation therapy.

1.4 11q23 Abnormalities: MLL (KMT2A) Rearrangements

The 11q23 abnormalities are interesting recurrent cytogenetic aberrations observed in both AML and acute lymphoblastic leukemia (ALL), resulting from chromosomal translocation between 11q23 and various translocation partners. Rearrangements of the *MLL (KMT2A)* gene located on 11q23 have been identified at molecular level and are detected in about 5% of AML [3, 31]. Median age of onset is between 40 and 60 and its incidence is significantly lower from thereafter. Etiology of *MLL* rearrangements is mostly unknown but factors such as ionizing radiation, chemical agents, and chemotherapeutic agents including alkylating agents and topoisomerase II inhibitors are correlated with increased risk of development of *MLL* rearrangement [32]. *MLL*-rearranged AML morphologically correlates with M4 and M5 (FAB) subtypes with prominent monocytic lineage involvement [33]. Common clinical characteristics include organomegaly, leukocytosis, and central nervous system involvement. Presence of *MLL* rearrangement is associated with poor outcome in general but differs among subtypes according to translocation partners, phenotype, age, and etiologic nature of leukemia [34].

The *MLL* gene was first identified in 1991 which has been implicated in numerous genetic aberrations. The *MLL* rearrangements have been identified to mainly occur through 11q23 terminal deletions, 11q inversions, and reciprocal translocations with about 80 different fusion partner genes [35]. The spectrum of partner genes is broader in AML than in ALL, comprising of t(9;11)(p22;q23) (*MLLT3*), t(10;11)(p12;q23) (*M LLT10*), t(11;19)(q23;p13.1) (*MLLT1*), t(11;19)(q23;p13.3) (*ELL*), t(11;17)(q23;q21) (*MLLT6*), t(1;11)(q21;q23) (*MLLT11*), t(X;11)(q24;q23) (*SEPT6*), etc. The common partner genes account for most of the leukemia while the remaining partner genes are infrequent [36]. Identification of fusion partner gene is important for risk stratification and decision of therapeutic plan as different partner genes display different prognosis [37].

Like other leukemia, diagnostic of *MLL* rearrangements includes conventional cytogenetic analysis, FISH, and RT-PCR. However, conventional cytogenetic analysis is unable to detect nearly one-third of *MLL* rearrangements in cryptic *MLL* rearrangements. FISH is one of the current methods for the detection of *MLL* rearrangements irrespective of the involved fusion partner gene [38]. FISH analysis using break-apart probe has the advantage of high specificity that can detect nucleotide sequences of short length. Therefore, FISH screening for *MLL* rearrangements is now incorporated in most AML protocols. Combined analysis of FISH and RT-PCR is successful in detecting known *MLL* rearrangements but different method is required to identify unknown translocation partner genes. The long-distance inverse-PCR (LDI-PCR) is a genomic breakpoint analysis that successfully detects unknown translocation partner genes and also complex translocations involving the *MLL* gene [37]. It is also particularly useful for MRD monitoring using patient-specific DNA sequences.

Pathogenesis of *MLL* rearranged leukemia involves other complementary mutations such as *RAS*, *BRAF*, and *NF1* mutations. *FLT3* is highly expressed while *RAS* pathway signaling is also an important cofactor in pathogenesis of AML. Understanding these cooperative mutations provides basis for an improved targeted therapy for *MLL* rearranged leukemia [39].

Treatment of the *MLL* rearranged leukemia usually involves standard to intensified treatment despite the heterogeneity of disease entity and the prognosis is intermediate to poor. Intensive therapeutic modalities are applicable for high-risk group leukemia and optimized regimens have improved the outcome of *MLL* rearrangements [39]. Targeted therapy of certain specific biologic markers such as the *FLT3* inhibitor (e.g., *PKC412*) is available [40] while directly targeting the *MLL* complex is another potential therapeutic approach [41].

2 Rare Chromosomal Translocations

2.1 t(1;3)(p36;q21)

About 50 cases of AML with t(1;3)(p36;q21) (Fig. 4) have been reported to date [42, 43]. The t(1;3) was first described in myelodysplastic syndrome (MDS) in 1984 and found in AML as well later on [44, 45]. The t(1;3) is rare but recurrent chromosomal abnormality detected in myeloid neoplasms such as MDS, myeloproliferative neoplasm (MPN), and AML. The 2008 WHO classification categorizes AML with t(1;3) into a distinct disease entity [1]. The gene rearrangement and the involved partner genes of t(1;3) were ambiguous. The t(1;3) triggers promoter swapping of the housekeeping gene *RPN 1*, which induces a transcriptional upregulation of the *PRDM16* gene. Like other 1p36/*PRDM16* rearrangements, the overexpression of *PRDM16* is the key functional outcome of t(1;3) [43].

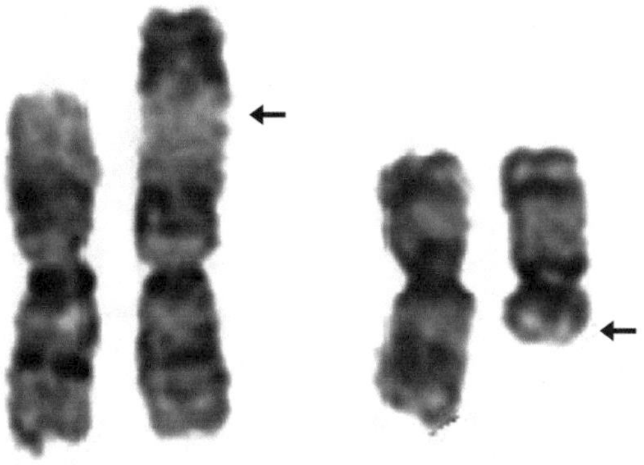

Fig. 4 Partial karyogram showing t(1;3)(p36;q21). *Arrows* indicate the breakpoints

Occurrence of t(1;3) is almost equal among both sexes, with a reported median age at the late 50s. The t(1;3) occurs as a sole chromosomal abnormality in most cases whereas del(5q) is the most common secondary chromosomal abnormality. Complex karyotype is also frequently seen as well. A few cases of APL with t(1;3) are reported [46]. Severe anemia, macrocytosis, and relatively high platelet count are usually found in AML/MDS with t(1;3) [47]. A review of 37 publications including 58 cases with t(1;3) confirms this finding as 29.7% showed thrombocytosis, while reporting an unusual case of extreme thrombocytosis as high as 2,000,000/μL [46]. The prognosis of t(1;3) positive AML is poor, complete remission achieved only in a limited number of patients. A retrospective analysis of 36 patients had a median survival period of 21.3 months and most t(1;3) cases are unresponsive to conventional chemotherapy [43, 46].

2.2 der(1;7)(q10;p10)

The der(1;7)(q10;p10) is a representative acquired whole arm translocation mostly detected in myeloid neoplasms such as AML, MDS, and MPN [48]. The der(1;7) is an unbalanced whole arm translocation formed between the long arm of chromosome 1 and short arm of chromosome 7, resulting in derivative chromosome der(1;7) and causing gain of 1q and loss of 7q (Fig. 5). Detection rate of der(1;7) in AML is about 0.2–2%, with a male predominance [43, 48]. It is rare in childhood AML and usually detected in elderly AML. This abnormality is detected as a sole chromosomal abnormality in about 60% while the most common secondary chromosomal aberration is trisomy 8 [43]. Most MDS/AML patients bearing this abnormality are associated with history of chemotherapy or radiotherapy and with poor prognosis [43, 48]. Recent studies report that *IDH1* and *IDH2* mutations are concurrently detected among therapy-related MDS/AML (t-MDS/AML) with der(1;7) [49].

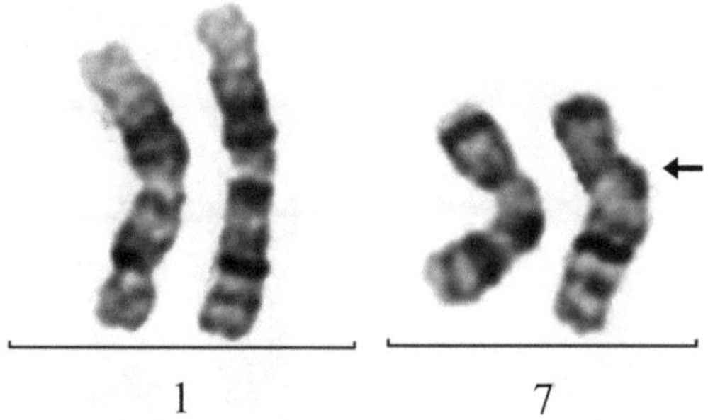

Fig. 5 Partial karyogram showing +1 and der(1;7)(q10;p10). *Arrow* indicates der which whole long arm of chromosome 1 and whole short arm of chromosome 7 are fused together

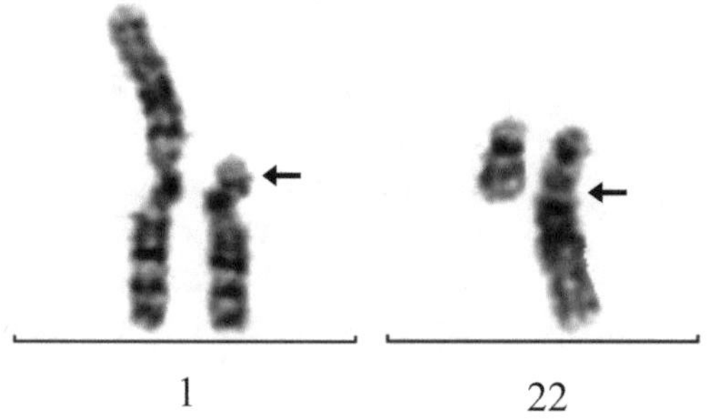

Fig. 6 Partial karyogram showing t(1;22)(p13;q13). *Arrows* indicate the breakpoints

2.3 t(1;22)(p13;q13): RMB15-MKL1 Rearrangement

The t(1;22)(p13;q13) (Fig. 6) has been reported in about 40 cases of AML according to the Mitelman database and is an uncommon but recurrent chromosomal aberration detected in less than 1% in AML [1, 42]. It is interesting that nearly all reported cases of AML with t(1;22) are classified as morphologic subtype of acute megakaryoblastic leukemia (AML-M7), showing a strong pathognomonic association between morphology and genetic subtype. It was first reported as an infant AML at the Fourth International Workshop on Chromosomes in Leukemia in 1982, the t(1;22) was later identified as a novel chimeric fusion gene (*RMB15-MKL1*) formed between *RBM15* gene located on 1p13 and *MKL1* gene located on 22q13 in 2001 by different research groups [50–52]. About 80% of AML with t(1;22) exists as a sole chromosomal aberration and some patients carry secondary chromosomal abnormalities in the forms of high hyperdiploidy [43]. AML with t(1;22) is mostly found in infants and young children under 3 years of age, with a female predominance [1, 42]. Unlike acute megakaryoblastic leukemia associated with Down syndrome, *GATA 1* mutation is rarely accompanied. Immunophenotyping analysis shows positivity for myeloid markers of CD13, CD33 and also megakaryoblastic markers of CD41 and CD61. Initial studies linked poor prognosis to AML with t(1;22), whereas recent studies report long disease-free survival and relatively fair response to intensive chemotherapy [1].

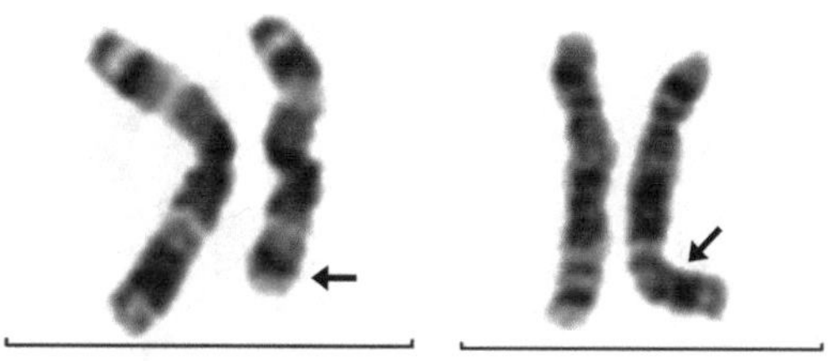

Fig. 7 Partial karyogram showing t(3;5)(q25;q34). *Arrows* indicate the breakpoints

2.4 t(3;5)(q25;q34): NPM1-MLF1 Rearrangement

Breakpoints of chromosomal translocation t(3;5) are known to be extremely variable. More than 70 cases of AML with t(3;5) have been reported in the Mitelman database, with breakpoints ranging broadly t(3;5)(q21~25;q31~35) (Fig. 7) [42]. The *NPM1-MLF1* rearrangement in AML and MDS is a chimeric fusion gene between 5′ region of *NPM1* gene from 5q34 and 3′ region of *MLF1* gene from 3q25 [53]. Most t(3;5) are de novo AML cases associated with morphologic subtypes of AML-M2, M4, and M6 (FAB) [43, 54]. AML with t(3;5) is closely associated with diagnosis of AML-Myelodysplasia Related Changes (AML-MRC) under the WHO classification [1]. The incidence of t(3;5) among AML is less than 1% [55], which most frequently occurs as a sole chromosomal abnormality and +8 being the most common secondary chromosomal abnormality [43, 54]. Interestingly, the t(3;5) is a cytogenetic aberration mostly found in male at the age of mid-30s. There are reports of t(3;5) in complex karyotypes [54], in which case confirmation of *NPM1-MLF1* rearrangement at a molecular level using FISH or multiplex RT-PCR can be helpful. Although high percentage of AML patients with t(3;5) achieve complete remission, early relapse and relatively short median survival time classifies t(3;5) as an intermediate risk group in AML [43, 54].

2.5 t(3;12)(q26;p13): ETV6-MECOM Rearrangement

The t(3;12)(q26;p13) (Fig. 8) is rare but recurrent chromosomal aberration that has been reported in about 50 cases of AML so far [42, 43]. Massad et al. [56] first reported the t(3;12) at chromosome level in 1990, which was confirmed later at gene level the *ETV6-MDS1-EVI1* (*ETV6-MECOM*) rearrangement by Peeters et al. [57]. The t(3;12) is associated with myeloid neoplasm especially in AML but also in MDS and chronic myeloid leukemia (CML) in rare cases [42]. Most cases of t(3;12) are detected in adult AML with no known gender difference regarding incidence [42, 43]. No morphologic subtype is specific to AML with t(3;12) but reports have been found in AML-M0, M2, M4, and M7. Recent study suggests that multilineage dysplasia is a common feature. About 60% of AML with t(3;12) exist as sole chromosomal abnormality and 40% accompany with structural aberrations of the chromosome 7 and monosomy 7 [42, 43, 58]. Since AML with t(3;12) is rare, additional studies regarding their therapeutic

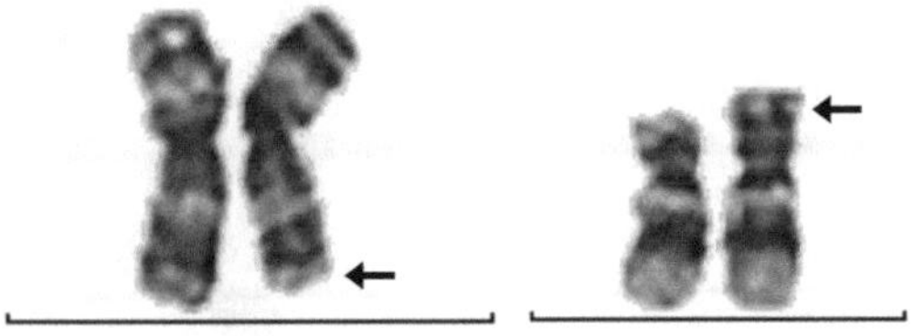

Fig. 8 Partial karyogram showing t(3;12)(q26;p13). *Arrows* indicate the breakpoints

response and prognostic impact are required in the future. However, an aggressive clinical course is expected based on eight cases of AML/MDS with t(3;12) accompanied with high rate of *FLT3*-ITD mutation [58].

2.6 t(3;21)(q26;q22): RUNX1-MECOM Rearrangement

The t(3;21)(q26;q22) (Fig. 9) is a rare chromosomal aberration in MDS or AML that occurs mostly in therapy-related conditions. This recurring translocation constitutes about 3 % of the 3q abnormalities detected in 4–5 % of AML [59, 60]. The t(3;21) appeared as a sole abnormality in 25 % of cases among the 146 cases listed on the Mitelman database while the common secondary abnormalities were monosomy 7 and trisomy 8. Isolated t(3;21) is mostly detected in AML while others are detected in blast phase of MPN [42]. Incidence is equal among both sexes and the median age is usually around 60 years of age [61].

Morphologic subtype is variable but appears mostly in AML-M2, M4 (FAB) and refractory anemia with excess of blasts (RAEB) in MDS. Commonly observed myelodysplastic feature is megakaryocytic hypoplasia causing decrease of platelet counts and megakaryocytes with the presence of micromegakaryocytes [62].

The t(3;21) produces the *RUNX1-MECOM* (*MDS1-EVI1* complex locus) fusion transcript, a chimeric oncoprotein that plays a major role in leukemogenesis [63]. Detection of t(3;21) using conventional cytogenetics, FISH, and RT-PCR analysis can be helpful for establishing the diagnosis of AML-MRC. Unlike the other members of 3q abnormality, *FLT3, NPM1, CEBPA, KIT, KRAS*, and *MLL-PTD* have not been reported in t(3;21) [60]. Prognosis of AML with t(3;21) is poor with short median survival and unfavorable response to intensive chemotherapy and stem cell transplantation [64].

2.7 t(6;9)(p22;q34): DEK-NUP214 Rearrangement

The t(6;9)(p22;q34) (Fig. 10) is one of the recurrent genetic abnormalities of AML according to WHO classification [1]. It was first reported by Rowley et al. at chromosome level in 1976. The chimeric fusion gene (*DEK-NUP214*) was identified by von Lindern et al. in 1992. It was formed between *DEK* gene located on 6p22 and *NUP214* gene located on 9q34 [65, 66]. Incidence of t(6;9)

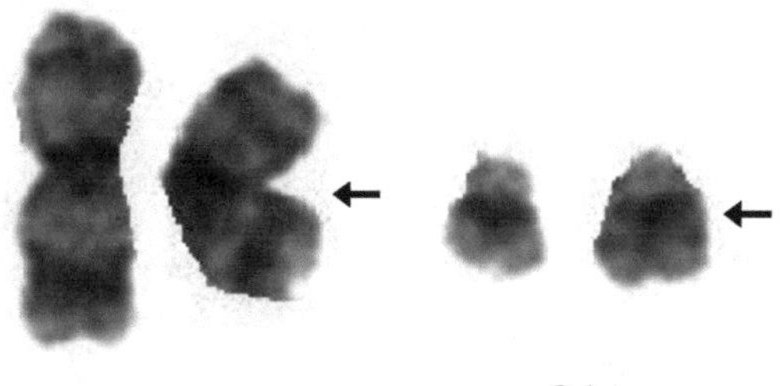

Fig. 9 Partial karyogram showing t(3;21)(q26;q22). *Arrows* indicate the breakpoints

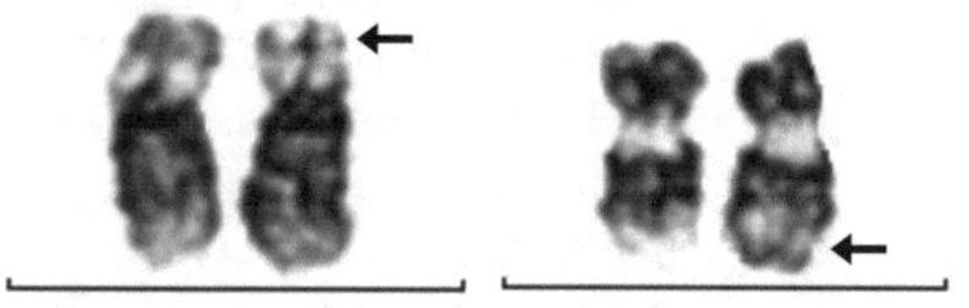

Fig. 10 Partial karyogram showing t(6;9)(p22;q34). *Arrows* indicate the breakpoints

in AML is known to be about 0.7–1.8 %, mostly occurs at early first decade and mid 30s [1]. About two thirds of AML with t(6;9) exist as sole chromosomal abnormality while the common additional chromosomal abnormalities include +8 and +13 [43, 67, 68]. In morphologic perspective, the AML with t(6;9) closely correlates to AML-M2 and M4 (FAB) classification. Basophilia is often observed in adult AML with t(6;9) but not apparent in pediatric patients [67, 68]. Any predilection of sex regarding occurrence is yet unknown, but a recent international collaborative study by Sandahl et al. describes a higher incidence from boys than girls [68]. A higher frequency of *FLT3*-I TD mutation is reported in AML with t(6;9), which presumably correlates with the dismal prognosis of AML with t(6;9) [43, 67]. It is generally categorized into high-risk group and patients receiving allogenic stem cell transplantation tend to show better overall survival compared to those who did not.

2.8 t(7;11)(p15;p15): NUP98-HOXA9 Rearrangement

The t(7;11)(p15;p15) (Fig. 11) was suggested the association with myeloid neoplasms since its first report from a CML patient in 1982 and eight additional cases of Japanese AML [69, 70]. Up to date about 80 cases of AML with t(7;11) are reported and two research groups have identified the *NUP98-HOXA9* chimeric fusion gene generated between *NUP98* located on 11p15 and *HOXA9* gene located on 7p15 [71, 72]. The t(7;11) in AML mostly exists as sole chromosomal abnormality, rarely to be accompanied by +8. According to two large-scale single institution based

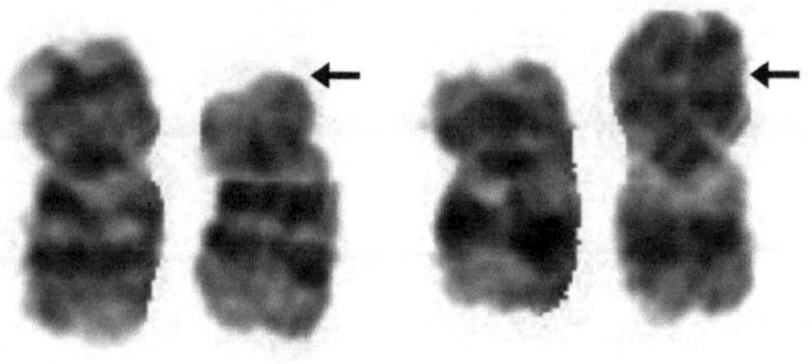

Fig. 11 Partial karyogram showing t(7;11)(p15;p15). *Arrows* indicate the breakpoints

studies from the Asia region, the incidence of AML with t(7;11) is estimated at 0.7–2.2% (17 out of 2506 AML cases and 11 out of 493 AML cases, respectively) [73, 74]. The t(7;11) is reported with ethnic predilection, mostly in Asian population including Japan and China. The age at diagnosis ranges from 7 to 80 years with a median age of late 30s. Two recent studies describe female predominance with significance [73, 74]. AML with t(7;11) correspond to M2 (FAB) classification, observed occasionally with Auer rods and trilineage dysplasia. Class I mutations of *KRAS* and *FLT3* are accompanied with relevance to *WT1* mutation. The prognosis of AML with t(7;11) is poor despite achieving morphological complete remission and associates with high relapse rate ultimately [73]. Lack of targeted chemotherapy for AML with t(7;11) results in poor overall survival and shorter relapse-free survival. Aggressive therapeutic approaches including stem cell transplantation are considered.

2.9 t(9;22)(q34;q11.2): BCR-ABL1 Rearrangement

The t(9;22)(q34;q11.2) is a characteristic aberration of CML and about a quarter of adult ALL. Philadelphia positive (Ph+) AML refers to AML harboring t(9;22) seen in about 1% of AML [75]. It is important that the presence of Ph+ chromosome is further investigated by differentiation between blastic phase of CML and Ph+ AML. There are discriminating points suggesting that Ph+ AML has the presence of minor *BCR-ABL1* breakpoint which are *NPM1* exon 12 mutation, and 19p chromosome gain based on array analysis [76, 77].

In morphologic aspect, the t(9;22) exhibits association with AML-M1, M2 (FAB). It is important for the diagnosis of Ph+ acute leukemia (AML or ALL). The leukemic blasts observed in peripheral blood or bone marrow should be analyzed by immunophenotyping for lineage determination. Complements of conventional cytogenetics, FISH, and RT-PCR are also essential for confirmatory detection of t(9;22) or *BCR-ABL1* rearrangement.

The t(9;22) is found as a sole chromosomal aberration in about 40% of AML patients and the common secondary abnormalities include trisomy 8, monosomy 7, and +der(22)t(9;22). Although dismal prognosis was reported for Ph+ AML regarding poor response to conventional chemotherapy, use of tyrosine kinase inhibitor can be effective, similar to their use in CML and Ph+ ALL patients [78].

2.10 t(16;21)(p11;q22): FUS-ERG Rearrangement

The t(16;21)(p11;q22) (Fig. 12) in AML was first reported in 1985 [79], later to be delineated at molecular level as the *FUS-ERG* fusion gene between the N terminal of *FUS* gene located on 16p11 and the DNA binding domain of *ERG* gene located on 21q22. About 60 cases of t(16;21) were mostly reported in AML, MDS, blastic phases of CML and ALL [43, 80]. More than half occurs as sole abnormality in AML with +8, +10, and +12 as the common additional chromosomal abnormalities [80]. A recent single institution study of 1277 AML found that 12 cases harbored t(16;21), with the incidence rate of about 1% [81]. The age at diagnosis ranges widely from 1 to 80 but the median age is known to be at late 20s. Similar to t(7;11)(p15;p15), AML cases with t(16;21) are frequently reported from Asian population including Korea and Japan, suggesting presence of an ethnic predilection which requires further research. The following are the distinctive morphologic features found in AML with t(16;21) [43, 80]. Firstly, t(16;21) is reported in all FAB classification except for M3 and usually with monocytoid features. Secondly, it is frequently observed with hemophagocytic feature. An association between eosinophilia and vacuolization of leukemic blast is also reported. A positive correlation between percentage of CD56-positive cells and the percentage of hemophagocytosis and vacuolization has been reported as well [81]. The prognosis of AML with t(16;21) is generally poor on accounts of failure to achieve complete remission after induction chemotherapy. It is possible to use RT-PCR of *FUS-ERG* fusion gene for MRD monitoring in which four main fusion transcripts (A, B, C, and D) are known to exist.

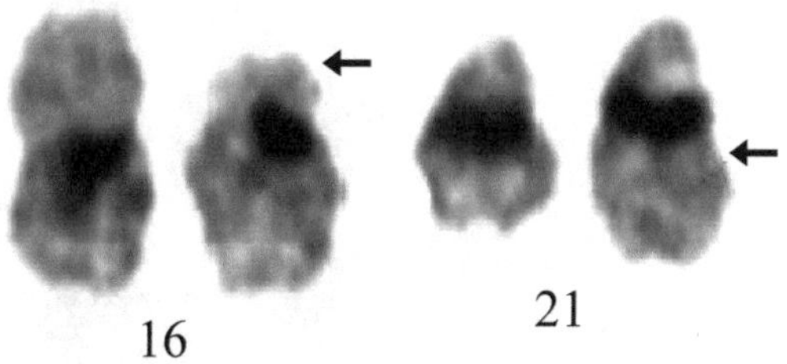

Fig. 12 Partial karyogram showing t(16;21)(p11;q22). *Arrows* indicate the breakpoints

3 Other Structural Abnormalities

3.1 inv(3)(q21q26)/t(3;3)(q21;q26)

The inv(3)(q21q26)/t(3;3)(q21;q26) (Fig. 13) is one of the notable chromosomal aberrations that WHO classification categorizes under AML with recurrent genetic abnormalities, detected in about 1–2% of AML [1]. It is known that inv(3) occurs more frequently than t(3;3) in AML [43]. It can be detected in de novo AML and also secondary AML patients previously diagnosed with MDS [1]. The inv(3) or t(3;3) results in the *RPN1* gene located on 3q21 inducing deregulated expression of the *MECOM* gene on 3q26, which ultimately leads to leukemogenesis [82, 83]. AML with inv(3)/t(3;3) is detected as a sole chromosomal abnormality in about 40% of cases, with the common additional chromosomal aberration of monosomy 7 that is detected in about 40–50% of the patients [1, 43]. It is usually reported in adult AML over 50 years of age and pediatric AML patients with this abnormality are extremely rare [43]. No difference of incidence between sex was reported.

The inv(3)/t(3;3) was reported in all morphologic subtypes of AML except for APL (M3) and is strongly associated with multilineage dysplasia including abnormal bone marrow megakaryocytes with or without thrombocytosis. Aggressive clinical course and short survival was reported in AML patients with inv(3)/t(3;3) [43]. They are generally unresponsive to conventional chemotherapy but allogenic stem cell transplantation appears to be helpful based on latest data.

3.2 del(9q)

The del(9q) (Fig. 14) is a recurrent chromosomal abnormality detected in about 2% of AML [43, 84]. A quarter of del(9q) in AML exists as sole abnormality and about one third are detected with t(8;21). Interestingly, AML with sole del(9q) exhibits male predominance, and occurrence is concentrated between mid 40s and early 50s [42, 43]. It is most frequent in de novo AML and rarely in secondary AML or t-AML.

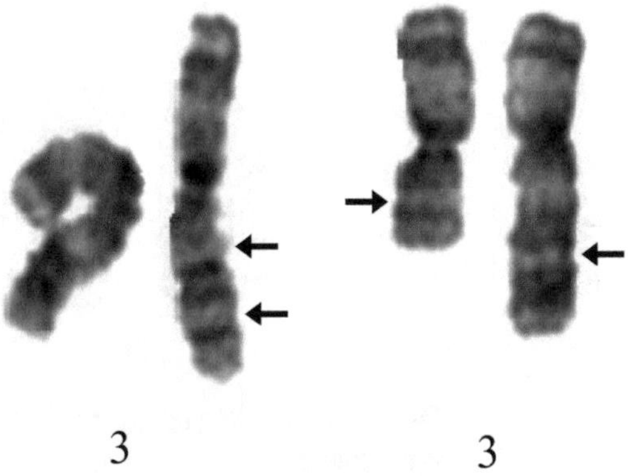

Fig. 13 Partial karyograms showing inv(3)(q21;q26) (*left panel*) and t(3;3)(q21;q26) (*right panel*). *Arrows* indicate the breakpoints

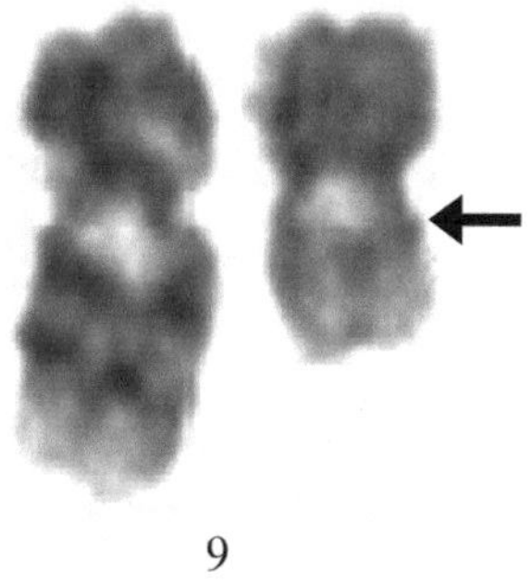

Fig. 14 Partial karyogram showing del(9)(q13q22). *Arrow* indicates the breakpoints

Sole deletion del(9q) has a strong association with characteristic morphologic features that are the presence of single, long, and slender Auer rod, vacuolization of granulocytic lineage and erythroid dysplasia [84]. Breakpoints of interstitial deletion of del(9q) are variable, but the mechanisms behind leukemogenesis involve haploinsufficiency caused by deletion of tumor suppressor genes located between critical region of 9q21-q22 [43, 84]. Prognosis of del(9q) is classified as intermediate as a sole abnormality but is favorable when accompanied with t(8;21) [43]. The *CEBPA* mutation is another indicator of favorable prognosis which is frequently found in patients with del(9q) [85].

3.3 del(17p)/ i(17) (q10)

The del(17p) (Fig. 15) is a chromosomal aberration mostly detected in myeloid neoplasms such as AML, MDS, and CML [86]. In 2–4% of AML, del(17p) is concurrently detected along with various numerical and structural abnormalities but rarely as a sole chromosomal aberration [43, 86]. Loss of the *TP53* gene and the mutation of the remaining *TP53* allele is common in AML with del(17p), which is the feature of t-AML.

The i(17)(q10) (Fig. 15) is a common cancer-related chromosomal abnormality detected in hematologic malignancies and solid tumors [43]. Based on the Mitelman database, about 160 cases of AML with i(17)(q10) are reported, 30% existing as sole chromosomal abnormality [42]. Numerical abnormalities such as monosomy (−5, −7) or trisomy (+8, +13) are the common secondary chromosomal aberrations. Contrary to del(17p), isolated i(17)(q10) is associated with de novo AML and diagnosis of AML-MRC [1]. AML with del(17p) or i(17)(q10) exhibits male predominance and occurs mostly in elderly patients. AML with i(17)(q10) exhibits haploinsufficiency of the *TP53* gene due to deletion of 17p region, but unlike del(17p), *TP53* mutation is infrequent [43]. However, prognosis of AML with i(17)(q10) is similarly poor as del(17p).

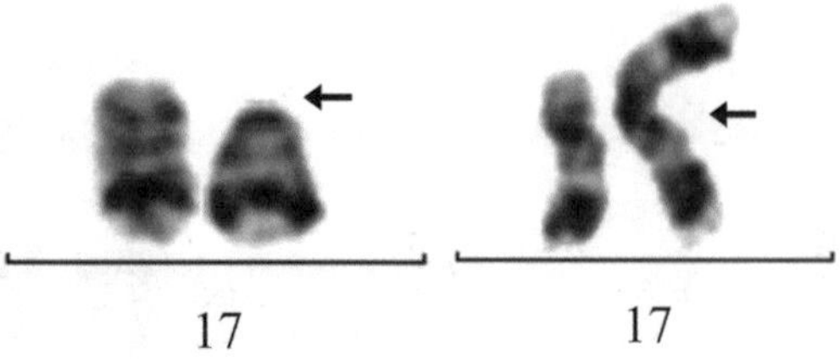

Fig. 15 Partial karyograms showing del(17)(p12) (*left panel*) and i(17)(q10) (*right panel*). *Arrows* indicate the breakpoints

4 Numerical Chromosomal Abnormalities

4.1 Trisomy 8

Trisomy 8 is the most common numerical chromosomal abnormality found in AML [42]. It occurs as a sole abnormality in about 5–6% of AML and more frequently with additional concurrent chromosomal abnormalities [87]. The presence of trisomy 8 is more frequent in the elderly, de novo AML and differs among morphologic subtypes [88]. Morphologic subtypes of AML-M4 and M5 (FAB) are strongly associated with trisomy 8 as a sole abnormality and in other subtypes of AML not otherwise specified (NOS). AML-M1 and M2 usually associate with additional abnormalities [89]. Trisomy 8 has not been associated with a specific immunophenotype [90]. Etiology of trisomy 8 in AML is unclear though regarded as an acquired abnormality. Association with prior exposure to chemotherapeutic agents, ionizing radiation, and topoisomerase inhibitors has not been reported. Conventional cytogenetic analysis is sufficient for the evaluation of trisomy 8 and utilizing FISH for detecting the presence of any cryptic chromosomal abnormalities accompanied with trisomy 8 is unsupported [91].

Despite the ubiquity of trisomy 8, prognostic impact of its presence or detailed mechanism in leukemogenesis remains uncertain [91] due to limited data of trisomy 8 as a sole abnormality. A recent array-based comparative genomic hybridization (array CGH) study on AML with sole trisomy 8 revealed that cryptic abnormalities are frequent among sole trisomy 8, supporting that this alone is insufficient for leukemogenesis [92].

Prognostic impact of trisomy 8 is controversial, different studies report intermediate to poor prognoses. AML with sole trisomy 8 is categorized as intermediate cytogenetic group although this may differ according to the diseases including MDS and MPN [93].

4.2 Trisomy 11

Trisomy 11 is a nonrandom chromosomal aberration found in about 2–3% of AML and 1% as isolated trisomy 11 [43, 94]. There are no difference between sex regarding incidence of AML with trisomy 11 and it occurs mostly among elderly AML patients at a median age of 60 [43, 95]. Trisomy 11 is usually detected in de novo AML but prior history of MDS is also possible, though its association with previous chemotherapy is minimal [43]. Its association with morphologic subtypes of AML-M1, M2, and M4 (FAB) is reported with a common feature of trilineage dysplasia [95]. Partial tandem duplication of the *MLL* gene (*MLL*-PTD) located on 11q23 is frequently detected in AML with trisomy 11. Response to chemotherapy in patients of AML with trisomy 11 is unfavorable and leads to dismal prognosis [43, 94, 95].

4.3 Trisomy 13

Trisomy 13 is detected in about 1–3% of AML patients [43, 96]. Sole trisomy 13 is detected in about a quarter and secondary chromosomal abnormality with t(6;9) is also frequently found [43]. AML with trisomy 13 is mostly found in elderly patients over 70 years of age with a male predominance [43, 96]. Morphologic features in AML with trisomy 13 are heterogeneous but usually associate with AML-M0 and M1 (FAB). Trisomy 13 cases are known to exhibit characteristic hand-mirror blasts with cytoplasmic blebs and tails, few or no granules in small blasts and trilineage dysplasia [97]. An association with *RUNX1* mutation and high expression of *FLT3* was also reported [43]. Clinical course is generally poor due to short period of remission and the low rate of complete remission [43, 96].

4.4 Trisomy 21

Trisomy 21 is the second most common trisomy and the third common karyotypic abnormality in AML, MDS, and MPN. About 3–6% of cytogenetically abnormal AML have trisomy 21 [42, 98]. However, it is rarely observed as a sole chromosomal abnormality and is commonly found with other trisomy or as a secondary change to inv(16) or t(16;16) [2]. No specific morphologic subtype has been associated with trisomy 21. Immunophenotype is usually positive for CD13, CD14, CD15, CD33, and MPO while aberrant CD7 expression appears to be a characteristic of AML with sole trisomy 21 [99]. Trisomy 21 is more often observed in men and in younger age with a median of 40 years [100].

Leukemogenic role of trisomy 21 is postulated from the findings that trisomy 21 is a common cytogenetic aberration in AML and ALL and the risk is 10-fold higher in Down syndrome. Trisomy 21 is often detected with gene mutations of *NPM1*, *RUNX1*, and *TET2*. However, the current understanding of myeloid malignancies with trisomy 21 is heterogenous and variable. Trisomy 21 as additional aberration does not modify the prognosis, AML with trisomy 21 was reported to have poor prognosis according to their short median survival period [101].

4.5 Trisomy 22

Trisomy 22 is a rare but recurrent chromosomal abnormality detected in about 2–3% of AML [43]. Sole trisomy 22 has shown male predominance in adult AML [42] and most frequently detected among young adults at their 30s, while reports of trisomy 22 in pediatric AML are very uncommon [42, 43]. Interestingly, trisomy 22 is the most frequently associated secondary chromosomal abnormality in AML with inv(16) detected in about 20% of cases [43, 102]. In this regard, considerable proportion of trisomy 22 was reported to be morphologically associated with AML-M4Eo. Cooperative mutations associated with trisomy 22 have not been reported yet. Xu et al. reported in a series of 19 AML patients with sole trisomy 22 harboring cryptic inv(16) and over half patients had cryptic rearrangements confirmed by FISH analysis [103]. It is recommendable for AML patients with trisomy 22 to be further evaluated with molecular methods of FISH or RT-PCR for the presence of cryptic inv(16) or *CBFB-MYH11* rearrangement. Prognosis of AML with trisomy 22 lacks any large-scale study but is categorized as an intermediate-risk group in general.

5 Normal Karyotype Acute Myeloid Leukemia (NK-AML)

Normal karyotype-acute myeloid leukemia (NK-AML) refers to the absence of any identifiable cytogenetic aberration that is found in about 40–50% of de novo AML and up to 10% of t-AML by conventional cytogenetic analysis [3, 42]. Cryptic aberrations may unintentionally fall into these categories such as inv(3), inv(16), t(5;11)(p35;p15.1), and t(11;19), but should not be considered cytogenetically "normal". NK-AML exhibits marked genetic heterogeneity by molecular genetic analysis, showing recurrent genetic aberrations of *FLT3, CEBPA, NPM1, RUNX1, TET2, IDH1/IDH2, DNMT3A, ASXL1, MLL,* and *WT1* mutations. *FLT3* mutation is associated with poor prognosis whereas presence of *NPM1* and *CEBPA* mutations associates with favorable prognosis under WHO classification [1]. Mutations of epigenetic modifier genes—*IDH1/IDH2, DNMT3A,* and *TET2*—are also known to be closely associated with NK-AML. *WT1, RUNX1,* and *BCOR* mutations are detected at variable frequency. Notably, the *CEBPA* mutation is reported in familial AML [104].

Although normal karyotype may not be associated with a specific morphologic subtype, prognosis of NK-AML can differ between morphologic subtypes (FAB) of M1/M2 and M4/M5 [105]. In addition to *FLT3-IT D, NPM1,* and *CEBPA* mutations, advancements in molecular genetics such as the next generation sequencing (NGS) are discovering more gene mutations of prognostic impact. A multigene approach is proposed for the prognostic determination of AML recently despite the fact that the prognostic impact of *IDH1/IDH2, DNMT3A,* and *TET 2* genes is still controversial [106].

Acknowledgments

This work was supported by the Basic Science Research Program through the National Research Foundation of Korea (NRF) funded by the Ministry of Science, ICT and Future Planning (2014R1A1A1002797). Dr. Claus Meyer kindly reviewed for 11q23 abnormality of chapter and Dr. Wall Meaghan provided the t(3;12)(q26;p13) partial karyotype shown in Fig. 8. We thank Jin-A Choi for her excellent technical support in the cytogenetics laboratory of Kyung Hee University Medical Center.

References

1. Arber DA, Vardiman JW, Brunning RD et al (2008) Acute myeloid leukemia and related precursor neoplasms. In: Swerdllow S, Campo E, Harris NL (eds) WHO classification of tumours of haematopoietic and lymphoid tissues, 4th edn. IARC Press, France
2. Harrison CJ, Hills RK, Moorman AV et al (2010) Cytogenetics of childhood acute myeloid leukemia: United Kingdom Medical Research Council Treatment trials AML 10 and 12. J Clin Oncol 28(16):2674–2681
3. Grimwade D, Hills RK, Moorman A et al (2010) Refinement of cytogenetic classification in acute myeloid leukaemia: Determination of prognostic significance of rarer recurring chromosomal abnormalities amongst 5,876 younger adult patients treated in the UK Medical Research Council trials. In 50th Annual Scientific Meeting of the British Society for Haematology, Edinburgh, UK. Br J Haematol S1:17. doi:10.1111/j.1365-2141.2010.08116.x
4. Berger R, Bernheim A, Daniel MT et al (1982) Cytologic characterization and significance of normal karyotypes in t(8; 21) acute myeloblastic leukemia. Blood 59(1):171–178
5. Farra C, Awwad J, Valent A et al (2004) Complex translocation (8;12;21): a new variant of t(8;21) in acute myeloid leukemia. Cancer Genet Cytogenet 155(2):138–142
6. Miyoshi H, Kozu T, Shimizu K et al (1993) The t(8;21) translocation in acute myeloid leukemia results in production of an AML1-MTG8 fusion transcript. EMBO J 12(7):2715
7. Ohki M (1993) Molecular basis of the t(8;21) translocation in acute myeloid leukaemia. Semin Cancer Biol 6:369–375
8. Hatlen MA, Wang L, Nimer SD (2012) AML1-ETO driven acute leukemia: insights into pathogenesis and potential therapeutic approaches. Front Med 6(3):248–262
9. Radtke I, Mullighan CG, Ishii M et al (2009) Genomic analysis reveals few genetic alterations in pediatric acute myeloid leukemia. Proc Natl Acad Sci U S A 106(31): 12944–12949
10. Micol JB, Duployez N, Boissel N et al (2014) Frequent ASXL2 mutations in acute myeloid leukemia patients with t(8;21)/RUNX1-RUNX1T1 chromosomal translocations. Blood 124(9):1445–1449
11. Park TS, Song J, Lee KA et al (2008) Paracentric inversion–associated t(8;21) variant in de novo acute myelogenous leukemia: characteristic patterns of conventional cytogenetics, FISH, and multicolor banding analysis. Cancer Genet Cytogenet 183(1):72–76
12. Zhang L, Li Q, Li W et al (2013) Monitoring of minimal residual disease in acute myeloid leukemia with t(8;21)(q22;q22). Int J Hematol 97(6):786–792
13. Kim HJ, Ahn HK, Jung CW et al (2013) KIT D816 mutation associates with adverse outcomes in core binding factor acute myeloid leukemia, especially in the subgroup with RUNX1/RUNX1T1 rearrangement. Ann Hematol 92(2):163–171
14. Gustafson SA, Lin P, Chen SS et al (2009) Therapy-related acute myeloid leukemia with t (8; 21)(q22; q22) shares many features with de novo acute myeloid leukemia with t (8; 21)(q22; q22) but does not have a favorable outcome. Am J Clin Pathol 131(5):647–655
15. Marcucci G, Mrózek K, Ruppert AS et al (2005) Prognostic factors and outcome of core binding factor acute myeloid leukemia patients with t (8; 21) differ from those of patients with inv (16): a Cancer and Leukemia Group B study. J Clin Oncol 23(24): 5705–5717

16. Warrell RP Jr, de The H, Wang ZY et al (1993) Acute promyelocytic leukemia. N Engl J Med 329(3):177–189
17. Huret J, Chomienne C (1998) t(15;17)(q22;q21). Atlas Genet Cytogenet Oncol Haematol 2(3):101–103. doi:10.4267/2042/37443
18. Kim MJ, Yang JJ, Meyer C et al (2012) Molecular methods for genomic analyses of variant PML-RARA or other RARA-related chromosomal translocations in acute promyelocytic leukemia. Korean J Hematol 47(4):307–308
19. Wan TS, So CC, Hui KC et al (2007) Diagnostic utility of dual fusion PML/RARα translocation DNA probe (D-FISH) in acute promyelocytic leukemia. Oncol Rep 17(4):799–805
20. Wang ZY, Chen Z (2008) Acute promyelocytic leukemia: from highly fatal to highly curable. Blood 111(5):2505–2515
21. Kim MJ, Cho SY, Kim MH et al (2010) FISH-negative cryptic PML–RARA rearrangement detected by long-distance polymerase chain reaction and sequencing analyses: a case study and review of the literature. Cancer Genet Cytogenet 203(2):278–283
22. Hillestad LK (1957) Acute promyelocytic leukemia. Acta Med Scand 159(3):189–194
23. Arthur DC, Bloomfield CD (1983) Partial deletion of the long arm of chromosome 16 and bone marrow eosinophilia in acute nonlymphocytic leukemia: a new association. Blood 61(5):994–998
24. Le Beau MM, Larson RA, Bitter MA et al (1983) Association of an inversion of chromosome 16 with abnormal marrow eosinophils in acute myelomonocytic leukemia: a unique cytogenetic–clinicopathological association. N Engl J Med 309(11):630–636
25. Schlenk RF, Benner A, Krauter J et al (2004) Individual patient data–based meta-analysis of patients aged 16 to 60 years with core binding factor acute myeloid leukemia: a survey of the German Acute Myeloid Leukemia Intergroup. J Clin Oncol 22(18):3741–3750
26. Claxton D, Liu P, Hsu H et al (1994) Detection of fusion transcripts generated by the inversion 16 chromosome in acute myelogenous leukemia. Blood 83(7):1750–1756
27. Park TS, Lee ST, Song J et al (2009) Detection of a novel CBFB/MYH11 variant fusion transcript (K-type) showing partial insertion of exon 6 of CBFB gene using two commercially available multiplex RT-PCR kits. Cancer Genet Cytogenet 189(2):87–92
28. Schwind S, Edwards CG, Nicolet D et al (2013) inv(16)/t(16;16) acute myeloid leukemia with non–type A CBFB-MYH11 fusions associate with distinct clinical and genetic features and lack KIT mutations. Blood 121(2):385–391
29. Merchant SH, Haines S, Hall B et al (2004) Fluorescence in situ hybridization identifies cryptic t(16;16)(p13;q22) masked by del(16)(q22) in a case of AML-M4 Eo. J Mol Diagn 6(3):271–274
30. Marcucci G, Caligiuri MA, Bloomfield CD (2003) Core binding factor (CBF) acute myeloid leukemia: is molecular monitoring by RT–PCR useful clinically? Eur J Haematol 71(3):143–154
31. Schoch C, Schnittger S, Klaus M et al (2003) AML with 11q23/MLL abnormalities as defined by the WHO classification: incidence, partner chromosomes, FAB subtype, age distribution, and prognostic impact in an unselected series of 1897 cytogenetically analyzed AML cases. Blood 102(7):2395–2402
32. Andersen MK, Johansson B, Larsen SO et al (1998) Chromosomal abnormalities in secondary MDS and AML. Relationship to drugs and radiation with specific emphasis on the balanced rearrangements. Haematologica 83(6):483–488
33. Cimino G, Rapanotti MC, Elia L et al (1995) ALL-1 gene rearrangements in acute myeloid leukemia: association with M4–M5 French-American-British classification subtypes and young age. Cancer Res 55(8):1625–1628
34. Balgobind BV, Raimondi SC, Harbott J et al (2009) Novel prognostic subgroups in childhood 11q23/MLL-rearranged acute myeloid leukemia: results of an international retrospective study. Blood 114(12):2489–2496
35. Meyer C, Hofmann J, Burmeister T et al (2013) The MLL recombinome of acute leukemias in 2013. Leukemia 27(11):2165–2176
36. Marschalek R (2011) Mechanisms of leukemogenesis by MLL fusion proteins. Br J Haematol 152(2):141–154
37. Meyer C, Schneider B, Reichel M et al (2005) Diagnostic tool for the identification of MLL rearrangements including unknown partner genes. Proc Natl Acad Sci U S A 102(2):449–454
38. Dyson MJ, Talley PJ, Reilly JT et al (2003) Detection of cryptic MLL insertions using a commercial dual-color fluorescence in situ hybridization probe. Cancer Genet Cytogenet 147(1):81–83
39. Balgobind B, Zwaan C, Pieters R et al (2011) The heterogeneity of pediatric MLL-rearranged acute myeloid leukemia. Leukemia 25(8):1239–1248

40. Stone RM, DeAngelo DJ, Klimek V et al (2005) Patients with acute myeloid leukemia and an activating mutation in FLT3 respond to a small-molecule FLT3 tyrosine kinase inhibitor, PKC412. Blood 105(1):54–60
41. Wong P, Iwasaki M, Somervaille TC et al (2007) Meis1 is an essential and rate-limiting regulator of MLL leukemia stem cell potential. Genes Dev 21(21):2762–2774
42. Mitelman F, Johansson B, Mertens F (2016) Mitelman database of chromosome aberrations and gene fusions in cancer. http://cgap.nci.nih.gov/Chromosomes/Mitelman. Accessed 1 Jan 2016
43. Johansson B, Harrison CJ (2015) Acute myeloid leukemia. In: Heim S, Mitelman F (eds) Cancer cytogenetics: chromosomal and molecular genetic aberrations of tumor cells, 4th edn. John Wiley & Sons, Hoboken, NJ
44. Moir D, Jones P, Pearson J et al (1984) A new translocation, t(1;3)(p36;q21), in myelodysplastic disorders. Blood 64(2):553–555
45. Bloomfield CD, Garson O, Volin L et al (1985) t(1;3)(p36;q21) in acute nonlymphocytic leukemia: a new cytogenetic-clinicopathologic association. Blood 66(6):1409–1413
46. Lim G, Kim MJ, Oh SH et al (2010) Acute myeloid leukemia associated with t(1;3)(p36;q21) and extreme thrombocytosis: a clinical study with literature review. Cancer Genet Cytogenet 203(2):187–192
47. Welborn JL, Lewis JP, Jenks H et al (1987) Diagnostic and prognostic significance of t (1; 3)(p36; q21) in the disorders of hematopoiesis. Cancer Genet Cytogenet 28(2):277–285
48. Bruyère H (2015) der(1;7)(q10;p10). In: Chronic Myeloproliferative Diseases (MPD). Atlas of genetics and cytogenetics in oncology and haematology. INIST. http://AtlasGeneticsOncology.org/Anomalies/t0107ID1003.html. Accessed 1 Jan 2016
49. Westman M, Pedersen-Bjergaard J, Andersen M et al (2013) IDH1 and IDH2 mutations in therapy-related myelodysplastic syndrome and acute myeloid leukemia are associated with a normal karyotype and with der(1;7)(q10;p10). Leukemia 27(4):957–959
50. Arthur DC (1984) Abnormalities of chromosome 22. Cancer Genet Cytogenet 11(3):316–318. doi:10.1016/S0165-4608(84)80018-7
51. Ma Z, Morris SW, Valentine V et al (2001) Fusion of two novel genes, RBM15 and MKL1, in the t(1;22)(p13;q13) of acute megakaryoblastic leukemia. Nat Genet 28(3):220–221
52. Mercher T, Busson-Le Coniat M, Monni R et al (2001) Involvement of a human gene related to the Drosophila spen gene in the recurrent t (1; 22) translocation of acute megakaryocytic leukemia. Proc Natl Acad Sci U S A 98(10):5776–5779
53. Yoneda-Kato N, Look AT, Kirstein MN et al (1996) The t(3;5)(q25. 1;q34) of myelodysplastic syndrome and acute myeloid leukemia produces a novel fusion gene, NPM-MLF1. Oncogene 12(2):265–275
54. Lim G, Choi JR, Kim MJ et al (2010) Detection of t (3; 5) and NPM1/MLF1 rearrangement in an elderly patient with acute myeloid leukemia: clinical and laboratory study with review of the literature. Cancer Genet Cytogenet 199(2):101–109
55. Aypar U, Knudson RA, Pearce KE et al (2014) Development of an NPM1/MLF1 D-FISH probe set for the detection of t(3;5)(q25;q35) identified in patients with acute myeloid leukemia. J Mol Diagn 16(5):527–532
56. Massaad L, Prieur M, Leonard C et al (1990) Biclonal chromosome evolution of chronic myelomonocytic leukemia in a child. Cancer Genet Cytogenet 44(1):131–137
57. Peeters P, Wlodarska I, Baens M et al (1997) Fusion of ETV6 to MDS1/EVI1 as a result of t (3; 12)(q26; p13) in myeloproliferative disorders. Cancer Res 57(4):564–569
58. Wang XI, Lu X, Zhao L et al. (2014) Myeloid neoplasms associated with t(3;12)(q26.2;p13) are clinically aggressive and frequently harbor FLT3 mutations: a report of 8 cases and review of literature. J Leuk (Los Angels) 2:161. doi:10.4172/2329-6917.1000161
59. Rubin CM, Larson RA, Anastasi J et al (1990) t(3;21)(q26;q22): a recurring chromosomal abnormality in therapy-related myelodysplastic syndrome and acute myeloid leukemia. Blood 76(12):2594–2598
60. Lugthart S, Gröschel S, Beverloo HB et al (2010) Clinical, molecular, and prognostic significance of WHO type inv(3)(q21q26.2)/t(3;3)(q21;q26.2) and various other 3q abnormalities in acute myeloid leukemia. J Clin Oncol 28(24):3890–3898
61. Li S, Yin CC, Medeiros LJ et al (2012) Myelodysplastic syndrome/acute myeloid leukemia with t(3;21)(q26.2;q22) is commonly a therapy-related disease associated with poor outcome. Am J Clin Pathol 138(1):146–152
62. Yin C, Cortes J, Barkoh B et al (2006) t(3;21)(q26;q22) in myeloid leukemia: an aggressive syndrome of blast transformation associated with hydroxyurea or antimetabolite therapy. Cancer 106(8):1730–1738
63. Maki K, Yamagata T, Mitani K (2008) Role of the RUNX1-EVI1 fusion gene in leukemogenesis. Cancer Sci 99(10):1878–1883

64. Park TS, Choi JR, Yoon SH et al (2008) Acute promyelocytic leukemia relapsing as secondary acute myelogenous leukemia with translocation t(3;21)(q26;q22) and RUNX1–MDS1–EVI1 fusion transcript. Cancer Genet Cytogenet 187(2):61–73
65. Rowley JD, Potter D (1976) Chromosomal banding patterns in acute nonlymphocytic leukemia. Blood 47(5):705–721
66. Von Lindern M, Fornerod M, Van Baal S et al (1992) The translocation (6;9), associated with a specific subtype of acute myeloid leukemia, results in the fusion of two genes, dek and can, and the expression of a chimeric, leukemia-specific dek-can mRNA. Mol Cell Biol 12(4):1687–1697
67. Oyarzo MP, Lin P, Glassman A et al (2004) Acute myeloid leukemia with t(6;9)(p23;q34) is associated with dysplasia and a high frequency of flt3 gene mutations. Am J Clin Pathol 122:348–358
68. Sandahl JD, Coenen EA, Forestier E et al (2014) t(6;9)(p22;q34)/DEK-NUP214 rearranged pediatric myeloid leukemia: an international study on 62 patients. haematologica. haematol. 2013.098517
69. Tomiyasu T, Sasaki M, Kondo K et al (1982) Chromosome banding studies in 106 cases of chronic myelogenous leukemia. Jpn J Hum Genet 27(3):243–258
70. Sato Y, Abe S, Mise K et al (1987) Reciprocal translocation involving the short arms of chromosomes 7 and 11, t(7p-;11p+), associated with myeloid leukemia with maturation. Blood 70(5):1654–1658
71. Borrow J, Shearman AM, Stanton VP et al (1996) The t(7;11)(p15;p15) translocation in acute myeloid leukaemia fuses the genes for nucleoporin NUP98 and class I homeoprotein HOXA9. Nat Genet 12(2):159–167
72. Nakamura T, Largaespada DA, Lee MP et al (1996) Fusion of the nucleoporin gene NUP98 to HOXA9 by the chromosome translocation t(7;11)(p15;p15) in human myeloid leukaemia. Nat Genet 12(2):154–158
73. Chou W, Chen C, Hou H et al (2009) Acute myeloid leukemia bearing t(7;11)(p15;p15) is a distinct cytogenetic entity with poor outcome and a distinct mutation profile: comparative analysis of 493 adult patients. Leukemia 23(7):1303–1310
74. Wei S, Wang S, Qiu S et al (2013) Clinical and laboratory studies of 17 patients with acute myeloid leukemia harboring t (7; 11)(p15; p15) translocation. Leuk Res 37(9):1010–1015
75. Soupir CP, Vergilio JA, Dal Cin P et al (2007) Philadelphia chromosome–positive acute myeloid leukemia. Am J Clin Pathol 127(4):642–650. doi:10.1309/B4NVER1AJJ84CTUU
76. Konoplev S, Yin CC, Kornblau SM et al (2013) Molecular characterization of de novo Philadelphia chromosome-positive acute myeloid leukemia. Leuk Lymphoma 54(1): 138–144
77. Nacheva EP, Grace CD, Brazma D et al (2013) Does BCR/ABL1 positive acute myeloid leukaemia exist? Br J Haematol 161(4):541–550
78. Shimizu H, Yokohama A, Hatsumi N et al (2014) Philadelphia chromosome-positive mixed phenotype acute leukemia in the imatinib era. Eur J Haematol 93(4):297–301
79. Mecucci C, Bosly A, Michaux JL et al (1985) Acute nonlymphoblastic leukemia with bone marrow eosinophilia and structural anomaly of chromosome 16. Cancer Genet Cytogenet 17(4):359–363
80. Kim J, Park TS, Song J et al (2009) Detection of FUS–ERG chimeric transcript in two cases of acute myeloid leukemia with t (16; 21) (p11. 2; q22) with unusual characteristics. Cancer Genet Cytogenet 194(2):111–118
81. Jekarl DW, Kim M, Lim J et al (2010) CD56 antigen expression and hemophagocytosis of leukemic cells in acute myeloid leukemia with t(16;21)(p11;q22). Int J Hematol 92(2):306–313
82. Fichelson S, Dreyfus F, Berger R et al (1992) Evi-1 expression in leukemic patients with rearrangements of the 3q25-q28 chromosomal region. Leukemia 6(2):93–99
83. Suzukawa K, Parganas E, Gajjar A et al (1994) Identification of a breakpoint cluster region 3′of the ribophorin I gene at 3q21 associated with the transcriptional activation of the EVI1 gene in acute myelogenous leukemias with inv(3)(q21q26). Blood 84(8):2681–2688
84. Peniket A, Wainscoat J, Side L et al (2005) Del (9q) AML: clinical and cytological characteristics and prognostic implications. Br J Haematol 129(2):210–220
85. Fröhling S, Schlenk RF, Krauter J et al (2005) Acute myeloid leukemia with deletion 9q within a noncomplex karyotype is associated with CEBPA loss-of-function mutations. Genes Chromosomes Cancer 42(4):427–432
86. Soenen-Cornu V, Preudhomme C, Laï JL et al (1999) del(17p) in myeloid malignancies. Atlas Genet Cytogenet Oncol Haematol 3(4):198–201. doi:10.4267/2042/37563
87. Heim S, Mitelman F (1992) Cytogenetic analysis in the diagnosis of acute leukemia. Cancer 70(S4):1701–1709

88. Paulsson K, Säll T, Fioretos T et al (2001) The incidence of trisomy 8 as a sole chromosomal aberration in myeloid malignancies varies in relation to gender, age, prior iatrogenic genotoxic exposure, and morphology. Cancer Genet Cytogenet 130(2):160–165
89. Johansson B, Mertens F, Mitelman F (1994) Secondary chromosomal abnormalities in acute leukemias. Leukemia 8(6):953–962
90. Hrusak O, Porwit-MacDonald A (2002) Antigen expression patterns reflecting genotype of acute leukemias. Leukemia 16(7): 1233–1258
91. Paulsson K, Johansson B (2007) Trisomy 8 as the sole chromosomal aberration in acute myeloid leukemia and myelodysplastic syndromes. Pathol Biol (Paris) 55(1):37–48
92. Paulsson K, Heidenblad M, Strömbeck B et al (2006) High-resolution genome-wide array-based comparative genome hybridization reveals cryptic chromosome changes in AML and MDS cases with trisomy 8 as the sole cytogenetic aberration. Leukemia 20(5): 840–846
93. Grimwade D, Walker H, Oliver F et al (1998) The importance of diagnostic cytogenetics on outcome in AML: analysis of 1,612 patients entered into the MRC AML 10 trial. Blood 92(7):2322–2333
94. Alseraye FM, Zuo Z, Bueso-Ramos C et al (2011) Trisomy 11 as an isolated abnormality in acute myeloid leukemia is associated with unfavorable prognosis but not with an NPM1 or KIT mutation. Int J Clin Exp Pathol 4(suppl 4):371–377
95. Desangles F (1997) +11 or trisomy 11 (solely). Atlas Genet Cytogenet Oncol Haematol 1(1):12. doi:10.4267/2042/32025
96. Lee R, Dal CP (2012) +13 or trisomy 13. Atlas Genet Cytogenet Oncol Haematol 16(8):572–573. doi:10.4267/2042/47494
97. Mehta A, Bain B, Fitchett M et al (1998) Trisomy 13 and myeloid malignancy-characteristic blast cell morphology: a United Kingdom Cancer Cytogenetics Group survey. Br J Haematol 101(4):749–752
98. Cortes J, Kantarjian H, O'Brien S et al (1995) Clinical and prognostic significance of trisomy 21 in adult patients with acute myelogenous leukemia and myelodysplastic syndromes. Leukemia 9(1):115–117
99. Yamamoto K, Nagata K, Hamaguchi H (2002) A new case of CD7-positive acute myeloblastic leukemia with trisomy 21 as a sole acquired abnormality. Cancer Genet Cytogenet 133(2):183–184
100. Larsson N, Lilljebjörn H, Lassen C et al (2012) Myeloid malignancies with acquired trisomy 21 as the sole cytogenetic change are clinically highly variable and display a heterogeneous pattern of copy number alterations and mutations. Eur J Haematol 88(2):136–143
101. Wan TS, Au WY, Chan JC et al (1999) Trisomy 21 as the sole acquired karyotypic abnormality in acute myeloid leukemia and myelodysplastic syndrome. Leuk Res 23(11): 1079–1083
102. Paschka P, Du J, Schlenk RF et al (2013) Secondary genetic lesions in acute myeloid leukemia with inv(16) or t(16;16): a study of the German-Austrian AML Study Group (AMLSG). Blood 121(1):170–177
103. Xu W, Zhou HF, Fan L et al (2008) Trisomy 22 as the sole abnormality is an important marker for the diagnosis of acute myeloid leukemia with inversion 16. Onkologie 31(8-9):440–444
104. Smith ML, Cavenagh JD, Lister TA et al (2004) Mutation of CEBPA in familial acute myeloid leukemia. N Engl J Med 351(23):2403–2407
105. Bullinger L, Döhner K, Bair E et al (2004) Use of gene-expression profiling to identify prognostic subclasses in adult acute myeloid leukemia. N Engl J Med 350(16):1605–1616
106. Patel JP, Gönen M, Figueroa ME et al (2012) Prognostic relevance of integrated genetic profiling in acute myeloid leukemia. N Engl J Med 366(12):1079–1089

Chapter 20

Recurrent Cytogenetic Abnormalities in Myeloproliferative Neoplasms and Chronic Myeloid Leukemia

John Swansbury

Abstract

The commonest types of myeloproliferative neoplasm (MPN) have remarkably similar recurrent chromosome abnormalities, but with varying incidence and prognostic implications. After a clear decade of treatment of chronic myeloid leukemia (CML) with tyrosine kinase inhibitors, the differing prognostic implications of abnormalities additional to the Ph chromosome are being revealed. This chapter provides a description of the main chromosome abnormalities in MPN and CML and their clinical implications in a time of rapid changes in both the application of new diagnostic techniques and the introduction of targeted therapies.

Key words Chromosome, Cytogenetics, Myeloproliferative, Chronic myeloid leukemia

1 Introduction

This chapter describes the chromosome abnormalities associated with disorders that are characterized by an excess of one or more myeloid cell types, usually have a chronic course, have a clonal origin, and are malignant or pre-malignant. The major types are:

1. Polycythemia vera (PV) with an excess of red blood cells; also called polycythemia rubra vera (PRV);
2. Essential thrombocythemia (ET) with an excess of platelets; also call thrombocytosis;
3. Primary myelofibrosis (PMF) with an excess of fibrous tissue replacing the bone marrow; also called idiopathic myelofibrosis or agnogenic myeloid metaplasia;
4. Chronic myelogenous leukemia (CML). Strictly speaking, this should be called chronic granulocytic leukemia (CGL) as the term refers to an excess of granulocytes, as distinct from CNL, CBL, and CEL (*see* Subheadings 2.4–2.6);

Thomas S.K. Wan (ed.), *Cancer Cytogenetics: Methods and Protocols*, Methods in Molecular Biology, vol. 1541,
DOI 10.1007/978-1-4939-6703-2_20, © Springer Science+Business Media LLC 2017

5. Chronic neutrophilic leukemia (CNL) with an excess of neutrophils;
6. Chronic basophilic leukemia (CBL) with an excess of basophils;
7. Hypereosinophilic syndrome (HES) and chronic eosinophilic leukemia (CEL), with an excess of eosinophils;
8. Chronic myelomonocytic leukemia (CMML) with an excess of monocytes; and
9. Systemic mastocytosis (SM) with an excess of mast cells.

Of these disorders, CML is distinctive in that practically all cases have a *BCR-ABL1* gene fusion that is present in almost all cells at diagnosis, and usually produces the Philadelphia chromosome (*see* Subheading 3). In all the other disorders, chromosomally abnormal clones are seen much more rarely; are usually present in a much lower proportion of the dividing cell population; and the abnormalities are much less disease-specific.

CMML is deemed to be one of the myelodysplastic syndromes (MDS) and therefore will not be described further in this chapter.

Excluding CML, the other disorders are collectively known as the myeloproliferative neoplasms (MPN, formerly called myeloproliferative disorders). The predominant cell type that gives each MPN its name can change during the course of a disease, so, for example, PV can progress to PMF. And in addition to all these being serious disorders in their own right, there is also the further risk of transformation to acute myeloid leukemia in a small proportion of cases.

For chromosome studies of MPN, a bone marrow aspirate is necessary, as a blood sample is very unlikely to be informative. The only exception is PMF, in which the replacement of bone marrow by fibrotic tissue results in extramedullary hematopoiesis and this may result in clonal cells being in circulation. An aspirate is also best for CML, though at diagnosis up to 50% of blood samples have produced divisions for chromosome study in the author's laboratory. A blood sample is very unlikely to be informative in CML once treatment has started.

For more information than can be included in this chapter, the reader is referred to the online Mitelman database of chromosome aberrations and gene fusions in cancer [1], and the summaries in the online Atlas of genetics and cytogenetics in oncology and hematology [2], the World Health Organization (WHO) classification of tumors of hematopoietic and lymphoid tissues [3], and the publication by Heim and Mitelman [4]. All of these are slightly out of date, however, and the classification of MPN has changed in recent years, so the next edition of the WHO publication should be consulted when it is published, for an update on the current understanding of these disorders.

2 Chromosome Studies in MPN

Chromosome studies in malignancy generally have two principal functions: to aid in diagnosis, and to indicate prognosis. MPN are a group of chronic disorders that can resemble relatively benign disorders, often secondary or reactive, so confirming the diagnosis can be important. However, chromosomally abnormal clones are relatively rare in some kinds of MPN, occurring in about 15% of PV, and 7% of ET. Therefore, confirming a diagnosis of these MPN is better done in other ways: for example, molecular techniques using multiplex polymerase chain reaction (PCR) for mutations in genes such as *JAK2*, *CALR*, and *MPL* will give an informative result in over 90% of cases. Additionally, PCR for *BCR-ABL1* fusion is useful to distinguish between ET and CML. For these reasons, many cytogenetics laboratories no longer offer a routine diagnostic service for PV and ET; it is more efficient to reserve chromosome studies for those rare cases where PCR has not been informative and the clinician still seeks diagnostic clarification.

2.1 Polycythemia Vera (PV)

Although the incidence of cytogenetics abnormalities at diagnosis of PV is low (15%), it does increase as the disease progresses, and in advanced, treated disease it has reached 80% in some series. The most common abnormality at diagnosis is an interstitial deletion of the long arms of a chromosome 20 [5], and this was the second abnormality, after the Ph chromosome to be historically associated with a hematologic malignancy. The other common abnormalities, as listed in Table 1, are +8, +9, gain of 1q and deletion of 13q. Two of these abnormalities are illustrated in Fig. 1. Progression of PV to other diagnoses, such as PMF or AML, often involves the acquisition of further abnormalities, especially gain of 1q if not already present, but also deletion of 5q, 7q, or 17p.

2.2 Essential Thrombocythemia (ET)

It can be clinically difficult to distinguish between ET and CML, and so excluding the presence of the Ph chromosome or a *BCR-ABL1* fusion is diagnostically useful. In addition, if a del(5q13~q35) is detected, or any abnormality involving the *MECOM* gene at band 3q26.2, then a diagnosis of MDS becomes likely.

The same common abnormalities occur in ET as in PV [6] but at a lower incidence. ET is a relatively benign disease, with few cases progressing to overt leukemia; this is often associated with the acquisition of abnormalities such as deletion of 7q or 17p. Unusual abnormalities can occur in ET as in all other disorders; Figure 2 illustrates the common gain of 1q in a patient with ET, but arising from a translocation that is unusual in myeloid disorders.

Table 1
Principal recurrent chromosome abnormalities in common myeloproliferative neoplasms

Diagnosis	PV	ET	PMF	HES	SM
Approximate prevalence of visible, clonal chromosome abnormalities	15%	5–7%	30–50%	15%	35%
Trisomy 1q	X	X	X		
del(7)(q21~36)		X	X		X
Trisomy 8	X	X	X		X
Trisomy 9	X	X	X		X
del(13)(q13~q21)	X	X	X		
del(17)(p11~13)		X	X		
i(17q)		X	X		
del(20)(q11.2q13.1) and del(20)(q11.2q13.3)	X	X	X		X
Other				See text	See text

PV Polycythemia vera, *ET* Essential thrombocythemia, *PMF* Primary myelofibrosis, *HES* Hypereosinophilic syndrome, *SM* Systemic mastocytosis

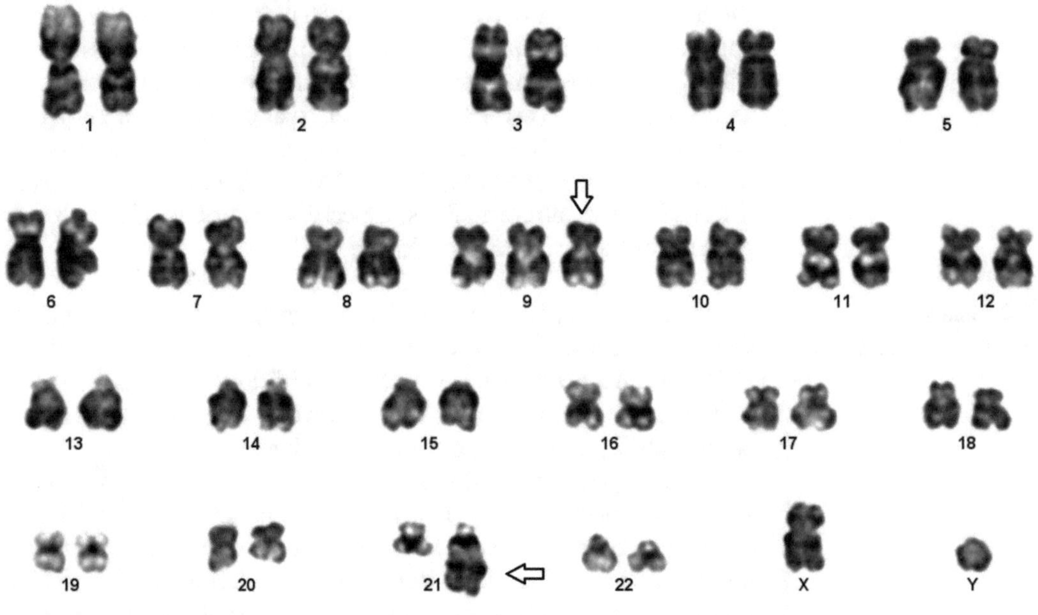

Fig. 1 A karyogram showing 47,XY,+9,der(21)t(1;21)(q21;q22). This clone is from a patient with *JAK2*+ve polycythemia vera. It has the gain of a chromosome 9 (trisomy 9) that is one of the most common findings in this disorder. In addition, there is an unbalanced translocation between chromosomes 1 and 21 that has resulted in gain of the long arm of the chromosome 1 (+1q). Translocations resulting in +1q occur in a wide variety of malignancies

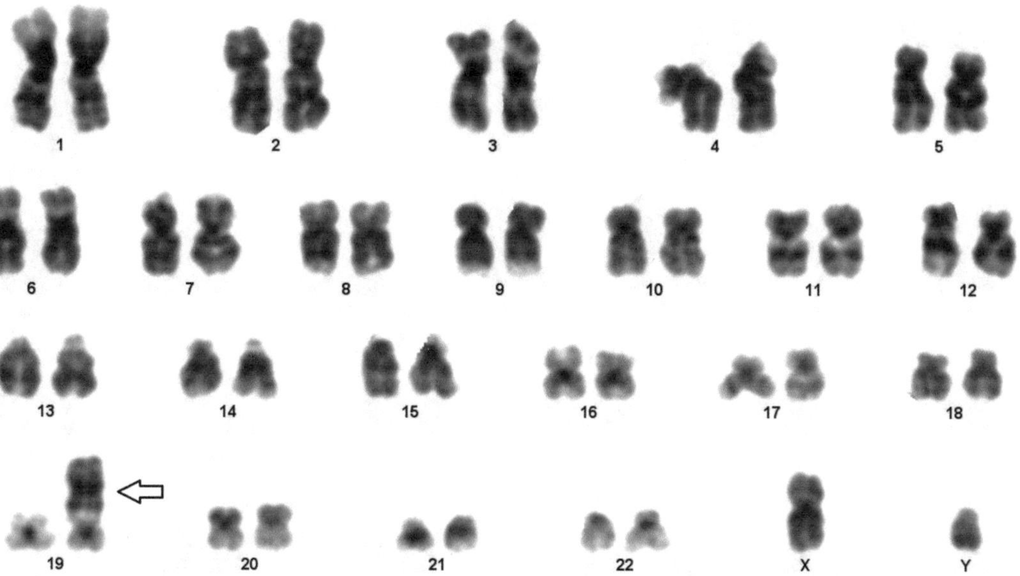

Fig. 2 A karyogram showing 46,XY,der(19)t(1;19)(q21;p13). This patient had a long history of poorly controlled thrombocythemia; at the time of this study, the platelet count was 644×10^9/L. The clone had an unbalanced translocation between a chromosome 1 and a 19 that has resulted in gain of the long arms of the 1 (+1q). The translocation in this case resembles the translocation that is associated with B-lineage acute lymphoblastic leukemia and is rare in other disorders

2.3 Primary Myelofibrosis (PMF)

In PMF it is technically difficult to get an adequate bone marrow aspirate for a chromosome study but if material is obtained then an abnormal clone can be found in 30–40% of cases, rising to 50% and more in those with advanced disease.

Unlike other types of MPN, some chromosome abnormalities found at diagnosis of PMF do have a clear prognostic significance. Inversion of 3q, loss of a chromosome 5 or a 7, deletion of their long arms (5q-, 7q-), gain of a chromosome 8, translocations involving 11q, deletion of 12p, or any complex clone (Fig. 3) are regarded as high risk; other single abnormalities (the commonest being deletion from the long arm of chromosome 13 or 20) are standard risk [7].

Most common in PMF, but also occurring in other myeloid disorders, is an unbalanced whole arm translocation der(1;7)(q10;p10), which in the presence of two normal #1 chromosomes results in a combination of two common abnormalities: gain of an extra copy of the long arms of chromosome 1 and loss of the long arms of a chromosome 7 (Fig. 4).

2.4 Chronic Neutrophilic Leukemia (CNL)

Twenty-three percent of cases of this rare disorder have been reported to have a chromosomally abnormal clone. The abnormalities have been much the same as those reported to occur in other MPN, with no one abnormality being specific for CNL, or

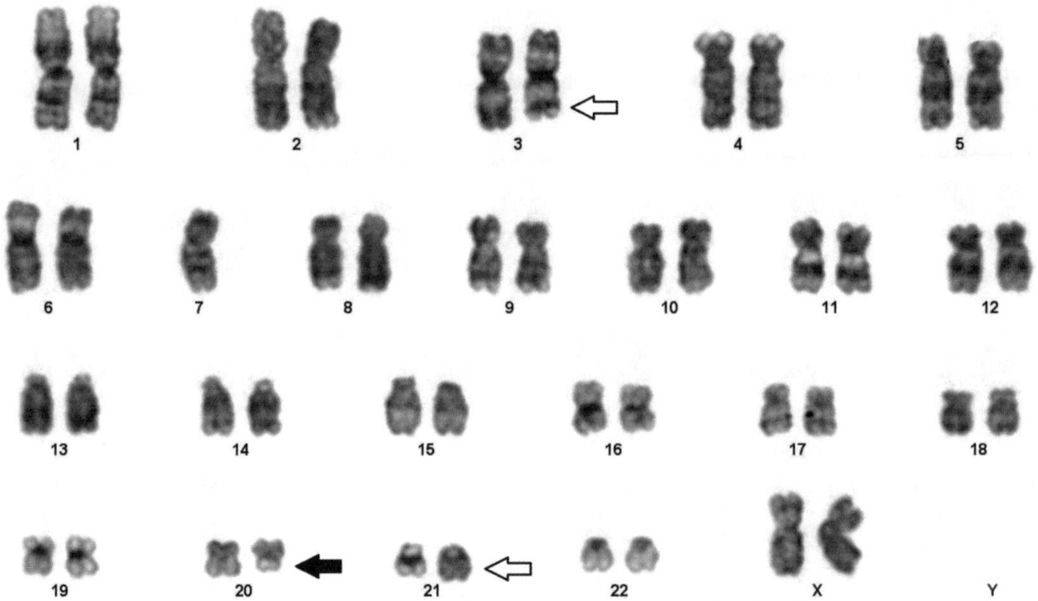

Fig. 3 A karyogram showing 45,XX,t(3;21)(q26.2;q22),-7,del(20)(q11.2q13.3). In 2013, this patient had primary myelofibrosis and an abnormal clone with isolated del(20)(q11.2q13.3). Two years later the disease had transformed to AML with 53 % blasts, and the clone had evolved with the acquisition of further abnormalities: as well as the del(20q) (black arrow), there was monosomy for chromosome 7, and a translocation between a chromosome 3 and a 21 (white arrows). A FISH study confirmed involvement of the *MECOM* gene (formerly called *EVI1*) at 3q26.2. This translocation is particularly associated with dysmegakaryopoiesis

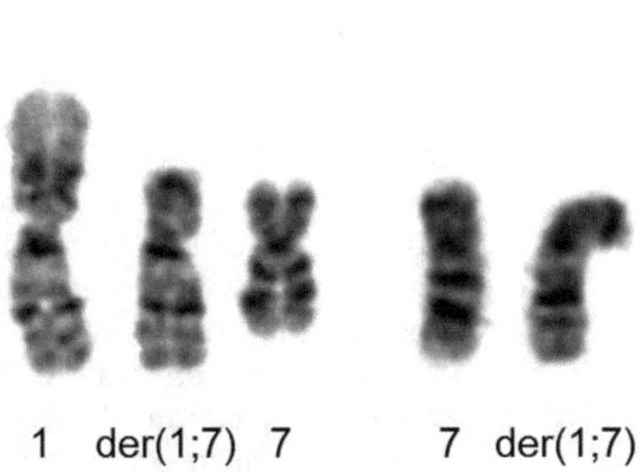

Fig. 4 Partial karyograms showing der(1;7)(q10;p10). On the left is a normal chromosome 1 and the third chromosome is a normal 7. In between these two is the derivative chromosome that is composed of the short arm of chromosome 7 and the long arm of chromosome 1. This abnormality usually occurs with 2 normal #1 chromosomes, so as well as deletion of the long arm of the 7 (7q-) there is gain of the long arm of a chromosome 1. The pair of chromosomes on the right illustrate that the abnormality can be less obvious in poorer-quality cells, and it can be missed by an inexperienced analyst

being known to have a different prognostic significance in this disorder compared to others.

2.5 Chronic Basophilic Leukemia (CBL)

This is a particularly rare condition, with correspondingly very few reported cytogenetic studies. There is little evidence so far for a specific cytogenetic abnormality that is associated with particular clinical characteristics.

2.6 Hypereosinophilic Syndrome (HES) and Chronic Eosinophilic Leukemia (CEL)

Eosinophilia is frequently the normal result of infection and it therefore resolves when the infection has ended. However, there are some clonal disorders characterized by abnormal eosinophils [8]. Among these is HES, which is rare but has major clinical implications, so a test that can give a positive diagnosis is welcome. Visible clonal chromosome abnormalities have been reported to occur in up to 15% of cases. However, an abnormality that occurs in 40–60% of HES is a deletion in 4q12 that is cryptic by chromosome study but can be detected by fluorescence in situ hybridization (FISH) with a probe for the *PDGFRA* gene at this location. An alternative approach is to use PCR primers for *FIPIL1-PDGFRA*. Confirming involvement of *PDGFRA* does more than help to confirm the diagnosis: these patients have a good response to imatinib, the tyrosine kinase inhibitor originally used for the treatment of CML.

The *PDGFRB* gene at 5q33 is also frequently involved in HES, often as a translocation t(5;12)(q31~33;p12). However, there are at least 15 known translocation partners with *PDGFRB* and so a PCR-based assay is not so widely used as is FISH. Again, this disorder often responds to treatment with imatinib.

Translocations involving a third gene, *FGFR1* at 8p11, are also recurrent in HES. Unlike the case with *PDGFRA* and *PDGFRB*, translocations involving *FGFR1* are not associated with responsiveness to imatinib.

In view of the cryptic deletion of 4q12 and the multiplicity of translocation partners with both 5q31~33 and 8p11, it is logical for the cytogenetics laboratory to have a policy of using FISH as a primary assay whenever HES is suspected, using probes for *PDGFRA*, *PDGFRB*, and *FGFR1*.

Note that the presence of abnormalities of any of these genes in the absence of eosinophilia can identify a rare, different MPN listed by the WHO [3].

A diagnosis of CEL is difficult to confirm, and its criteria include the absence of any translocation involving the genes present in other types of MPN, including *PDGFRA*, *PDGFRB*, *FGFR1*, and *BCR-ABL1*. The incidence of visible clonal abnormalities is low (around 15%). There is no specific chromosome abnormality that identifies CEL; those that do occur include +8 and i(17q) and these are also seen in many other kinds of myeloid disorders.

2.7 Systemic Mastocytosis (SM)

SM is one of various kinds of mastocytosis. Very few cytogenetics studies have been reported in any kind; most are in SM, and even these amount to very few cases. None of the abnormalities seen is specific for SM. They include those that are common to most types of MPN, such as 7q-, +8, +9, and 20q-, but 11q- and +14 have also been reported. Their clinical implications in SM are unknown. Far more common in SM are point mutations in genes such as *KIT*.

3 Chromosome Studies in CML

The development of tyrosine kinase inhibitors (TKI) such as imatinib has transformed the treatment of CML. A disease that was previously almost incurable even with the most intensive chemotherapy has now become manageable for most people in a way that is much more readily tolerated. In some places, a chromosome study is no longer used to confirm the diagnosis: detection of a *BCR-ABL1* gene fusion by FISH or PCR is considered to be sufficient to commence treatment. However, chromosome studies do add clinically useful information [9, 10].

The association between CML and the Philadelphia chromosome (Ph, a small chromosome 22 arising from a translocation with a chromosome 9) dates back to 1960. Other abnormalities that are additional to the Ph at the diagnosis of CML do not currently affect the choice of first-line treatment with TKI, though some have been associated with an adverse prognosis, including -7, del(7q), translocations involving 3q26.2, i(17)(q10), and the presence of two or more additional chromosome abnormalities. Some other common additional abnormalities, such as –Y, +8, and +Ph, do not appear to have an adverse effect compared to clones with the Ph as the sole abnormality [10]. However, any further abnormalities emerging post-diagnosis (cytogenetic clonal evolution) are an indication of disease progression (Fig. 5), failure of response to the current treatment, and the need to move to a different therapy [9].

Some current treatment trials use chromosome studies to assess initial response to TKI. The usual requirement is to assess at least 20 metaphases, at 3, 6, and 12 months until a "complete cytogenetic response" (CCyR) is achieved, which is no Ph positive divisions in at least 20 divisions assessed. If there has not been substantial clearance of Ph+ve cells from the dividing cell population (specifically a "partial cytogenetic response" is needed, which is less than 35% of the divisions being Ph+ve) after 3 months of treatment [9] or 6 months [11], then it is likely that a different TKI will be needed.

After achievement of a CCyR, further assessment of residual CML is usually better made at a higher level of sensitivity by PCR. However, in most centers a full chromosome study is undertaken every 12 months to look for Ph-negative clones. The effect of TKI on the dynamics of bone marrow activity seems to

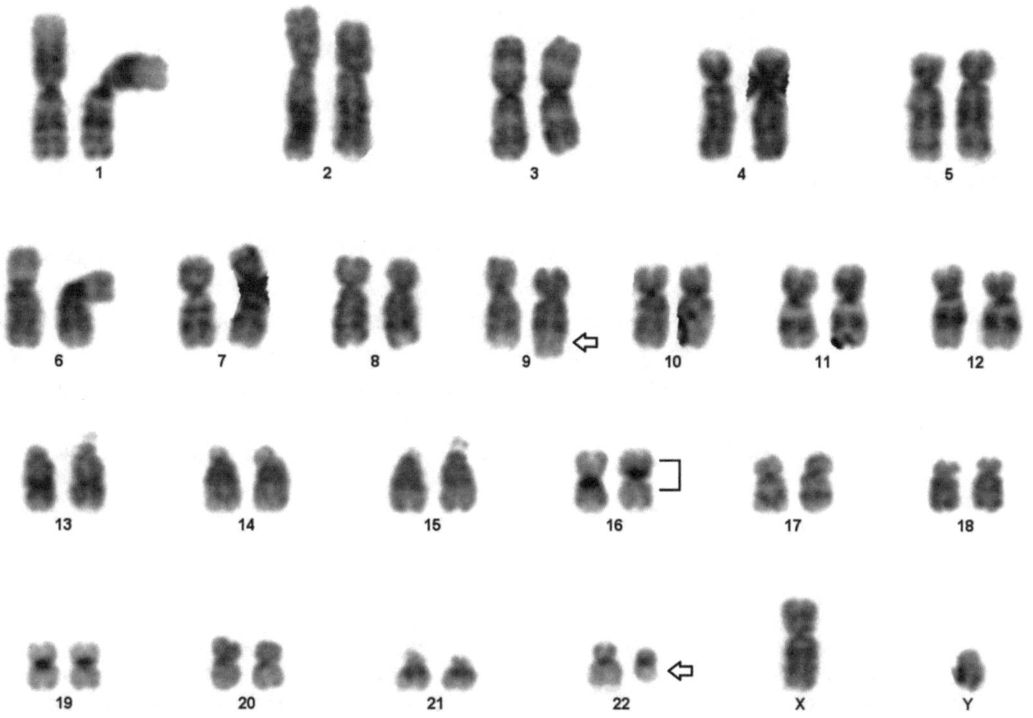

Fig. 5 A karyogram showing 46,XX,t(9;22)(q34;q11.2),inv(16)(p13q22). The translocation t(9;22)(q34;q11.2), indicated by *arrows*, produces the diminutive Ph (Philadelphia) chromosome that occurs in the great majority of cases of CML. As well as the common further abnormalities described in the text, occasionally there are also the translocations that define types of acute myeloid leukemia. In this case, at diagnosis of CML there was only the Ph chromosome seen; at later blast crisis there was also the inversion of chromosome 16 that is normally associated with AML. A FISH study confirmed *CBFB-MYH11* fusions in 98 % of the cells scored

predispose to the establishment of such clones and they occur in 5–10% of patients. The natural history of Ph-negative clones occurring after treatment with TKI is still to be determined. Most of the clones seem to have little clinical significance unless there is dysplasia, and some prove to be transient. However, a clone with monosomy 7 or 7q- indicates a high risk of MDS or acute leukemia, so active follow-up is indicated.

4 Conclusion

This chapter is a brief synopsis of current knowledge about the implications of chromosome abnormalities in MPN and CML. However, the advent of new diagnostic assays, such as sequencing, and the development of new types of treatment, such as therapy targeted at specific genetic abnormalities, is resulting in rapid changes in the clinical management of hematologic disorders. Identifying the genetic make-up of a patient's malignancy has been used to identify broad prognostic groups, but it is becoming increasingly important in determining exactly which therapeutic agents will and will not be effective.

Acknowledgments

I am grateful to all the members of the team in the Cytogenetics Laboratory at the Royal Marsden Hospital and to the many colleagues past and present who have directly or indirectly contributed their experience to the diagnostic service of this laboratory and to the preparation of this chapter. Marianne Wall did the primary analysis for the clone shown in Fig. 1, Paul Kotzampaltiris (Figs. 2 and 5), Claudia Walter (Fig. 3), and Julie Howard-Reeves (Fig. 4).

References

1. Mitelman F, Johansson B, Mertens F (eds) Mitelman database of chromosome aberrations in cancer. http://cgap.nci.nih.gov/Chromosomes/Mitelman
2. Atlas of genetics and cytogenetics in oncology and haematology. http://www.atlasgeneticsoncology.org/
3. Swerdlow SH, Campo E, Harris NL et al (eds) (2008) WHO classification of tumours of hematopoietic and lymphoid tissues. IARC, Lyon
4. Heim S, Mitelman F (eds) (2015) Cancer cytogenetics, 4th edn. Wiley, Hoboken, NJ
5. Nacheva E, Holloway T, Carter N et al (1995) Characterization of 20q deletions in patients with myeloproliferative disorders or myelodysplastic syndromes. Cancer Genet Cytogenet 80:87–94
6. Third International Workshop on Chromosomes in Leukemia (1981) Report on essential thrombocythemia. Cancer Genet Cytogenet 4:138–142
7. Caramazza D, Begna KH, Gangat N et al (2011) Refined cytogenetic-risk categorization for overall and leukemia-free survival in primary myelofibrosis: a single center study of 433 patients. Leukemia 25(1): 82–88
8. Gotlib J (2015) World Health Organization-defined eosinophilic disorders: 2015 update on diagnosis, risk stratification, and management. Am J Haematol 90:1078–1089
9. Baccarani M, Deininger MW, Rosti G et al (2013) European LeukemiaNet recommendations for the management of chronic myeloid leukemia. Blood 122(6):872–884
10. Wang W, Cortes JE, Tang G et al (2016) Risk stratification of chromosomal abnormalities in chronic myelogenous leukemia in the era of tyrosine kinase inhibitor therapy. Blood 127:2742–2750
11. U.S. National Comprehensive Cancer Network guidelines. https://www.nccn.org/

Chapter 21

Recurrent Cytogenetic Abnormalities in Acute Lymphoblastic Leukemia

Mary Shago

Abstract

Both B-cell and T-cell acute lymphoblastic leukemia (ALL) exhibit recurrent cytogenetic alterations, many with prognostic implications. This chapter overviews the major recurrent categories of cytogenetic abnormalities associated with ALL, with an emphasis on the detection and characterization of these cases by G-band and FISH analyses.

Key words Cytogenetics, Fluorescence in situ hybridization (FISH), Acute lymphoblastic leukemia, Chromosome abnormalities

1 Introduction

Acute lymphoblastic leukemia (ALL), the most common childhood cancer, results from an overproduction of immature lymphoid hematopoietic cells [1]. Based on knowledge accumulated by numerous studies dating back more than 50 years, both B-cell ALL and T-cell ALL are associated with characteristic and recurrent cytogenetic changes [2, 3]. More recently, the application of expression and genomic microarray technologies and next generation sequencing have revealed many additional recurrent submicroscopic abnormalities associated with ALL [4]. There are a number of techniques that can detect the copy number changes and recurrent gene fusions that occur in ALL, including multiplex ligation-dependent probe amplification (MLPA), genomic microarray analysis, reverse transcriptase polymerase chain reaction (RT-PCR), RNA sequencing, and next generation sequencing targeted gene panels. Currently, cytogenetic analysis remains an essential component in the diagnostic evaluation of a patient with ALL, often complemented with molecular technologies. This review will focus on recurrent categories of chromosome abnormalities in childhood ALL that can be detected by G-banding and fluorescence in situ hybridization (FISH) analysis.

Thomas S.K. Wan (ed.), *Cancer Cytogenetics: Methods and Protocols*, Methods in Molecular Biology, vol. 1541, DOI 10.1007/978-1-4939-6703-2_21,

The lymphoblasts of ALL patients derive from the B cell lineage in 80–85% of cases, and display a precursor B cell immunophenotype [1]. There are multiple well-established cytogenetic subgroups in B-cell acute lymphoblastic leukemia, those associated with a favorable prognosis, including hyperdiploidy, and t(12;21)(p13;q22), and those that predict an adverse prognosis, including t(9;22), hypodiploidy, *KMT2A* (*MLL*) gene rearrangements, iAMP21, and Philadelphia chromosome-like ALL (Ph-like ALL) [1, 5]. Results of cytogenetic analysis are incorporated into treatment stratification [4]. In adolescents and young adults, many of the high-risk childhood cytogenetic subgroups occur with a much higher frequency.

T-cell ALL constitutes approximately 15% of childhood ALL [1]. The most common cytogenetic abnormalities observed in T-ALL are translocations involving the T cell receptor genes, *TCR alpha/delta* (14q11.2), and *TCR beta* (7q34). The translocation partners are transcription factors that are upregulated by the *TCR* gene enhancer regions. Examples of the most frequently observed *TCR* and non-*TCR* T-ALL translocations will be discussed in Subheading 3. Cytogenetic alterations do not currently play a role in risk stratification in the treatment of T-ALL; however, there are prognostic implications and potential therapeutic options for some of the recurrent abnormalities [6].

The chromosomal abnormalities summarized in this review are listed in Table 1, along with the frequencies and prognostic significance of these abnormalities in childhood ALL.

2 B-cell Acute Lymphoblastic Leukemia

2.1 Hyperdiploidy

With a frequency of 30%, hyperdiploidy is the most common recurrent abnormality in childhood B-ALL. Hyperdiploid B-ALL cases typically have a chromosome count of 51–65 chromosomes [7, 8]. The pattern of gains is nonrandom, with one additional copy of chromosomes X, 4, 6, 10, 14, 17, 18, and two additional copies of 21 being the most frequently observed alterations in hyperdiploid clones. High hyperdiploidy with specific gains of chromosomes 4, 10, 17, and 18 has been associated with an excellent prognosis in pediatric B-ALL [7, 9]. In addition to the common gains, karyotypes with 57–60 chromosomes typically also have trisomies of chromosomes 5, 8, 11, and 12, while karyotypes with 63–67 chromosomes frequently also have gains of chromosomes 2, 3, 9, 16, and 22 [8]. Hyperdiploid clones may display structural abnormalities in addition to the chromosome gains, but these structural alterations generally do not alter the prognosis. However, it should be noted that some recurrent cytogenetic abnormalities such as the t(9;22), the t(1;19), or *KMT2A* (*MLL*) gene rearrangements may occasionally be seen in the context of a

Table 1
Recurrent chromosomal abnormalities in acute lymphoblastic leukemia

Section	Cytogenetic abnormality	Frequency (%)[a]	Outcome
B-cell acute lymphoblastic leukemia			
2.1	Hyperdiploidy	30	Good
2.2	t(12;21)(p13;q22)(*ETV6-RUNX1*)	25	Good
2.3	Ph-/*BCR-ABL1*-like	10–15	Poor
2.4	*KMT2A* (*MLL*) gene rearrangements (11q23)	4	Poor
2.5	t(1;19)(q23;p13.3)(*TCF3-PBX1*)	5	Intermediate
2.6	t(9;22)(q34;q11.2) (*BCR-ABL1*)	3	Poor
2.7	Hypodiploidy	2	Poor
2.8	iAMP21 (21q)	2	Poor
2.9	*ZNF384* gene rearrangements (12p13)	1–2	Unknown
2.10	Dicentric (9;20)	2	Intermediate
2.11	t(17;19)(q22;p13.3)(*TCF3-HLF*)	<1	Poor
2.12	*IGH* gene rearrangements (14q32)	5	Intermediate
2.13	*MYC* gene rearrangements (8q24)	<1	Intermediate
T-cell acute lymphoblastic leukemia			
3.1	*TAL1* gene rearrangements (1p32)	20	Good
3.2	*TLX1* (*HOX11*) gene rearrangements (10q24)	8	Good
3.3	*LMO2* (*RBTN2*) gene rearrangements (11p13)	15	Unknown
3.4	t(5;14)(q35;q32)(*TLX3-BCL11B*)	20	Poor
3.5	*MYB* gene rearrangements (6q23)	1	Unknown
3.6	*MYC* gene rearrangements (8q24)	1	Unknown
3.7	t(10;11)(p12;q14)(*PICALM-MLLT10*)	10	Poor
3.8	*NUP214-ABL1* fusion and amplification	6	Poor
3.9	*KMT2A* (*MLL*) gene rearrangements (11q23)	6	Unknown[b]

[a]Frequencies in childhood leukemia
[b]t(11;19)(q23;p13.3) associated with a good outcome in T-ALL; outcome of other *KMT2A* gene rearrangements uncertain

hyperdiploid karyotype [10]. These cases may also include trisomies of chromosomes 2 and 19, which are rare in typical hyperdiploid cases. Although some chromosomes, such as 21 and 14, tend to be present in tetrasomic form in hyperdiploid B-ALL, a clone with a number of tetrasomic chromosomes, and with few or no trisomies may in fact represent a "hidden" doubled near-haploid or doubled hypodiploid clone (*see* Subheading 2.7).

2.2 t(12;21)(p13;q22) (ETV6-RUNX1)

The translocation t(12;21)(p13;q22), resulting in fusion of the *ETV6* (12p13) and *RUNX1* (21q22) genes, is the most common recurrent translocation in pediatric B-ALL. It is estimated to occur in ~25% of pediatric B-ALL and is generally associated with a favorable prognosis. The t(12;21) translocation is cryptic by routine G-banding and requires FISH analysis for cytogenetic detection [11]. Commercial FISH probe strategies include dual color/dual fusion and extra signal dual color translocation designs. Both of these probe types will also detect the additional secondary changes common to chromosomes 12 and 21 in t(12;21) cases such as: gain of an extra copy of the derivative chromosome (21), gain of an additional copy of chromosome 21, and deletion of the *ETV6* locus from the non-translocated chromosome 12 [12]. Deletions and duplications of variable sizes can also be observed across the derivative (12)t(12;21) breakpoint [13]. With current treatment strategies, the additional karyotypic alterations do not have an apparent impact on the good prognosis associated with the t(12;21). The *ETV6-RUNX1* fusion is present on the derivative chromosome 21 in most cases of t(12;21) B-ALL. Occasionally, the *ETV6-RUNX1* fusion may be localized on the derivative chromosome 12, often by interstitial insertion of *RUNX1* sequence into the *ETV6* allele [14]. Subtelomeric FISH analysis using probes for 12pter and 21qter may be helpful to further characterize insertion cases. Although the t(12;21) itself is cryptic, the majority of cases have additional cytogenetically visible chromosomal abnormalities. Common secondary abnormalities of chromosomes other than 12 and 21 in t(12;21) cases include del(6q), del(8p), del(9p), del(11q), del(13q), gain of chromosomes 10 and 16, and rarely, tetraploidy [15–17].

2.3 Philadelphia Chromosome-like Acute Lymphoblastic Leukemia (Ph-like ALL)

Gene expression analysis was initially used to demonstrate that approximately half of *BCR-ABL1*-negative high risk B-ALL cases without other recurrent cytogenetic abnormalities had a gene expression signature similar to t(9;22)-ALL [18, 19]. Ph-like B-ALL (also called *BCR-ABL1*-like ALL) has a prevalence of approximately 10% in children, rising to approximately 25% in adolescents and young adults [20]. Ph-like ALL has subsequently been shown to include a large number of recurrent rearrangements that primarily result in the fusion of a kinase-encoding gene to a partner gene [20, 21]. Although there are multiple gene partners in this category of leukemia, the consistent activation of a kinase pathway implies that treatment with kinase inhibitors may be an option in these patients. The kinase-encoding genes reported to be rearranged in Ph-like ALL are *JAK2* (9p24.1), *ABL1* (9q34), *PDGFRB* (5q32), *ABL2* (1q25.2), *PTK2B* (8p21.2), *EPOR* (19p13.2), *TSLP* (5q22.1), *CSF1R* (5q32), *DGKH* (13q14), *NTRK* (15q25.3), *TYK2* (19p13.2), and *IL2RB* (22q12.3). Other than the *ABL1* gene coverage provided by the commonly used *BCR-ABL1* FISH probe (Fig. 1), many cytogenetics laboratories may not have FISH probes for these kinase gene regions, although probes for some of these loci are available commercially. However, some of the rearrangements can be detected by G-banding analysis, which may subsequently be followed up with FISH analysis or molecular methods (Table 2). Also noted in Table 2 are rearrangements where the gene orientations will not allow fusion by simple translocation or deletion mechanisms. It would be expected that these fusions are formed by complex rearrangements involving more than two breakpoints.

Deregulation of the cytokine receptor-like factor 2 (*CRLF2*) gene, located within the pseudoautosomal region 1 (PAR1) of the X and Y chromosomes (Xp22.3/Yp11.3), also results in the Ph-like gene expression signature and activation of kinase pathways, and may account for up to 50% of the Ph-like ALL patients [22]. The most common rearrangement resulting in the upregulation of *CRLF2* gene expression is a submicroscopic interstitial deletion in Xp22.3 or Yp11.3 resulting in the fusion of *CRLF2* to the promoter of the *P2RY8* gene, which is ~250 kb centromeric to *CRLF2* on Xp22.3/Yp11.3 (Table 2). Alternatively, a translocation t(X or Y;14)(p22.3 or p11.3;q32) between the *IGH* locus and *CRLF2* gene activates *CRLF2* gene expression. Both *IGH-CRLF2* and *P2RY8-CRLF2* may be detected using commercial FISH probes.

CRLF2 gene rearrangements are also found at a particularly high frequency in Down syndrome patients with ALL. In Down

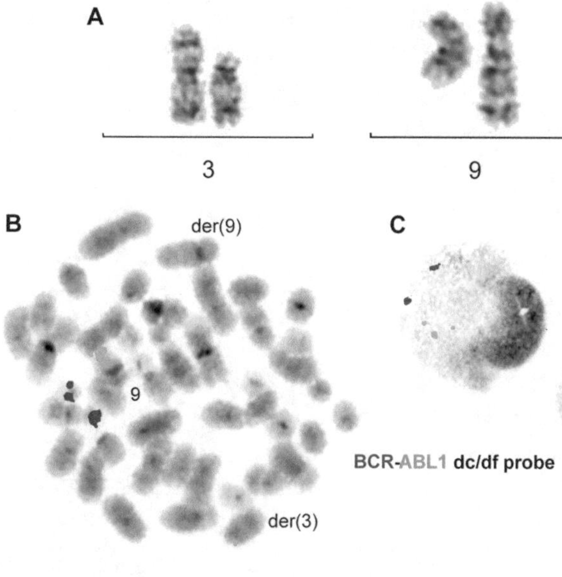

Fig. 1 (**a**) Partial karyogram of translocation t(3;9)(p13;q34) resulting in fusion of the *FOXP1* and *ABL1* genes. Metaphase (**b**) and interphase (**c**) cells showing the splitting of the *ABL1* signal on the derivative chromosomes 3 and 9. The FISH images are displayed with inverted DAPI

Table 2
Ph-like ALL gene fusions and cytogenetic rearrangements

Kinase/signaling receptor gene	Partner	Partner location	Rearrangement	Visible by G-banding[a]
JAK2 (9p24.1)	*TPR*	1q31.1	t(1;9)(q31.1;p24.1)	Yes
	SSBP2	5q14.1	t(5;9)(q14.1;p24.1)	Yes
	EBF1	5q33.3	t(5;9)(q33.3;p24.1)	No
	PCM1	8p22	t(8;9)(p22;p24.1)	?Yes
	PAX5	9p13.2	del(9)(p13.2p24.1)[b]	Yes
	PPFIBP1	12p11.2	t(9;12)(p24.1;p11.2)	Yes
	ETV6	12p13	t(9;12)(p24.1;p13)	No
	ATF7IP	12p13.1	t(9;12)(p24.1;p13.1)	No
	STRN3	14q12	t(9;14)(p24.1;q12)	Yes
	TERF2	16q22.1	t(9;16)(p24.1;q22.1)	?Yes
	SPAG9	17q21.3	t(9;17)(p24.1;q21.3)	Yes
	BCR	22q11.2	t(9;22)(p24.1;q11.2)[c]	?Yes
	OFD1	Xp22.2	t(X;9)(p22.2;p24.1)	No
ABL1 (9q34)	*SFPQ*	1p34.3	t(1;9)(p34.3;q34)	Yes
	RCSD1	1q24.2	t(1;9)(q24.2;q34)	Yes
	RANBP2	2q12.3	t(2;9)(q12.3;q34)	Yes
	FOXP1	3p13	t(3;9)(p13;q34)	Yes
	SNX2	5q23.2	t(5;9)(q23.2;q34)	Yes
	ZMIZ1	10q22.3	t(9;10)(q34;q22.3)	Yes
	ETV6	12p13	t(9;12)(q34;p13)[c]	No
PDGFRB (5q32)	*ZEB2*	2q22.3	t(2;5)(q22.3;q32)	Yes
	TNIP1	5q33.1	del(5)(q32q33.1)	No
	EBF1	5q33.3	del(5)(q32q33.1)	No
	ATF7IP	12p13.1	t(5;12)(q32;p13.1)	Yes
ABL2 (1q25.2)	*RCSD1*	1q24.2	del(1)(q24.2q25.2)[b]	No
	ZC3HAV1	7q34	t(1;7)(q25.2;q34)	?Yes
	PAG1	8q21.1	t(1;8)(q25.2;q21.1)	Yes
PTK2B (8p21.2)	*KDM6A*	Xp11.3	t(X;8)(p11.3;p21.2)	Yes
	STAG2	Xq25	t(X;8)(q25;p21.2)[c]	Yes

(continued)

Table 2
(continued)

Kinase/signaling receptor gene	Partner	Partner location	Rearrangement	Visible by G-banding[a]
CRLF2 (Xp22.3 and Yp11.3)	*P2RY8*	Xp22.3 or Yp11.3	del(X)(p22.3p22.3) or del(Y)(p11.3p11.3)	No
	IGH	14q32	t(X or Y;14)(p22.3 or p11.3;q32)	No
EPOR (19p13.2)	*IGH*	14q32	t(14;19)(q32;p13.2)	No
	IGK	2p11.2	t(2;19)(p11.2;p13.2)	Yes
TSLP (5q22.1)	*IQGAP2*	5q13.3	del(5)(q13.3q22.1)	Yes
CSF1R (5q32)	*SSBP2*	5q14.1	del(5)(q14.1q32)[b]	Yes
DGKH (13q14.1)	*ZFAND3*	6p21.2	t(6;13)(p21.2;q14.1)[c]	Yes
NTRK3 (15q25.3)	*ETV6*	12p13	t(12;15)(p13;q25.3)	No
TYK2 (19p13.2)	*MYB*	6q23.3	t(6;19)(q23.3;p13.2)	?Yes
IL2RB (22q12.3)	*MYH9*	22q12.3	del(22)(q12.3q12.3)[b]	No

References: [20, 24–29]
[a]Ability to detect by G-banding will depend on quality of chromosome morphology and banding
[b]On same chromosome arm, however, complex rearrangement required as genes not oriented correctly for fusion by simple deletion
[c]Requires complex rearrangement due to opposite orientation of genes with respect to chromosome arms

syndrome patients, the rearrangements may have a less adverse prognosis, as the submicroscopic *IKZF1* gene deletions/mutations that often accompany Ph-like ALL karyotypes are less common in this patient population [23].

2.4 KMT2A (MLL) Gene Rearrangements (11q23)

The *KMT2A* gene, located at 11q23, is recurrently rearranged in both ALL and acute myeloid leukemia (AML) [30]. The *KMT2A* gene encodes a transcriptional coactivator with methyltransferase activity. Over 50 partner fusion genes have been identified [31]. The rearrangements result in the fusion of the 5′ portion of *KMT2A*, including the methyltransferase domain, to the 3′ region of the partner genes. Many of the *KMT2A* gene rearrangements are very rare, with a small proportion of the partner genes identified in the majority of cases. In B-cell ALL, the most commonly detected translocations/partners are the t(4;11)(q21;q23) (*KMT2A-AFF1*), the t(11;19)(q23;p13.3)(*KMT2A-MLLT1*), the t(10;11)(p12;q23)(*KMT2A-MLLT10*), and the t(9;11)(p21;q23) (*KMT2A-MLLT3*). *KMT2A* gene rearrangements are observed in ~80% of infant leukemia cases and are associated with a particularly poor prognosis in this patient group [32]. The translocations are visible by G-band analysis, and can be detected by FISH analysis with a commercial dual color break-apart probe for the *KMT2A* gene. Of the common translocations, the t(10;11) often does not present as a straightforward translocation, instead appearing as an inverted insertion of 11q into 10p, or a dicentric (10;11) chromosome (Fig. 2). The *KMT2A* and *MLLT10* genes are oppositely oriented on their respective chromosome arms, and complex mechanisms are required to create the fusion [33].

Secondary chromosome abnormalities observed in ALL with *MLL* gene rearrangement include gain of an X chromosome, alterations of 12p and 9p, and del(6q). No prognostic effects of these secondary chromosomal changes have been associated with 11q23 abnormalities in childhood ALL [34].

2.5 t(1;19)(q23;p13.3)(TCF3-PBX1)

The translocation t(1;19)(q23;p13.3) is observed in approximately 5% of pediatric B-ALL patients, and results in the fusion of the *PBX1* gene at 1q23 with the *TCF3* (*E2A*) gene at 19p13.3 [35, 36]. The oncogenic *TCF3-PBX1* fusion gene is expressed from the derivative chromosome 19. In approximately one third of patients the translocation appears in the balanced form, whereas two thirds of patients harbor the unbalanced form with the derivative chromosome 19 and two normal chromosomes 1 [37]. Common secondary chromosome abnormalities in *TCF3-PBX1* B-ALL include del(6q), del(9p), i(9q), and del(13q). A proportion of cases have hyperdiploid chromosome content in addition to the t(1;19)/der(19)t(1;19) [37, 38]. However, cases with hyperdiploidy and an apparent t(1;19)/der(19)t(1;19) should be assessed by FISH or molecular methods for the presence of the *TCF3-PBX1* gene rearrangement, as the t(1;19) rearrangements in these cases may not involve the *TCF3* and *PBX1* genes [10]. In several recent studies,

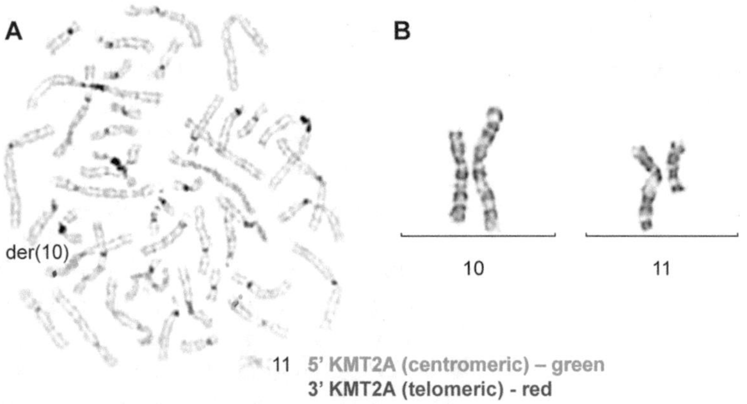

Fig. 2 (**a**) Metaphase FISH image of a complex rearrangement involving 10p and 11q, resulting in a *KMT2A-MLLT10* gene rearrangement. The FISH image is displayed with inverted DAPI. (**b**) Partial karyogram of the rearrangement between chromosomes 10 and 11. The nomenclature for the derivative chromosomes is der(10)(11qter->11q23::11q13->11q23::10p12->10qter) and der(11)t(10;11)(p12;q13)

no differences in outcome have been identified for the balanced versus the unbalanced form of the translocation [37, 39, 40]. The translocation may be confirmed with a dual color/dual fusion translocation probe set, or a dual color break-apart probe directed to *TCF3*. The latter probe strategy may be used to detect additional *TCF3* gene rearrangements including the t(17;19)(p22;p13.3)(*TCF3-HLF*) (*see* Subheading 2.11) or the t(12;19)(p13;p13.3)(*TCF3-ZNF384*) (*see* Subheading 2.9).

2.6 t(9;22)(q34;q11.2)(BCR-ABL1)

The translocation t(9;22)(q34;q11.2) is present in approximately 3% of pediatric patients with B-ALL. The translocation, also observed in a number of other hematological malignancies, results in the fusion of the *BCR* gene at 22q11.2 to the *ABL1* kinase gene at 9q34. The majority of pediatric ALL patients with a *BCR-ABL1* gene fusion have a breakpoint in the minor breakpoint cluster region on chromosome 22, resulting in a protein product with a molecular weight of 190 kDa. The t(9;22) is a adverse prognostic indicator in precursor B ALL; however, recent treatment regimens incorporating tyrosine kinase inhibitors may improve the outcome [41]. Secondary chromosome abnormalities are seen in approximately two thirds of patients with the t(9;22), and may have a negative impact on outcome [41, 42]. Recurrent secondary abnormalities include gain of an additional copy of the derivative chromosome 22, loss of chromosome 7, del(7p), del(9p), trisomy 8, and hyperdiploidy. Deletions at or near the breakpoint on the derivative chromosome 9 occur in a proportion of patients, and may be observed with FISH analysis as loss of part or all of the fusion signal on the derivative chromosome 9 [43].

2.7 Hypodiploidy

Hypodiploidy, characterized by less than 44 (43 or fewer) chromosomes, occurs with an overall frequency of 2% in childhood B-ALL. Three cytogenetic subgroups of hypodiploidy have been defined: near haploidy, with 24–31 chromosomes; low hypodiploid, with 32–39 chromosomes; and high hypodiploid, with 40–43 chromosomes [44]. The near haploidy and low hypodiploidy subgroups are associated with an adverse prognosis in B-ALL [44–46]. In the near haploid cases, the chromosomes usually retained in two copies are chromosomes 14, 18, 21, and the sex chromosomes. In the low hypodiploid karyotypes, the most frequent monosomic chromosomes are chromosomes 3, 4, 7, 13, 15, 16, and 17. Patients with 40–43 chromosome high hypodiploid karyotypes are very rare, and the majority of these patients may not have the clinical features associated with hypodiploidy [44].

Sequence analysis of the low hypodiploid B-ALL subgroup has shown that the majority of these cases harbor *TP53* mutations [47, 48]. The *TP53* mutations are also present in non-tumor cells in approximately half of the patients, indicating possible germline inheritance and an association with Li-Fraumeni syndrome.

Doubling of the hypodiploid clone is not uncommon, and consequently cases may present with the doubled hypodiploid clone appearing as either a subclone, or as the sole clone identifiable by G-band analysis [48, 49]. Distinguishing the latter situation, in which only the "doubled hypodiploid" clone is present, from hyperdiploidy can be a challenge for cytogenetics laboratories. In general, a doubled hypodiploid clone will have more chromosomes present in tetrasomic form rather than as trisomies. However, the doubling of the hypodiploid clone is rarely an exact duplicate of the original hypodiploid clone, and the presence of gains and losses subsequent to the doubling can further mask the hypodiploid origin of the karyotype. The laboratory should pay careful attention to the results of interphase FISH analysis in cases with suspected doubled hypodiploidy; the nondividing cells may harbor both the original clone and the subclone. For truly masked potential doubled hypodiploid clones, it is important to assess the case with molecular methods such as microsatellite analysis (by comparing a diagnostic and a remission sample) or single-nucleotide polymorphism (SNP) microarray analysis to determine whether there is evidence of whole chromosome uniparental/copy neutral loss of heterozygosity allelic patterns [50].

2.8 Intrachromosomal Amplification of Chromosome 21 (iAMP21)

Intrachromosomal amplification of chromosome 21 or iAMP21 is estimated to occur in ~2% pediatric B-ALL and is defined as the presence of three or more additional copies of *RUNX1* on a structurally abnormal chromosome 21. The iAMP21 chromosome is often initially detected by *ETV6-RUNX1* FISH analysis [51–53]. Although the presence of multiple *RUNX1* signals in the interphase cells may be initially suggestive of the chromosome 21 gains commonly seen in hyperdiploid karyotypes, the *RUNX1* signals cluster on a single chromosome when metaphase cells from these cases are examined by FISH (Fig. 3). Exact quantification of the number of *RUNX1* signals in the nuclei may be difficult because of the clustering of signals. In the karyotypes of these patients, one chromosome 21 is replaced by a structurally abnormal chromosome 21 or a "marker" chromosome of variable morphology. The "marker" chromosome is usually much larger than a normal chromosome 21, and may be submetacentric or metacentric in appearance. Ring iAMP21 chromosomes or iAMP21 chromosomes composed of chromosome 21 and material from an additional chromosome have also been reported [54]. The karyotypes may be complex, with gain of an X chromosome, gain of chromosomes 10 or 14, loss of chromosome 7, del(7q), del(11q), and del(12p) reported as secondary chromosome abnormalities [54]. Genomic microarray analysis indicates complex structural rearrangements including chromothripsis underlying the formation of the iAMP21 chromosome [55]. FISH and genomic array analyses have indicated that iAMP21 chromosomes frequently have deletions of the subtelomeric region of 21q [55].

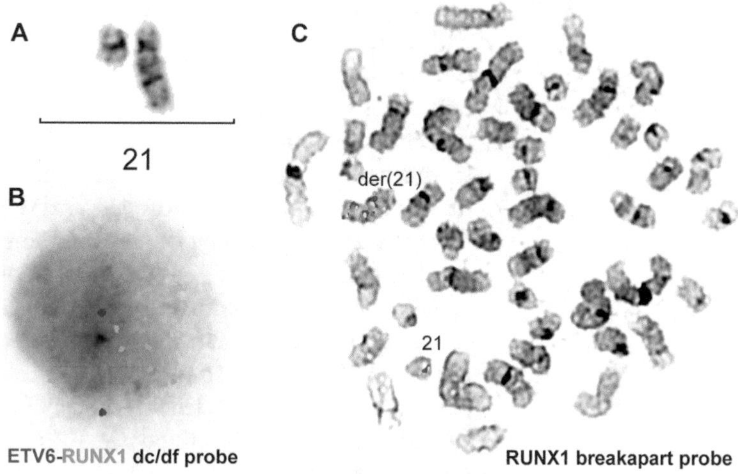

Fig. 3 (**a**) Partial karyogram of an iAMP21 chromosome replacing a normal chromosome 21. (**b**) FISH analysis of an interphase cell with a dual color/dual fusion *ETV6-RUNX1* probe showing multiple copies of the *RUNX1* signal and two copies of the *ETV6* signal. (**c**) Metaphase FISH image with a dual color break-apart probe for the *RUNX1* gene showing the localization of the *RUNX1* signals on the iAMP21 chromosome. FISH images are displayed with inverted DAPI

Identification of patients with an iAMP21 is essential, as these patients have an improved outcome when treated on high-risk protocols with more intensive chemotherapy [56–58]. For situations in which metaphase cells are not available but interphase cells have multiple *RUNX1* signals and lack the interphase FISH profile for chromosomes 4, 10, and 17 typical of a hyperdiploid case, FISH analysis with a subtelomeric probe for 21q may be useful.

Of note, individuals who have the rare germline Robertsonian translocation der(15;21)(q10;q10) have been identified to have a 2700-fold increased risk of developing iAMP21 ALL as compared to the general population [59].

2.9 ZNF384 Gene Rearrangements (12p13)

The *ZNF384* gene (previously called *CIZ* or *NMP4*), located telomeric to the *ETV6* gene at 12p13.31, encodes a putative zinc finger transcription factor and is recurrently rearranged in acute leukemia. There are four known fusion partners: *TAF15* (17q12), *EWSR1* (22q12), *TCF3* (*E2A*, 19p13.3), and *EP300* (22q13.2) [60–67]. With the exception of the t(12;17)(p13;q12)(*TAF15-ZNF384*), the rearrangements are difficult to detect by G-banding as the *ZNF384* gene and its partners are located in the distal regions of their respective chromosomes. The majority of the reported cases have a CD10-negative immunophenotype similar to that seen in *MLL* gene rearrangement cases, as well as myeloid marker gene expression. The prognosis associated with *ZNF384* gene rearrangements is unknown.

2.10 Dicentric (9;20)

Karyotypes with a dicentric chromosome dic(9;20)(p13;q11), with breakpoints in the proximal short arm of chromosome 9 and the proximal long arm of chromosome 20, are observed in approximately 2% of pediatric B-ALL patients [68, 69]. The dicentric chromosome consists of the entire chromosome 9 long arm, centromere, and part of the short arm of chromosome 9 attached to part of the long arm, centromere, and the entire short arm of chromosome 20. Monosomy of chromosome 20 is usually observed in B-ALL with dic(9;20), with resultant loss of chromosome region 9p13-pter and loss of chromosome region 20q11-qter. Monosomy of chromosome 20 is an important indicator of this karyotype, as the dic(9;20) chromosome is difficult to distinguish from a normal chromosome 9 or a del(9p) [70]. The dicentric chromosome (9;20) can be characterized by FISH analysis using probes for *CDKN2A* (9p13), centromeric probes for chromosomes 9 and 20, subtelomeric probes for 20pter/20qter, or whole chromosome paint probes [71]. Genomic and molecular analyses of dic(9;20) cases have suggested breakpoint heterogeneity, and it is uncertain whether the oncogenic mechanism underlying the dic(9;20) is a gene fusion at the breakpoint, or loss of 9p and 20q material. *PAX5* gene fusions may result from the rearrangement in a proportion of the cases [72, 73]. Karyotypes with a derivative chromosome (9)t(9;20)(p11~13;q11) may represent an alternative form of this rearrangement.

2.11 t(17;19)(q22;p13.3)(TCF3-HLF)

The translocation t(17;19)(q22;p13.3) results in fusion of the *TCF3* (*E2A*) gene at 19p13.3 and the *HLF* gene at 17q22 [74, 75]. This translocation, very rare in pediatric B-ALL, is associated with a dismal prognosis [76, 77]. The t(17;19) is visible by G-band analysis (Fig. 4). The involvement of the *TCF3* gene may be confirmed by FISH analysis with a dual color break-apart probe for *TCF3* or with a dual color/dual fusion probe set for *TCF3-HLF* loci [76].

2.12 IGH Gene Rearrangements (14q32)

Translocations involving the immunoglobulin heavy chain gene (*IGH* at 14q32) and a partner gene are estimated to occur in approximately 5% of childhood B-ALL, with a higher incidence in adolescent and young adult patients [78]. The most prevalent partner gene is *CRLF2*, followed by CCAAT/enhancer-binding protein (*CEBP*) family member genes *CEBPA* (19q13.1), *CEBPB* (20q13.1), *CEBPD* (8q11.2), *CEBPE* (14q11.2), *CEBPG* (19q13.1), the *ID4* gene (6p22.3), and the *BCL2* gene (18q21) [78–80]. *IGH-CRLF2* gene rearrangements are discussed in Subheading 2.3.

Based on the percentage of lymphoblast cells in which the *IGH*-partner gene rearrangements were detected, *IGH-CEBPE* and *IGH-ID4* are secondary chromosome rearrangements in a proportion of patients, whereas *IGH-BCL2*, *IGH-CEBPA*, *IGH-CEBPB*, and *IGH-CRLF2* are usually the primary rearrangements

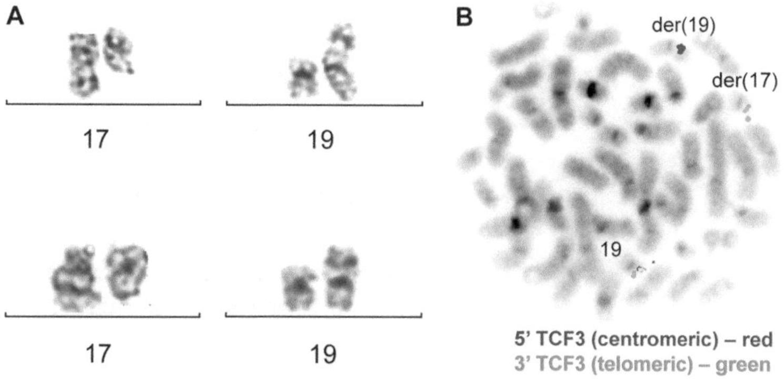

Fig. 4 (**a**) Partial karyograms from two metaphase cells with a t(17;19)(q22;p13.3). (**b**) Metaphase FISH image in inverse DAPI showing the rearrangement of the *TCF3* dual color break-apart probe, with transfer of the 3′ *TCF3* signal to the derivative chromosome 17. The t(17;19) results in *TCF3-HLF* gene fusion

[78]. The presence of an *IGH* gene rearrangement along with other recurrent abnormalities such as the t(9;22) has been reported in a number of patients [81]. Analogous to *IGH-CRLF2* gene rearrangements, a significant proportion of the B-ALL patients with t(8;14)(q11.2;q32)(*IGH-CEBPD*) have Down syndrome [82, 83]. The prognosis of *IGH* gene rearrangements in childhood ALL is uncertain, although the outcome in young adult patients with these rearrangements may be poor [78].

2.13 MYC Gene Rearrangements (8q24)

MYC (8q24) gene rearrangements are a rare but recurrent finding in pediatric B-ALL. Cases involving rearrangement of the *MYC* gene and the *IGH*, *IGK*, and *IGL* at 14q32, 2p12, and 22q11.2, respectively, have been reported [84–86]. The lymphoblasts typically exhibit a precursor B cell immunophenotype, with a FAB L2 or L3 morphology, with no expression of surface immunoglobulin and kappa or lambda light chains. Concurrent *MYC* gene rearrangement along with an additional cytogenetic rearrangement such as *IGH-BCL2* or the t(12;21) has also been observed [85, 87]. Cytogenetic identification and FISH confirmation of *MYC* gene rearrangement is important, as a mature B leukemia/lymphoma treatment protocol may be the appropriate treatment for these patients.

3 T Cell Acute Lymphoblastic Leukemia

3.1 TAL1 Gene Rearrangements (1p32)

The *TAL1* gene is a basic helix loop helix transcription factor that plays a key role in T cell development, and is frequently rearranged in T-ALL. In approximately 20% of T-ALL patients, a 90 kb deletion positions *TAL1* adjacent to the *STIL* gene promoter, resulting

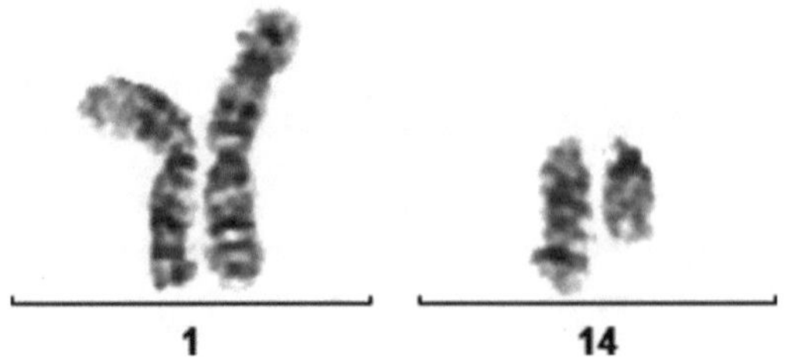

Fig. 5 Partial karyogram of the T-ALL recurrent rearrangement t(1;14)(p32;q11.2) resulting in juxtaposition of the *TCR alpha/delta* and *TAL1* genes

in overexpression of *TAL1*. The deletion is not visible by G-banding, but can be detected by FISH analysis or molecular methods [88, 89]. An additional 6% of patients have the translocations t(1;14)(p32;q11.2) (Fig. 5) or t(1;7)(p32;q34), localizing the *TAL1* gene next to the *TCR alpha/delta* and *TCR beta* genes respectively. T-ALL patients with *TAL1* gene rearrangements have a relatively good outcome [90]. Commercial dual color/dual fusion FISH probes are available for the *TCR alpha/delta* (14q11.2) and *TCR beta* (7q34) genes and these probes can be very useful in the characterization of T-ALL cytogenetic abnormalities [91].

3.2 TLX1 (HOX11) Gene Rearrangements (10q24)

The translocations t(7;10)(q34;q24) and t(10;14)(q24;q11.2) result in the positioning of the *TLX1* homeobox gene (10q24) adjacent to the regulatory regions of the *TCR alpha/delta* gene at 14q11.2 or, less frequently, the *TCR beta* gene at 7q34. The translocation is estimated to occur in approximately 8% of T-ALL cases, and may be associated with a good prognosis [92].

3.3 LMO2 (RBTN2) Gene Rearrangements (11p13)

The *LMO2* gene is a member of the LIM-domain only family of proteins, located at 11p13. Rearrangements involving *LMO2* and the *TCR alpha/delta* and *TCR beta* genes yield the t(11;14)(p13;q11.2) (Fig. 6) and the t(7;11)(q34;p13) [91, 93]. Related genes *LMO1* (11p15) and *LMO3* (12p12) are also recurrently rearranged with the *TCR* genes in T-ALL [6]. Small deletions in 11p12-p13 upstream and centromeric to the *LMO2* gene also result in *LMO2* gene overexpression in approximately 4% of T-ALL patients; however, these deletions are not visible by G-band analysis [94]. The prognosis associated with these *LMO2*, *LMO1*, and *LMO3* gene rearrangements is uncertain.

3.4 t(5;14)(q35;q32)(TLX3-BCL11B)

The translocation t(5;14)(q35;q32) is present in approximately 20% of childhood T-cell ALL [95]. The rearrangement juxtaposes the *TLX3* (*HOX11L2*) gene at 5q35 downstream of the *BCL11B* gene at 14q32, resulting in overexpression of *TLX3*. FISH analysis with a break-apart FISH probe for the *TLX3* gene is required for the detection of the t(5;14), as the rearrangement is not visible by

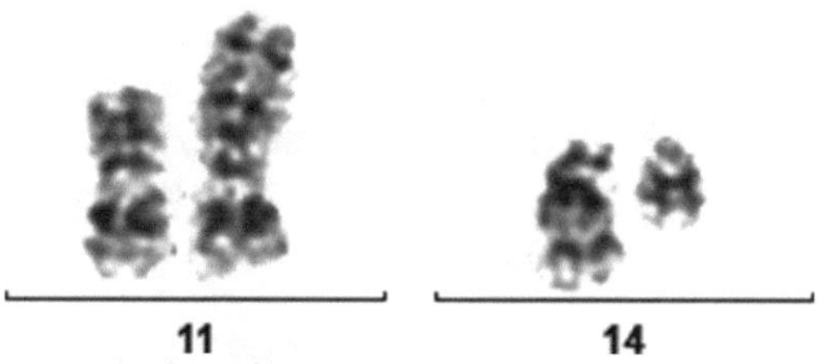

Fig. 6 Partial karyogram of the T-ALL recurrent rearrangement t(11;14)(p13;q11.2) resulting in juxtaposition of the *TCR alpha/delta* and *LMO2* genes

G-band analysis. In a variant t(5;14) rearrangement, the breakpoint on chromosome 5 involves the nearby *NKX2-5* gene, also located at 5q35 [96]. Both the *TLX3* and *NKX2-5* genes are homeobox family transcription factors. Overexpression of the *TLX3* gene has been identified as a poor prognostic indicator and these patients may benefit from more intensive chemotherapy regimens [97].

3.5 MYB Gene Rearrangements (6q23)

The translocation t(6;7)(q23;q34) places the *MYB* oncogene adjacent to the *TCR beta* gene, and occurs with a frequency of approximately 1% in T-ALL [98, 99]. The t(6;7) presents earlier than usual in childhood ALL, at a median age of 2.2 years.

3.6 MYC Gene Rearrangements (8q24)

The t(8;14)(q24.1;q11.2), resulting in the fusion of the *TCR alpha/delta* and the *MYC* genes, is a rare but recurrent abnormality in T-ALL [100]. Rearrangement of *MYC* with non-TCR partners has also been observed in T-ALL patients, as well as the *MYC* gene rearrangements co-occurring with an additional primary T-ALL cytogenetic/molecular genetic abnormality [100].

3.7 t(10;11)(p12;q14)(PICALM-MLLT10, CALM-AF10)

One of the most frequently detected translocations in T-ALL is the recurring t(10;11)(p12;q14) rearrangement resulting in fusion of the *PICALM* (*CALM*;11q14) and *MLLT10* (*AF10*;10p12) genes [101]. This translocation is not specific to T-ALL and may be observed in AML, eosinophilic leukemia, and granulocytic sarcoma [102]. The t(10;11)(*PICALM-MLLT10*) rearrangement has been associated with a poor prognosis in T-ALL [103].

3.8 NUP214-ABL1 Fusion on Amplified Episomes

The *NUP214* gene is located approximately 500 kb distal to the *ABL1* gene at 9q34, and is oriented in the same telomere to centromere direction as the *ABL1* gene. Fusion of the 5′ region of *NUP214* to the 3′ region of the *ABL1* gene occurs by a mechanism that involves a deletion of the 500 kb segment between the genes, with subsequent circularization of the DNA segment and episomal amplification of the resulting fusion gene [104]. The *NUP214-ABL1* gene rearrangement is not detectable by G-banding, but can be observed as *ABL1* gene episomal amplification using commercial *BCR-ABL1* FISH probes. The percentage of nuclei with the episomal amplification can be highly variable, and in some patients the amplified sequence is reintegrated as a homogeneously staining region (hsr) [105].

3.9 KMT2A (MLL) Gene Rearrangements (11q23)

Many of the *KMT2A* gene rearrangements reported in precursor B-ALL and in AML can also be observed in T-ALL [30]. The estimated frequency of *KMT2A* gene rearrangements in T-ALL is 6% [106]. With the exception of the t(11;19), the prognosis for these patients is uncertain. The t(11;19)(q23;p13.3)(*KMT2A-MLLT1*) is the *KMT2A* gene rearrangement most frequently documented in T-ALL, and the prognosis of children with T lineage ALL and the t(11;19) is relatively good [107].

4 Conclusions

Cytogenetic analysis plays a crucial role in the management of ALL patients. Karyotyping combined with FISH analysis identifies recurrent chromosomal abnormalities in ALL, many of which have prognostic and treatment implications. Commercial FISH probes are available for the detection and confirmation of many of the cytogenetic subgroups. Rapid FISH screening with a limited number of probes to detect the principle recurrent cytogenetic categories is a common practice. Follow-up FISH testing for less common chromosomal abnormalities may also be possible based on the results of G-band analysis.

Acknowledgments

I thank Ms. Lindsey Barbieto for assistance with artwork.

References

1. Swerdlow SH, Campo E, Harris NL et al (eds) (2008) WHO classification of tumours of haematopoietic and lymphoid tissues. IARC, Lyon
2. Bloomfield CD, Lindquist LL, Arthur D et al (1981) Chromosomal abnormalities in acute lymphoblastic leukemia. Cancer Res 41(11 Pt 2):4838–4843
3. Harrison CJ (2009) Cytogenetics of paediatric and adolescent acute lymphoblastic leukaemia. Br J Haematol 144(2):147–156. doi:10.1111/j.1365-2141.2008.07417.x
4. Moorman AV (2016) New and emerging prognostic and predictive genetic biomarkers in B-cell precursor acute lymphoblastic leukemia. Haematologica 101(4):407–416. doi:10.3324/haematol.2015.141101
5. Arber DA, Orazi A, Hasserjian R et al (2016) The 2016 revision to the World Health Organization (WHO) classification of myeloid neoplasms and acute leukemia. Blood. doi:10.1182/blood-2016-03-643544
6. Van Vlierberghe P, Ferrando A (2012) The molecular basis of T cell acute lymphoblastic leukemia. J Clin Invest 122(10):3398–3406. doi:10.1172/JCI61269
7. Moorman AV, Richards SM, Martineau M et al (2003) Outcome heterogeneity in childhood high-hyperdiploid acute lymphoblastic

leukemia. Blood 102(8):2756–2762. doi:10.1182/blood-2003-04-1128

8. Heerema NA, Raimondi SC, Anderson JR et al (2007) Specific extra chromosomes occur in a modal number dependent pattern in pediatric acute lymphoblastic leukemia. Genes Chromosomes Cancer 46(7):684–693. doi:10.1002/gcc.20451
9. Sutcliffe MJ, Shuster JJ, Sather HN et al (2005) High concordance from independent studies by the Children's Cancer Group (CCG) and Pediatric Oncology Group (POG) associating favorable prognosis with combined trisomies 4, 10, and 17 in children with NCI Standard-Risk B-precursor Acute Lymphoblastic Leukemia: a Children's Oncology Group (COG) initiative. Leukemia 19(5):734–740. doi:10.1038/sj.leu.2403673
10. Paulsson K, Harrison CJ, Andersen MK et al (2013) Distinct patterns of gained chromosomes in high hyperdiploid acute lymphoblastic leukemia with t(1;19)(q23;p13), t(9;22)(q34;q22) or MLL rearrangements. Leukemia 27(4):974–977. doi:10.1038/leu.2012.263
11. Douet-Guilbert N, Morel F, Le Bris MJ et al (2003) A fluorescence in situ hybridization study of TEL-AML1 fusion gene in B-cell acute lymphoblastic leukemia (1984-2001). Cancer Genet Cytogenet 144(2):143–147
12. Attarbaschi A, Mann G, Konig M et al (2004) Incidence and relevance of secondary chromosome abnormalities in childhood TEL/AML1+ acute lymphoblastic leukemia: an interphase FISH analysis. Leukemia 18(10):1611–1616. doi:10.1038/sj.leu.2403471
13. Al-Shehhi H, Konn ZJ, Schwab CJ et al (2013) Abnormalities of the der(12)t(12;21) in ETV6-RUNX1 acute lymphoblastic leukemia. Genes Chromosomes Cancer 52(2):202–213. doi:10.1002/gcc.22021
14. Reddy KS, Yang X, Mak L et al (2000) A child with ALL and ETV6/AML1 fusion on a chromosome 12 due to an insertion of AML1 and loss of ETV6 from the homolog involved in a t(12;15)(p13;q15). Genes Chromosomes Cancer 29(2):106–109
15. Forestier E, Andersen MK, Autio K et al (2007) Cytogenetic patterns in ETV6/RUNX1-positive pediatric B-cell precursor acute lymphoblastic leukemia: a Nordic series of 245 cases and review of the literature. Genes Chromosomes Cancer 46(5):440–450. doi:10.1002/gcc.20423
16. Attarbaschi A, Mann G, Konig M et al (2006) Near-tetraploidy in childhood B-cell precursor acute lymphoblastic leukemia is a highly specific feature of ETV6/RUNX1-positive leukemic cases. Genes Chromosomes Cancer 45(6):608–611. doi:10.1002/gcc.20324
17. Raimondi SC, Zhou Y, Shurtleff SA et al (2006) Near-triploidy and near-tetraploidy in childhood acute lymphoblastic leukemia: association with B-lineage blast cells carrying the ETV6-RUNX1 fusion, T-lineage immunophenotype, and favorable outcome. Cancer Genet Cytogenet 169(1):50–57. doi:10.1016/j.cancergencyto.2006.04.006
18. Mullighan CG, Su X, Zhang J et al (2009) Deletion of IKZF1 and prognosis in acute lymphoblastic leukemia. N Engl J Med 360(5):470–480. doi:10.1056/NEJMoa0808253
19. Den Boer ML, van Slegtenhorst M, De Menezes RX et al (2009) A subtype of childhood acute lymphoblastic leukaemia with poor treatment outcome: a genome-wide classification study. Lancet Oncol 10(2):125–134. doi:10.1016/S1470-2045(08)70339-5
20. Roberts KG, Li Y, Payne-Turner D et al (2014) Targetable kinase-activating lesions in Ph-like acute lymphoblastic leukemia. N Engl J Med 371(11):1005–1015. doi:10.1056/NEJMoa1403088
21. Roberts KG, Morin RD, Zhang J et al (2012) Genetic alterations activating kinase and cytokine receptor signaling in high-risk acute lymphoblastic leukemia. Cancer Cell 22(2):153–166. doi:10.1016/j.ccr.2012.06.005
22. Harvey RC, Mullighan CG, Chen IM et al (2010) Rearrangement of CRLF2 is associated with mutation of JAK kinases, alteration of IKZF1, Hispanic/Latino ethnicity, and a poor outcome in pediatric B-progenitor acute lymphoblastic leukemia. Blood 115(26):5312–5321. doi:10.1182/blood-2009-09-245944
23. Buitenkamp TD, Pieters R, Gallimore NE et al (2012) Outcome in children with Down's syndrome and acute lymphoblastic leukemia: role of IKZF1 deletions and CRLF2 aberrations. Leukemia 26(10):2204–2211. doi:10.1038/leu.2012.84
24. Kobayashi K, Mitsui K, Ichikawa H et al (2014) ATF7IP as a novel PDGFRB fusion partner in acute lymphoblastic leukaemia in children. Br J Haematol 165(6):836–841. doi:10.1111/bjh.12834
25. Reiter A, Walz C, Watmore A et al (2005) The t(8;9)(p22;p24) is a recurrent abnormality in chronic and acute leukemia that fuses PCM1 to JAK2. Cancer Res 65(7):2662–2667. doi:10.1158/0008-5472.CAN-04-4263
26. Yano M, Imamura T, Asai D et al (2015) Identification of novel kinase fusion transcripts in paediatric B cell precursor acute lymphoblastic leukaemia with IKZF1 dele-

tion. Br J Haematol 171(5):813–817. doi:10.1111/bjh.13757
27. De Braekeleer E, Douet-Guilbert N, Rowe D et al (2011) ABL1 fusion genes in hematological malignancies: a review. Eur J Haematol 86(5):361–371. doi:10.1111/j.1600-0609.2011.01586.x
28. Ernst T, Score J, Deininger M et al (2011) Identification of FOXP1 and SNX2 as novel ABL1 fusion partners in acute lymphoblastic leukaemia. Br J Haematol 153(1):43–46. doi:10.1111/j.1365-2141.2010.08457.x
29. Kawamura M, Taki T, Kaku H et al (2015) Identification of SPAG9 as a novel JAK2 fusion partner gene in pediatric acute lymphoblastic leukemia with t(9;17)(p24;q21). Genes Chromosomes Cancer 54(7):401–408. doi:10.1002/gcc.22251
30. Meyer C, Hofmann J, Burmeister T et al (2013) The MLL recombinome of acute leukemias in 2013. Leukemia 27(11):2165–2176. doi:10.1038/leu.2013.135
31. Huret J (2003) 11q23 rearrangements in leukaemia. Atlas Genet Cytogenet Oncol Haematol 7(4):255–259
32. Hilden JM, Dinndorf PA, Meerbaum SO et al (2006) Analysis of prognostic factors of acute lymphoblastic leukemia in infants: report on CCG 1953 from the Children's Oncology Group. Blood 108(2):441–451. doi:10.1182/blood-2005-07-3011
33. Van Limbergen H, Poppe B, Janssens A et al (2002) Molecular cytogenetic analysis of 10;11 rearrangements in acute myeloid leukemia. Leukemia 16(3):344–351. doi:10.1038/sj.leu.2402397
34. Moorman AV, Raimondi SC, Pui CH et al (2005) No prognostic effect of additional chromosomal abnormalities in children with acute lymphoblastic leukemia and 11q23 abnormalities. Leukemia 19(4):557–563. doi:10.1038/sj.leu.2403695
35. Kamps MP, Murre C, Sun XH et al (1990) A new homeobox gene contributes the DNA binding domain of the t(1;19) translocation protein in pre-B ALL. Cell 60(4):547–555
36. Nourse J, Mellentin JD, Galili N et al (1990) Chromosomal translocation t(1;19) results in synthesis of a homeobox fusion mRNA that codes for a potential chimeric transcription factor. Cell 60(4):535–545
37. Andersen MK, Autio K, Barbany G et al (2011) Paediatric B-cell precursor acute lymphoblastic leukaemia with t(1;19)(q23;p13): clinical and cytogenetic characteristics of 47 cases from the Nordic countries treated according to NOPHO protocols. Br J Haematol 155(2):235–243. doi:10.1111/j.1365-2141.2011.08824.x
38. Secker-Walker LM, Berger R, Fenaux P et al (1992) Prognostic significance of the balanced t(1;19) and unbalanced der(19)t(1;19) translocations in acute lymphoblastic leukemia. Leukemia 6(5):363–369
39. Felice MS, Gallego MS, Alonso CN et al (2011) Prognostic impact of t(1;19)/ TCF3-PBX1 in childhood acute lymphoblastic leukemia in the context of Berlin-Frankfurt-Munster-based protocols. Leuk Lymphoma 52(7):1215–1221. doi:10.3109/10428194.2011.565436
40. Asai D, Imamura T, Yamashita Y et al (2014) Outcome of TCF3-PBX1 positive pediatric acute lymphoblastic leukemia patients in Japan: a collaborative study of Japan Association of Childhood Leukemia Study (JACLS) and Children's Cancer and Leukemia Study Group (CCLSG). Cancer Med 3(3):623–631. doi:10.1002/cam4.221
41. Schultz KR, Carroll A, Heerema NA et al (2014) Long-term follow-up of imatinib in pediatric Philadelphia chromosome-positive acute lymphoblastic leukemia: Children's Oncology Group study AALL0031. Leukemia 28(7):1467–1471. doi:10.1038/leu.2014.30
42. Heerema NA, Harbott J, Galimberti S et al (2004) Secondary cytogenetic aberrations in childhood Philadelphia chromosome positive acute lymphoblastic leukemia are nonrandom and may be associated with outcome. Leukemia 18(4):693–702. doi:10.1038/sj.leu.2403324
43. Robinson HM, Martineau M, Harris RL et al (2005) Derivative chromosome 9 deletions are a significant feature of childhood Philadelphia chromosome positive acute lymphoblastic leukaemia. Leukemia 19(4):564–571. doi:10.1038/sj.leu.2403629
44. Harrison CJ, Moorman AV, Broadfield ZJ et al (2004) Three distinct subgroups of hypodiploidy in acute lymphoblastic leukaemia. Br J Haematol 125(5):552–559. doi:10.1111/j.1365-2141.2004.04948.x
45. Heerema NA, Nachman JB, Sather HN et al (1999) Hypodiploidy with less than 45 chromosomes confers adverse risk in childhood acute lymphoblastic leukemia: a report from the children's cancer group. Blood 94(12):4036–4045
46. Raimondi SC, Zhou Y, Mathew S et al (2003) Reassessment of the prognostic significance of hypodiploidy in pediatric patients with acute lymphoblastic leukemia. Cancer 98(12):2715–2722. doi:10.1002/cncr.11841
47. Holmfeldt L, Wei L, Diaz-Flores E et al (2013) The genomic landscape of hypodiploid acute lymphoblastic leukemia. Nat Genet 45(3):242–252. doi:10.1038/ng.2532

48. Muhlbacher V, Zenger M, Schnittger S et al (2014) Acute lymphoblastic leukemia with low hypodiploid/near triploid karyotype is a specific clinical entity and exhibits a very high TP53 mutation frequency of 93%. Genes Chromosomes Cancer 53(6):524–536. doi:10.1002/gcc.22163
49. Safavi S, Forestier E, Golovleva I et al (2013) Loss of chromosomes is the primary event in near-haploid and low-hypodiploid acute lymphoblastic leukemia. Leukemia 27(1):248–250. doi:10.1038/leu.2012.227
50. Baughn LB, Biegel JA, South ST et al (2015) Integration of cytogenomic data for furthering the characterization of pediatric B-cell acute lymphoblastic leukemia: a multi-institution, multi-platform microarray study. Cancer Genet 208(1-2):1–18. doi:10.1016/j.cancergen.2014.11.003
51. Busson-Le Coniat M, Nguyen Khac F, Daniel MT et al (2001) Chromosome 21 abnormalities with AML1 amplification in acute lymphoblastic leukemia. Genes Chromosomes Cancer 32(3):244–249
52. Niini T, Kanerva J, Vettenranta K et al (2000) AML1 gene amplification: a novel finding in childhood acute lymphoblastic leukemia. Haematologica 85(4):362–366
53. Harewood L, Robinson H, Harris R et al (2003) Amplification of AML1 on a duplicated chromosome 21 in acute lymphoblastic leukemia: a study of 20 cases. Leukemia 17(3):547–553. doi:10.1038/sj.leu.2402849
54. Harrison CJ, Moorman AV, Schwab C et al (2014) An international study of intrachromosomal amplification of chromosome 21 (iAMP21): cytogenetic characterization and outcome. Leukemia 28(5):1015–1021. doi:10.1038/leu.2013.317
55. Rand V, Parker H, Russell LJ et al (2011) Genomic characterization implicates iAMP21 as a likely primary genetic event in childhood B-cell precursor acute lymphoblastic leukemia. Blood 117(25):6848–6855. doi:10.1182/blood-2011-01-329961
56. Robinson HM, Broadfield ZJ, Cheung KL et al (2003) Amplification of AML1 in acute lymphoblastic leukemia is associated with a poor outcome. Leukemia 17(11):2249–2250. doi:10.1038/sj.leu.2403140
57. Attarbaschi A, Mann G, Panzer-Grumayer R et al (2008) Minimal residual disease values discriminate between low and high relapse risk in children with B-cell precursor acute lymphoblastic leukemia and an intrachromosomal amplification of chromosome 21: the Austrian and German acute lymphoblastic leukemia Berlin-Frankfurt-Munster (ALL-BFM) trials. J Clin Oncol 26(18):3046–3050. doi:10.1200/JCO.2008.16.1117
58. Heerema NA, Carroll AJ, Devidas M et al (2013) Intrachromosomal amplification of chromosome 21 is associated with inferior outcomes in children with acute lymphoblastic leukemia treated in contemporary standard-risk children's oncology group studies: a report from the children's oncology group. J Clin Oncol 31(27):3397–3402. doi:10.1200/JCO.2013.49.1308
59. Li Y, Schwab C, Ryan SL et al (2014) Constitutional and somatic rearrangement of chromosome 21 in acute lymphoblastic leukaemia. Nature 508(7494):98–102. doi:10.1038/nature13115
60. Martini A, La Starza R, Janssen H et al (2002) Recurrent rearrangement of the Ewing's sarcoma gene, EWSR1, or its homologue, TAF15, with the transcription factor CIZ/NMP4 in acute leukemia. Cancer Res 62(19):5408–5412
61. La Starza R, Aventin A, Crescenzi B et al (2005) CIZ gene rearrangements in acute leukemia: report of a diagnostic FISH assay and clinical features of nine patients. Leukemia 19(9):1696–1699. doi:10.1038/sj.leu.2403842
62. Zhong CH, Prima V, Liang X et al (2008) E2A-ZNF384 and NOL1-E2A fusion created by a cryptic t(12;19)(p13.3; p13.3) in acute leukemia. Leukemia 22(4):723–729. doi:10.1038/sj.leu.2405084
63. Nyquist KB, Thorsen J, Zeller B et al (2011) Identification of the TAF15-ZNF384 fusion gene in two new cases of acute lymphoblastic leukemia with a t(12;17)(p13;q12). Cancer Genet 204(3):147–152. doi:10.1016/j.cancergen.2011.01.003
64. Grammatico S, Vitale A, La Starza R et al (2013) Lineage switch from pro-B acute lymphoid leukemia to acute myeloid leukemia in a case with t(12;17)(p13;q11)/TAF15-ZNF384 rearrangement. Leuk Lymphoma 54(8):1802–1805. doi:10.3109/10428194.2012.753450
65. Gocho Y, Kiyokawa N, Ichikawa H et al (2015) A novel recurrent EP300-ZNF384 gene fusion in B-cell precursor acute lymphoblastic leukemia. Leukemia 29(12):2445–2448. doi:10.1038/leu.2015.111
66. Krance RA, Raimondi SC, Dubowy R et al (1992) t(12;17)(p13;q21) in early pre-B acute lymphoid leukemia. Leukemia 6(4):251–255
67. Barber KE, Harrison CJ, Broadfield ZJ et al (2007) Molecular cytogenetic characterization of TCF3 (E2A)/19p13.3 rearrangements in B-cell precursor acute lymphoblastic

leukemia. Genes Chromosomes Cancer 46(5):478–486. doi:10.1002/gcc.20431

68. Forestier E, Gauffin F, Andersen MK et al (2008) Clinical and cytogenetic features of pediatric dic(9;20)(p13.2;q11.2)-positive B-cell precursor acute lymphoblastic leukemias: a Nordic series of 24 cases and review of the literature. Genes Chromosomes Cancer 47(2):149–158. doi:10.1002/gcc.20517
69. Pichler H, Moricke A, Mann G et al (2010) Prognostic relevance of dic(9;20)(p11;q13) in childhood B-cell precursor acute lymphoblastic leukaemia treated with Berlin-Frankfurt-Munster (BFM) protocols containing an intensive induction and post-induction consolidation therapy. Br J Haematol 149(1):93–100.doi:10.1111/j.1365-2141.2009.08059.x
70. Clark R, Byatt SA, Bennett CF et al (2000) Monosomy 20 as a pointer to dicentric (9;20) in acute lymphoblastic leukemia. Leukemia 14(2):241–246
71. Heerema NA, Maben KD, Bernstein J et al (1996) Dicentric (9;20)(p11;q11) identified by fluorescence in situ hybridization in four pediatric acute lymphoblastic leukemia patients. Cancer Genet Cytogenet 92(2):111–115
72. Schoumans J, Johansson B, Corcoran M et al (2006) Characterisation of dic(9;20)(p11-13;q11) in childhood B-cell precursor acute lymphoblastic leukaemia by tiling resolution array-based comparative genomic hybridisation reveals clustered breakpoints at 9p13.2 and 20q11.2. Br J Haematol 135(4):492–499. doi:10.1111/j.1365-2141.2006.06328.x
73. An Q, Wright SL, Moorman AV et al (2009) Heterogeneous breakpoints in patients with acute lymphoblastic leukemia and the dic(9;20)(p11-13;q11) show recurrent involvement of genes at 20q11.21. Haematologica 94(8):1164–1169. doi:10.3324/haematol.2008.002808
74. Inaba T, Roberts WM, Shapiro LH et al (1992) Fusion of the leucine zipper gene HLF to the E2A gene in human acute B-lineage leukemia. Science 257(5069):531–534
75. Hunger SP, Ohyashiki K, Toyama K et al (1992) Hlf, a novel hepatic bZIP protein, shows altered DNA-binding properties following fusion to E2A in t(17;19) acute lymphoblastic leukemia. Genes Dev 6(9):1608–1620
76. Yeung J, Kempski H, Neat M et al (2006) Characterization of the t(17;19) translocation by gene-specific fluorescent in situ hybridization-based cytogenetics and detection of the E2A-HLF fusion transcript and protein in patients' cells. Haematologica 91(3):422–424
77. Minson KA, Prasad P, Vear S et al. (2013) t(17;19) in children with acute lymphocytic leukemia: a report of 3 cases and a review of the literature. Case Rep Hematol 2013: 563291. doi:10.1155/2013/563291
78. Russell LJ, Enshaei A, Jones L et al (2014) IGH@ translocations are prevalent in teenagers and young adults with acute lymphoblastic leukemia and are associated with a poor outcome. J Clin Oncol 32(14):1453–1462. doi:10.1200/JCO.2013.51.3242
79. Akasaka T, Balasas T, Russell LJ et al (2007) Five members of the CEBP transcription factor family are targeted by recurrent IGH translocations in B-cell precursor acute lymphoblastic leukemia (BCP-ALL). Blood 109(8):3451–3461. doi:10.1182/blood-2006-08-041012
80. Chapiro E, Radford-Weiss I, Cung HA et al (2013) Chromosomal translocations involving the IGH@ locus in B-cell precursor acute lymphoblastic leukemia: 29 new cases and a review of the literature. Cancer Genet 206(5):162–173. doi:10.1016/j.cancergen.2013.04.004
81. Jeffries SJ, Jones L, Harrison CJ et al (2014) IGH@ translocations co-exist with other primary rearrangements in B-cell precursor acute lymphoblastic leukemia. Haematologica 99(8):1334–1342. doi:10.3324/haematol.2014.103820
82. Lundin C, Heldrup J, Ahlgren T et al (2009) B-cell precursor t(8;14)(q11;q32)-positive acute lymphoblastic leukemia in children is strongly associated with Down syndrome or with a concomitant Philadelphia chromosome. Eur J Haematol 82(1):46–53. doi:10.1111/j.1600-0609.2008.01166.x
83. Messinger YH, Higgins RR, Devidas M et al (2012) Pediatric acute lymphoblastic leukemia with a t(8;14)(q11.2;q32): B-cell disease with a high proportion of Down syndrome: a Children's Oncology Group study. Cancer Genet 205(9):453–458. doi:10.1016/j.cancergen.2012.07.016
84. Navid F, Mosijczuk AD, Head DR et al (1999) Acute lymphoblastic leukemia with the (8;14)(q24;q32) translocation and FAB L3 morphology associated with a B-precursor immunophenotype: the Pediatric Oncology Group experience. Leukemia 13(1):135–141
85. Loh ML, Samson Y, Motte E et al (2000) Translocation (2;8)(p12;q24) associated with a cryptic t(12;21)(p13;q22) TEL/AML1 gene rearrangement in a child with acute lymphoblastic leukemia. Cancer Genet Cytogenet 122(2):79–82
86. Gupta AA, Grant R, Shago M et al (2004) Occurrence of t(8;22)(q24.1;q11.2) involving the MYC locus in a case of pediatric acute lymphoblastic leukemia with a precursor B cell immunophenotype. J Pediatr Hematol Oncol 26(8):532–534

87. Liu W, Hu S, Konopleva M et al (2015) De novo MYC and BCL2 double-hit B-cell precursor acute lymphoblastic leukemia (BCP-ALL) in pediatric and young adult patients associated with poor prognosis. Pediatr Hematol Oncol 32(8):535–547. doi:10.3109/08880018.2015.1087611
88. van der Burg M, Smit B, Brinkhof B et al (2002) A single split-signal FISH probe set allows detection of TAL1 translocations as well as SIL-TAL1 fusion genes in a single test. Leukemia 16(4):755–761. doi:10.1038/sj.leu.2402432
89. D'Angio M, Valsecchi MG, Testi AM et al (2015) Clinical features and outcome of SIL/TAL1-positive T-cell acute lymphoblastic leukemia in children and adolescents: a 10-year experience of the AIEOP group. Haematologica 100(1):e10–e13. doi:10.3324/haematol.2014.112151
90. Bash RO, Crist WM, Shuster JJ et al (1993) Clinical features and outcome of T-cell acute lymphoblastic leukemia in childhood with respect to alterations at the TAL1 locus: a Pediatric Oncology Group study. Blood 81(8):2110–2117
91. Cauwelier B, Dastugue N, Cools J et al (2006) Molecular cytogenetic study of 126 unselected T-ALL cases reveals high incidence of TCRbeta locus rearrangements and putative new T-cell oncogenes. Leukemia 20(7):1238–1244. doi:10.1038/sj.leu.2404243
92. Ferrando AA, Neuberg DS, Dodge RK et al (2004) Prognostic importance of TLX1 (HOX11) oncogene expression in adults with T-cell acute lymphoblastic leukaemia. Lancet 363(9408):535–536. doi:10.1016/S0140-6736(04)15542-6
93. Schneider NR, Carroll AJ, Shuster JJ et al (2000) New recurring cytogenetic abnormalities and association of blast cell karyotypes with prognosis in childhood T-cell acute lymphoblastic leukemia: a pediatric oncology group report of 343 cases. Blood 96(7):2543–2549
94. Van Vlierberghe P, van Grotel M, Beverloo HB et al (2006) The cryptic chromosomal deletion del(11)(p12p13) as a new activation mechanism of LMO2 in pediatric T-cell acute lymphoblastic leukemia. Blood 108(10):3520–3529. doi:10.1182/blood-2006-04-019927
95. Bernard OA, Busson-LeConiat M, Ballerini P et al (2001) A new recurrent and specific cryptic translocation, t(5;14)(q35;q32), is associated with expression of the Hox11L2 gene in T acute lymphoblastic leukemia. Leukemia 15(10):1495–1504
96. Nagel S, Kaufmann M, Drexler HG et al (2003) The cardiac homeobox gene NKX2-5 is deregulated by juxtaposition with BCL11B in pediatric T-ALL cell lines via a novel t(5;14)(q35.1;q32.2). Cancer Res 63(17):5329–5334
97. Attarbaschi A, Pisecker M, Inthal A et al (2010) Prognostic relevance of TLX3 (HOX11L2) expression in childhood T-cell acute lymphoblastic leukaemia treated with Berlin-Frankfurt-Munster (BFM) protocols containing early and late re-intensification elements. Br J Haematol 148(2):293–300. doi:10.1111/j.1365-2141.2009.07944.x
98. Clappier E, Cuccuini W, Kalota A et al (2007) The C-MYB locus is involved in chromosomal translocation and genomic duplications in human T-cell acute leukemia (T-ALL), the translocation defining a new T-ALL subtype in very young children. Blood 110(4):1251–1261. doi:10.1182/blood-2006-12-064683
99. Le Noir S, Ben Abdelali R, Lelorch M et al (2012) Extensive molecular mapping of TCRalpha/delta- and TCRbeta-involved chromosomal translocations reveals distinct mechanisms of oncogene activation in T-ALL. Blood 120(16):3298–3309. doi:10.1182/blood-2012-04-425488
100. La Starza R, Borga C, Barba G et al (2014) Genetic profile of T-cell acute lymphoblastic leukemias with MYC translocations. Blood 124(24):3577–3582. doi:10.1182/blood-2014-06-578856
101. Asnafi V, Radford-Weiss I, Dastugue N et al (2003) CALM-AF10 is a common fusion transcript in T-ALL and is specific to the TCRgammadelta lineage. Blood 102(3):1000–1006. doi:10.1182/blood-2002-09-2913
102. Caudell D, Aplan PD (2008) The role of CALM-AF10 gene fusion in acute leukemia. Leukemia 22(4):678–685. doi:10.1038/sj.leu.2405074
103. van Grotel M, Meijerink JP, van Wering ER et al (2008) Prognostic significance of molecular-cytogenetic abnormalities in pediatric T-ALL is not explained by immunophenotypic differences. Leukemia 22(1):124–131. doi:10.1038/sj.leu.2404957
104. Graux C, Cools J, Melotte C et al (2004) Fusion of NUP214 to ABL1 on amplified episomes in T-cell acute lymphoblastic leukemia. Nat Genet 36(10):1084–1089. doi:10.1038/ng1425

105. Graux C, Stevens-Kroef M, Lafage M et al (2009) Heterogeneous patterns of amplification of the NUP214-ABL1 fusion gene in T-cell acute lymphoblastic leukemia. Leukemia 23(1):125–133. doi:10.1038/leu.2008.278

106. Karrman K, Forestier E, Heyman M et al (2009) Clinical and cytogenetic features of a population-based consecutive series of 285 pediatric T-cell acute lymphoblastic leukemias: rare T-cell receptor gene rearrangements are associated with poor outcome. Genes Chromosomes Cancer 48(9):795–805. doi:10.1002/gcc.20684

107. Pui CH, Chessells JM, Camitta B et al (2003) Clinical heterogeneity in childhood acute lymphoblastic leukemia with 11q23 rearrangements. Leukemia 17(4):700–706. doi:10.1038/sj.leu.2402883

Chapter 22

Recurrent Cytogenetic Abnormalities in Non-Hodgkin's Lymphoma and Chronic Lymphocytic Leukemia

Edmond S.K. Ma

Abstract

Characteristic chromosomal translocations are found to be associated with subtypes of B-cell non-Hodgkin lymphoma (NHL), for example t(8;14)(q24;q32) and Burkitt lymphoma, t(14;18)(q32;q21) and follicular lymphoma, and t(11;14)(q13;q32) in mantle cell lymphoma. Only few recurrent cytogenetic aberrations have been identified in the T-cell NHL and the best known is the *ALK* gene translocation t(2;5)(p23;q35) in anaplastic large cell lymphoma. Since lymph node or other tissue is seldom submitted for conventional cytogenetics study, alternative approaches for translocation detection are polymerase chain reaction (PCR) or fluorescence in situ hybridization (FISH). FISH is more sensitive than PCR in the detection of lymphoma translocations since directly labeled large FISH probes that span the translocation breakpoints are used. Although the recurrent chromosomal abnormalities in NHL are not completely sensitive and specific for disease entities, unlike the scenario in acute leukemia, cytogenetic and molecular genetic study is commonly used to aid lymphoma diagnosis and classification. Currently, the main clinical utility is in the employment of interphase FISH panels to predict disease aggressiveness to guide therapy, for example identification of double-hit lymphoma, or in prognostication, for example risk-stratification in chronic lymphocytic leukemia. The recent application of high-throughput sequencing to NHL not only advances the understanding of disease pathogenesis and classification, but allows the discovery of new drug targets, such as *BRAF* gene inhibition in hairy cell leukemia. Coupled with the increasing availability of novel molecular targeted therapeutic agents, the hope for the future is to translate the genetics and genomics information to achieve personalized medicine in NHL.

Key words Cytogenetics, Chromosomal translocation, Non-Hodgkin lymphoma, FISH, PCR, Diagnosis, Classification, Prognosis, Molecular targeted therapy, Personalized medicine

1 Introduction

The diagnosis and classification of non-Hodgkin lymphoma (NHL) requires the integration of clinical feature in conjunction with the results of morphology, immunophenotype, and genetic study [1]. Characteristic chromosomal translocations are found to be associated with subtypes of NHL, for example t(8;14)(q24;q32) and Burkitt lymphoma, t(14;18)(q32;q21) and follicular lymphoma, and t(11;14)(q13;q32) in mantle cell lymphoma. However,

Thomas S.K. Wan (ed.), *Cancer Cytogenetics: Methods and Protocols*, Methods in Molecular Biology, vol. 1541,
DOI 10.1007/978-1-4939-6703-2_22, © Springer Science+Business Media LLC 2017

unlike the situation in the acute leukemia in which chromosomal translocations define disease entities, such as t(15;17)(q22;q12) and acute promyelocytic leukemia, the chromosomal translocations in NHL are neither completely sensitive nor specific for a disease entity. For example, around 10% of follicular lymphoma is negative for t(14;18)(q32;q21) and around 5–10% of mantle cell lymphoma is negative for t(11;14)(q13;q32). The absence of the aforementioned translocations does not negate the corresponding NHL diagnosis if other features are compatible. Conversely, the t(14;18)(q32;q21) and t(8;14)(q24;q32) can be found in diffuse large B-cell lymphoma (DLBCL) and t(11;14)(q13;q32) can be found in plasma cell myeloma. This notwithstanding, detection of recurrent chromosomal abnormality is still an important investigation in NHL. This chapter is an update on the landscape of recurrent chromosomal abnormalities in NHL and their application in disease diagnosis, classification, and prognostication.

2 B-cell Lymphoma

The standard method to detect recurrent chromosomal translocations in B-cell lymphoma such as the t(14;18)(q32;q21) in follicular lymphoma or t(11;14)(q13;q32) in mantle cell lymphoma is by conventional cytogenetics. Nevertheless, lymph node or other tissue is seldom submitted for metaphase karyotype study. Alternative approaches for translocation detection are polymerase chain reaction (PCR) or fluorescence in situ hybridization (FISH). Even with standardized protocol, PCR assay is unable to cover all the translocation breakpoints. For example, FISH is more sensitive than PCR to detect t(14;18)(q32;q21) *IGH-BCL2* [2, 3] because the use of two upstream BCL2 primers can cover only around 75% of the translocations. Similarly, the use of one upstream *BCL1/*MTC primer can cover only around 41% of the t(11;14)(q13;q32) *IGH-BCL1* in mantle cell lymphoma [4]. The addition of other primers can improve the detection rate but also increases the complexity of testing. In contrast, the FISH probes that are utilized for diagnostic testing are typically directly labeled large probes that span the translocation breakpoints. Therefore, in the routine diagnostic setting, FISH is preferred over PCR for the detection of lymphoma translocations. Interphase FISH with a panel of probes is also commonly used for prognostication in chronic lymphocytic leukemia (CLL).

2.1 Chromosomal Abnormalities and Prognosis in CLL

Genetic aberrations in CLL are important independent predictors of disease progression and survival [5]. Conventional cytogenetics shows a low frequency of abnormalities but may be improved by the use of CpG-oligodeoxynucleotides and IL-2, which yields a detection rate of around one-third [6]. Although no chromosomal translocation is specific to CLL, patients having translocation show significantly shorter median treatment-free survival and significantly inferior overall survival [6]. The most frequent and clinically relevant chromosomal abnormalities in CLL are del(13q), trisomy 12, del(11q)/*ATM*, and del (17p)/*TP53*. Patients with a normal karyotype or deletion of 13q14 as a sole cytogenetic abnormality show a better prognosis than those with a complex karyotype or deletion of 11q23 or 17p13. The response to treatment is significantly higher in patients with normal karyotype than abnormal karyotypes, especially with complex changes.

In the routine diagnostic setting, an interphase FISH panel is applied to CLL and usually covers del(13q), trisomy 12, del(11q)/*ATM*, and del (17p)/*TP53* (Fig. 1). Among the categories of del(17p), del(11q), trisomy 12, normal karyotype, and del(13q) as the sole abnormality, the median survival times are 32, 79, 114, 111, and 133 months, respectively [5]. Patients in the del(17p) and del(11q) groups show more advanced disease than those in the other three groups. The shortest median treatment-free interval of 9 months is seen in del(17p) and the longest of 92

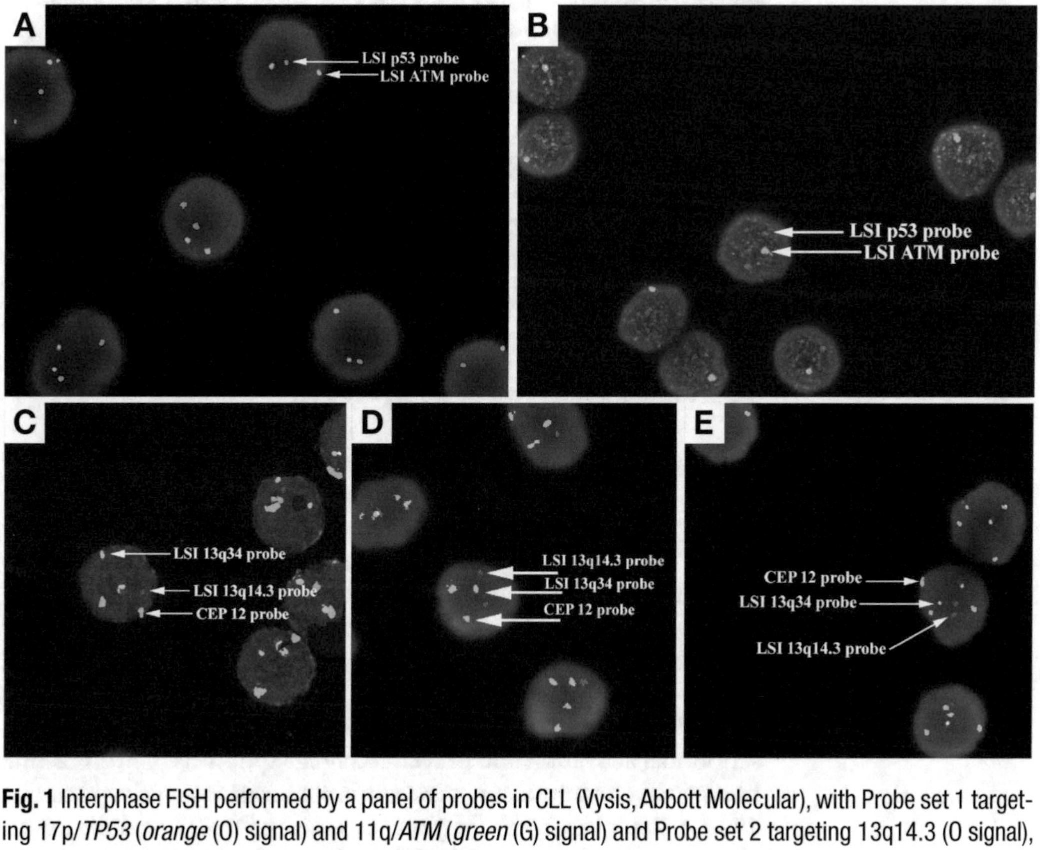

Fig. 1 Interphase FISH performed by a panel of probes in CLL (Vysis, Abbott Molecular), with Probe set 1 targeting 17p/*TP53* (*orange* (O) signal) and 11q/*ATM* (*green* (G) signal) and Probe set 2 targeting 13q14.3 (O signal), 13q34 (aqua (A) signal), and chromosome 12 (G signal). (**a**) Del(17p)/*TP53*, showing 1O2G signal pattern. (**b**) Del(11q)/*ATM*, showing 1G2O signal pattern. (**c**) Del(13q14), showing 1O2G2A signal pattern. (**d**) Del(13q34), showing 2O2G1A signal pattern. (**e**) Trisomy 12, showing 2O3G2A signal pattern

months is seen in del(13q). Response to rituximab also varies by cytogenetic group, which is 0% in del(17p), 66% in del(11q), 86% in del(13q), and 25% in +12 [7].

Deletion of chromosome 13q14 is the most frequent cytogenetic change in CLL, occurring in around 55% of cases and associated with a favorable prognosis in the absence of other high-risk genetic factors. There is apparently no prognostic difference between monoallelic and biallelic deletion of 13q, and both groups can be similarly categorized [8]. Trisomy 12 is detected in around 16% of cases and often associated with atypical morphological features but a neutral prognostic impact. Deletion of chromosome 11q23 involving the *ATM* gene, reported in around 18% of cases, identifies patients with extensive lymphadenopathy, rapid disease progression, and inferior survival. Deletion of 17p13 involving the *TP53* gene, seen in around 7% of cases, predicts for poor survival and resistance to treatment. Recently, it has been shown that *TP53* mutations carry a poor prognosis in CLL regardless of the presence of del(17p) when treated with fludarabine-based chemotherapy [9]. Therefore, evaluation of *TP53* status in CLL should include both del(17p) by FISH ± cytogenetics and *TP53* mutation study. Alemtuzumab may be an effective therapy for patients with CLL with TP53 mutations or deletions, or both [10].

These genetic markers are evaluated togther with other prognostic markers within the context of clinical trials. A comprehensive prognostic index for CLL is proposed that uses five independent factors to predict for overall survival, namely age, clinical stage, del(17p) and/or *TP53* mutation, *IGVH* mutation status, and β2-microglobulin [11]. However, this index is based on chemo-immunotherapy trials and may not be applicable to the advent of novel agents such as ibrutinib or idelalisib. From the laboratory perspective, it is important to cover del(17p), *TP53* mutation, and *IGVH* mutation testing in CLL patients.

2.2 Common Recurrent Chromosomal Translocations in B-cell Lymphoma

Recurrent chromosomal translocations in B-cell lymphoma commonly involve the *IGH* gene locus at chromosome 14q32 and fusion partner genes that play a role in important cell biology processes. Examples of common recurrent chromosomal translocations in B-cell lymphoma are listed in Table 1.

The t(14;18)(q32;q21) is the cytogenetic hallmark of follicular lymphoma (FL) and occurs in 80-90% of cases. The translocation results in the juxtaposition of the *BCL2* oncogene to the *IGH* locus, which results in overexpression of BCL2 because of transcriptional activation and prevents cellular apoptosis. Chromosome breakpoints mainly occur at two different locations on chromosome 18, the major breakpoint region accounting for 80% and the minor cluster region accounting for 10% of translocations respectively. At diagnosis, an isolated t(14;18) is uncommon and most cases show additional chromosomal changes. FL may undergo transformation

Table 1
Common recurrent chromosomal translocation in B-cell lymphoma

Lymphoma diagnosis	Translocation	Fusion genes
Burkitt lymphoma	t(8;14)(q24;q32) t(2;8)(p12;q24) t(8;22)(q24;q11)	*IGH-MYC* *IGκ-MYC* *IGλ-MYC*
Diffuse large B-cell lymphoma	t(14;18)(q32;q21) t(3;14)(q27;q32) t(2;3)(p12;q27) t(3;22)(q27;q11) t(3;v)(q27;v)	*IGH-BCL2* *IGH-BCL6* *IGκ-BCL6* *IGλ-BCL6* *BCL6* and other partners
Follicular lymphoma	t(14;18)(q32;q21)	*IGH-BCL2*
Mantle cell lymphoma	t(11;14)(q13;q32)	*IGH-BCL1*
Marginal zone B-cell lymphoma	t(11;18)(q21;q21) t(14;18)(q32;q21) t(1;14)(p22;q32) t(3;14)(p14;q32)	*API2-MALT1* *IGH-MALT1* *IGH-BCL10* *IGH-FOXP1*
Lymphoplasmacytic lymphoma	t(9;14)(p13;q32)	*IGH-PAX5*

into more aggressive high-grade lymphoma, is commonly associated with the accumulation of secondary genetic aberrations, such as *MYC* gene rearrangement, 17p/*TP53* deletion or mutation, *BCL2* mutation, and *BCL6* mutation. Around 10% of FL is negative for t(14;18) but shows other abnormalities, such as *BCL2* gene amplification and *BCL6* gene translocations [12]. A rare but distinctive subtype of t(14;18)-negative FL presenting with low clinical stage and large but localized inguinal tumors is characterized by predominantly diffused growth pattern and deletions in the chromosomal region 1p36 [13].

Mantle cell lymphoma (MCL) is characterized by t(11;14)(q13;q32) that results in the juxtaposition of the *BCL1* (*CCND1*) gene locus to the *IGH* gene and leads to over-expression of cyclin D1 on the lymphoma cells. Immunohistochemistry (IHC) detection of cyclin D1 expression is routinely employed for the diagnosis of MCL. Most cases of MCL show addition of cytogenetics abnormalities or complex karyotype. Common secondary abnormalities include del(13q14), del(17p), del(11q), del(6q), and +12. Note that the t(11;14)(q13;q32) or *IGH-BCL1(CCND1)* gene fusion is not specific to MCL but is also found in a subset of plasma cell myeloma [14] showing small lymphoplasmacytic morphology and CD20+ that enjoys a more favorable prognosis.

The t(9;14)(p13;q32) is found in around 50% of lymphoplasmacytic lymphoma (LPL) and involves the *PAX5* gene on chromosome 9, which encodes a B-cell-specific transcriptional factor controlling B-cell proliferation and differentiation. However, the diagnostic and predictive marker in LPL is currently focused on *MYD88* L265P mutation and more recently *CXCR4* mutation [15]. Likewise in hairy cell leukemia (HCL) in which no specific cytogenetic abnormality is found, the diagnostic marker is *BRAF* V600E mutation [16]. The *BRAF* gene mutation is highly sensitive and specific for HCL. Therefore in the two disease entities LPL and HCL, mutation detection has replaced cytogenetics in the routine diagnostic process.

The chromosomal changes in marginal zone B-cell lymphoma (MZL) include trisomy 3, t(1;14)(p22;q32) *IGH-BCL10*, t(14;18)(q32;q21) *IGH-MALT1*, t(11;18)(q21;q21) *API2-MALT1*, and t(3;14)(p13;q32) *IGH-FOXP1*. The translocations occur at varying frequency at different locations, are mutually exclusive, and are detectable in only around one quarter of all cases, the commonest being t(11;18)(q21;q21) *API2-MALT1* to be followed by t(14;18)(q32;q21) *IGH-MALT1*. Trisomy 3 is the most common numeric abnormality in gastric, thyroid, and parotid MZL. The t(11;18)(q21;q21) *API2-MALT-1* frequently involves MZL of the lung and gastrointestional tract but is very rare in splenic MZL. Notably, gastric mucosa-associated lymphoid tissue (MALT) lymphoma that harbors t(11;18)(q21;q21) is resistant to *Helicobacter pylori* eradication [17] and should be treated by chemotherapy or other modalities. The t(14;18)(q32;q21) *IGH-MALT1* is found in lung, liver, skin, ocular adnexae, and salivary gland, but not the spleen, stomach, and gastrointestinal tract. The t(1;14)(p22;q32) *IGH-BCL10* occurs more commonly in the high-grade MZL than in the low-grade disease. The t(3;14)(p13;q32) *IGH-FOXP1* is found in the thyroid, ocular adnexae, and skin, but not the stomach, spleen, and lung.

Diffuse large B-cell lymphoma (DLBCL) is the most common lymphoma in Western countries, accounting for around one third of all adult lymphoma cases. Cytogenetically, the most frequent chromosomal abnormality involves the *BCL6* gene at 3q27 in 30–40% of cases, to be followed by t(14;18)(q32;q21) *IGH-BCL2* in 15% and t(8;14)(q24;q32) *IGH-MYC* in 5–10%. By gene expression profiling [18], DLBCL can be categorized into germinal center B-cell (GCB) and activated B-cell (ABC) types based on the cell of origin, which predicts survival and response to chemotherapy. The t(14;18)(q32;q21) *IGH-BCL2* is associated with the GCB group, found in 45% of the GCB but not exclusively because the translocation is also found in 8% of the ABC group. However in the routine diagnostic setting the cell of origin designation in DLBCL is performed either by one of the IHC stratification algorithms [19] or more recently by the digital gene expression-based test on the Nanostring platform termed the Lymph2Cx assay [20]. The utilization of cytogenetic information as a marker of disease behavior in DLBCL is discussed in Subheading 2.3.

2.3 MYC Translocation and Double Hit Lymphoma

The *MYC* gene translocations with immunoglobulin gene (IG) partners, namely t(8;14)(q24;q32) *IGH-MYC*, t(2;8)(p12;q24) *IGκ-MYC*, and t(8;22)(q24;q11) *IGλ-MYC*, define Burkitt lymphoma (BL) [21]. The BL is a neoplasm of mature B-cells characterized by a uniform proliferation of medium sized lymphoid cells with high proliferation index and starry sky pattern, positive for CD10 and BCL6 expression but negative for BCL2 expression, and *MYC* rearrangement due to fusion with IG partners. However, there are cases in which phenotypic or genotypic features are atypical of BL, such as heterogeneous cell size, BCL2 expression, concurrent *MYC* and *BCL2* or *BCL6* translocations, and *MYC* translocation amid a complex karyotype. These imprecisely defined cases are group under the WHO 2008 category of B-cell lymphoma, unclassifiable, with features intermediate between DLBCL and BL (BCL-U) [22].

Routine karyotyping is not common practice in lymphoma and access to gene expression profiling or array comparative genomic hybridization is limited. Therefore, extensive FISH testing for *MYC*, *BCL2*, and *BCL6* translocations becomes imperative in the diagnosis of BL, DLBCL with high grade features and BCL-U, in addition to morphologic and immunophenotypic assessment. The term "double-hit" (DH) lymphoma as used in the literature typically refers to cases with MYC translocation in combination with either *BCL2* or *BCL6* or both ("triple-hit" lymphoma) (Fig. 2). DH lymphoma as currently defined is a heterogeneous entity that being variably reported to represent around 10% of DLBCL and ranging from one third to two thirds of BCL-U [23]. Other cases can include follicular lymphoma or transformation of low-grade lymphoma. The phenotype of DH lymphoma is germinal center (GC) B-cell showing expression of CD10 and BCL6 but usually not MUM1/IRF4. DH lymphoma generally runs an aggressive clinical course and alternative treatment to DLBCL is indicated.

Interphase FISH by *MYC*, *BCL2*, and *BCL6* gene break-apart probes is the most sensitive method to detect translocations but the partner gene is not identified. However even break-apart probes may not be able to detect all cases. For example *MYC* translocations may infrequently be missed if only the break-apart probe is used but detectable by *IGH-MYC* dual-fusion probe [24]. Also, specific fusion probes are required to positively identify the fusion partner. Therefore, the *MYC* break-apart and *IGH-MYC* dual-fusion probes can be performed together, so that *MYC* rearrangement if positive is known whether or not due to *IGH-MYC* and potential false negative can be minimized. In contrast to BL in which the *MYC* translocation partner is also the IG genes, DH lymphoma may show *MYC* gene fusion with non-IG partners such as *BCL6*, *BCL11A*, and *PAX5*. Although studies have shown that the *MYC* fusion with non-IG partners may be less aggressive in clinical behavior [25], the importance of *MYC* partner gene

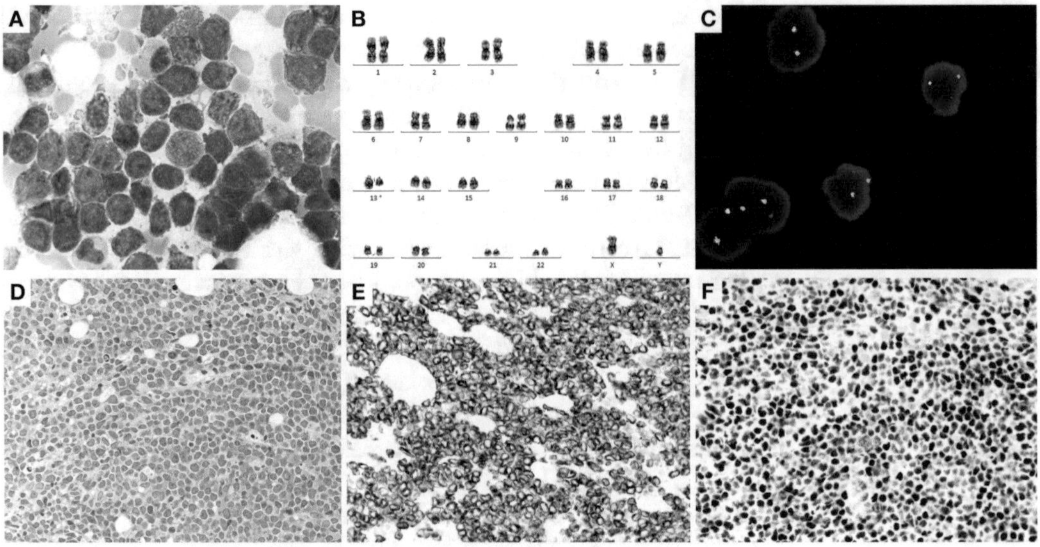

Fig. 2 Double-hit lymphoma. (**a**) Bone marrow aspirate showing heavy infiltration by medium to large-sized abnormal lymphoid cells. Wright-Giemsa × 1000. The lymphoid cells showed a mature B-cell phenotype: CD19+ CD20+ CD22+ FMC7+ cytoplasmic-CD79a + surface-IgM+ and kappa light chain restriction. (**b**) A representative karyotyping showing del(13)(q22). Note that chromosomes 8, 14, and 18 were morphologically normal. Karyotype was: 46,XY,del(13)(q22)[9]/46,XY[20]. (**c**) *MYC* gene rearrangement positive by dual-color split-apart probe. Normal cells showed two yellow (wild-type) yellow signals, whereas positive interphase cells showed split orange and green signals in addition to 1 yellow signal. *IGH-BCL2* fusion was positive by dual-color dual-fusion probe and *BCL6* rearrangement was negative by dual-color split-apart probe. (**d**) Trephine biopsy showing diffuse infiltration by abnormal lymphoid cells crowded together. H&E × 600. (**e**) BCL2+ by IHC. (**f**) Nuclear BCL6+ by IHC. The IHC phenotype was CD10+ CD20+ BCL2+ BCL6+ TdT- cyclin-D1- CD5-

remains to be clarified and there is no need to routinely determine the partner gene.

With the availability of MYC monoclonal antibodies for the IHC study [26], it is possible to enrich for *MYC* translocation cases by adopting a certain threshold of MYC protein expression by IHC, for example 40–50 % of cells, before FISH testing is performed to save cost. Laboratories should assess the performance of MYC IHC study and determine an appropriate cutoff to adopt. Nevertheless, currently, the laboratory strategy to maximize the detection of DH lymphoma should employ FISH testing in all aggressive DLBCL by *MYC* break-apart and *IGH-MYC* dual-fusion probes together with *BCL2* and *BCL6* break-apart probes. Of note, a related entity termed double-expressor (DE) DLBCL [27], usually defined on IHC basis as having ≥40 % MYC+ and ≥50–70 % BCL2+ lymphoma cells, is not equivalent to DH lymphoma. While 80–90 % of DH lymphoma is also DE, only <20 % of DE lymphoma is DH. DE is associated with an inferior survival in DLBCL but not as aggressive as DH lymphoma. Most *BCL6* rearranged DH lymphoma is excluded from DE and, unlike the GC predominance in DH, around two thirds of the DE DLBCL is of the non-GC type. There is currently considerable research effort to study the DH and DE lymphomas and in general to identify which are the extra-aggressive DLBCLs.

3 Peripheral T-cell Lymphoma

Peripheral T-cell lymphoma (PTCL) is a heterogeneous group of lymphoid malignancy derived from mature post-thyme T-cells and natural killer (NK) cells, altogether accounting for around 10% of all non-Hodgkin lymphoma in Western countries. Demonstration of T-cell clonality, unlike B-cells, cannot be performed by routine immunophenotyping for light chain restriction and requires molecular testing for T-cell receptor gene (TCR) rearrangement. Standardized protocol is available from BIOMED-2 and clinically useful [28]. The *TCR* gene is not rearranged in NK-cell disorders and demonstration of clonality is even more challenging. Clonality of NK-cells may be performed by demonstration of clonal cytogenetic abnormality, clonal EBV integration and detection of uniform expression of single (or multiple) killer-cell immunoglobulin receptor (KIR) isoform [29]. However, these tests are not applicable to all cases and the technique is not widely available.

In contrast to other hematological neoplasms in which cytogenetic abnormalities are important in disease pathogenesis and finding clinical applications in diagnosis and prognosis, only few recurrent cytogenetic aberrations have been identified in the T-cell NHL. The salient ones are *ALK* translocations in anaplastic large cell lymphoma (ALCL), translocations involving the *TCR* gene loci, t(5;9)(q33;q22) in PTCL, translocations involving the *IRF4* oncogene locus, isochromosome 7q in hepatosplenic T-cell lymphoma, *DUSP22* and *TP63* rearrangements in ALK-negative ALCL, and deletion 6q in NK/T-cell lymphoma.

3.1 Anaplastic Lymphoma Kinase (ALK) Gene Translocations

ALK-positive (+) ALCL is characterized by recurrent chromosomal translocations that involve the fusion between partner genes at the 5′-end to the *ALK* gene on chromosome 2p23 at the 3′-end and result in constitutive activation of the ALK tyrosine kinase. The *ALK* gene translocations are the best characterized genetic change in the T-cell NHL. ALK+ ALCL is currently the only PTCL entity in the WHO classification that is defined on genetic basis by *ALK* translocation and ALK overexpression. The most common *ALK* translocation is t(2;5)(p23;q35) that fuses the *ALK* to the nucleophosmin (*NPM1*) gene [30] on chromosome 5q35. Since then, other fusion partners are identified, namely t(1;2)(q25;p23) *TPM3-ALK* fusion, t(2;3)(p23;q11) *TFG-ALK* fusion, inv(2)(p23q35) *ATIC-ALK* fusion, and t(2;17)(p23;q23) *CLTC-ALK* fusion. Immunohistochemistry (IHC) is routinely used to detect lymphoma cells expressing ALK protein. Of interest, the subcellular distribution of the ALK staining differs by the translocation type. The most common t(2;5) is the only translocation that is associated with ALK staining in both the nucleus and cytoplasm, while the variant translocations show cytoplasmic only staining pattern.

Chromosomal translocation involving *ALK* breakpoint at 2p23 is detectable on conventional cytogenetics or by FISH with break-apart probes. RT-PCR assays commonly only target the *NPM1-ALK* fusion transcript and not the variant fusion partners. In the practical setting, however, IHC testing for ALK expression supersedes cytogenetic or molecular testing for the speed and cost effectiveness. In large cell lymphoma with a T-cell or null immunophenotype and CD30 expression, ALK IHC is mandatory to distinguish ALK+ ALCL from ALK-negative CD30+ T-cell lymphoma, which is clinically relevant since ALK+ ALCL irrespective of the translocation type is associated with a more favorable prognosis than both ALK-negative ALCL and PTCL, not otherwise specified (NOS) [31].

3.2 Translocations Involving the TCR Gene Loci

Three genetic loci exist, namely *TCR alpha* (*TRA*) and *TCR delta* (*TRD*) at chromosome 14q11, *TCR beta* (*TRB*) at 7q34, and *TCR gamma* (*TRG*) at 7p14. The *TRD* is located within the *TRA*. Since these genetic loci are active in T-cells, oncogenes that are fused to them as a result of chromosomal translocation are also upregulated through transcriptional activation.

The vast majority of T-prolymphocytic leukemia cases show translocations or inversion involving the *TRA* gene. The partner genes involved in rearrangement are the *TCL1* and *TCL1b* at chromosome 14q32 in the form of inv(14)(q11q32) or t(14;14)(q11;q32), and the *MTCP1* gene at chromosome Xq28 in the form of t(X;14)(q28;q11). Other TCR gene translocations are infrequent in PTCL and poorly understood since the translocation partner is often not identified [32].

3.3 Translocations Involving the IRF4 Oncogene Locus

Involvement of the multiple myeloma oncogene-1 (*MUM1*)/interferon regulatory factor-4 (*IRF4*) as the fusion gene partner of *TRA* in t(6;14)(p25;q11.2) is a rare but recurrent chromosomal translocation in PTCL, NOS associated with a cytotoxic phenotype and infiltration of the bone marrow and skin without significant lymphadenopathy or hepatosplenomegaly [33]. Subsequent FISH screening reveals non-*TCR* gene-related *IRF4* translocations, mostly ALK-negative ALCL of the systemic or primary cutaneous types. Among primary cutaneous T-cell lymphoma, FISH positivity for *IRF4* translocation is highly specific for primary cutaneous ALCL [34]. Since primary cutaneous ALCL may be difficult to distinguish from other CD30+ lymphoproliferations and correct diagnosis is important for management, FISH testing for *IRF4* translocation is clinically useful in the differential diagnosis of cutaneous T-cell lymphoid lesions.

3.4 DUSP22 and TP63 Rearrangements in ALK-negative ALCL

The genetic basis of ALCL lacking *ALK* rearrangement remains largely unknown until the recent identification of *DUSP22* [35] and *TP63* [36] rearrangements. The *DUSP22* gene is located at 6p25.3 and just telomeric to the *IRF4* gene at the same chromosomal location while the *TP63* gene, which is a homolog of the *TP53* gene, is located on 3q28. IHC and FISH screening study shows *DUSP22* rearrangement in 30% and *TP63* rearrangement in 8% of ALK-negative ALCL respectively. The rearrangements are mutually exclusive and absent in ALK+ ALCL. Patients with *DUSP22* rearrangement show favorable treatment outcome similar to ALK+ ALCL, whereas other genetic subtypes have inferior outcome [37].

3.5 Translocation (5;9)(q33;q22) in PTCL

The t(5;9)(q33;q22) translocation results in the fusion between IL-2 inducible T-cell kinase (*ITK*) gene on chromosome 5 and the spleen tyrosine kinase (*SYK*) gene on chromosome 9. This is the first recurrent translocation found in PTCL, NOS but only detected in a small subset of patients [38]. The translocation is associated with follicular PTCL in which the lymphoma cells show a follicular helper T-cell phenotype and a follicular growth pattern that may mimic follicular lymphoma, nodular lymphocyte predominant Hodgkin lymphoma, or nodal marginal zone lymphoma.

3.6 Isochromosome 7q in Hepatosplenic T-cell Lymphoma

Isochromosome 7q is a recurrent chromosomal abnormality in hepatosplenic T-cell lymphoma [39]. The i(7)(q10) results in the deletion of the short arm of chromosome 7 which may be associated with loss of tumor suppressor gene on 7p or the loss of *TRG* at 7p14, or conversely the duplication of the long arm of chromosome 7 may be associated with overexpression of oncogenes on 7q or gain of *TRB* at 7q34. Isochromosome 7q is detectable by conventional cytogenetics and FISH by a dual-color probe assay (Fig. 3). It should be noted that although i(7)(q10) is observed in the majority of hepatosplenic T-cell lymphoma, this abnormality is not specific for this lymphoma subtype.

3.7 Deletion 6q in NK/T-cell Lymphoma

Deletion at chromosome 6q21-q25 is the most common recurrent abnormality in extranodal nasal-type NK/T cell lymphoma, which is characterized by a proliferation of EBV-infected neoplastic NK cells usually in the nasopharynx and associated with a dismal prognosis. This type of lymphoma is prevalent in Asian countries. The del(6q) is seen in the majority of cases, in association with less frequent gains at chromosomes 1p, 6p, 11q, 12q, 17q, 20q and Xp, and losses at 11q, 13q and 17p, consistent with a complex karyotype [40, 41]. The critical deleted region at 6q21 harbors putative tumor suppressor genes *PRDM1*, *ATG5*, and *AIM1* [42], as well as *HACE1* [43]. Loss of function of these genes by mutations or methylations may play a role in the pathogenesis of this lymphoma subtype.

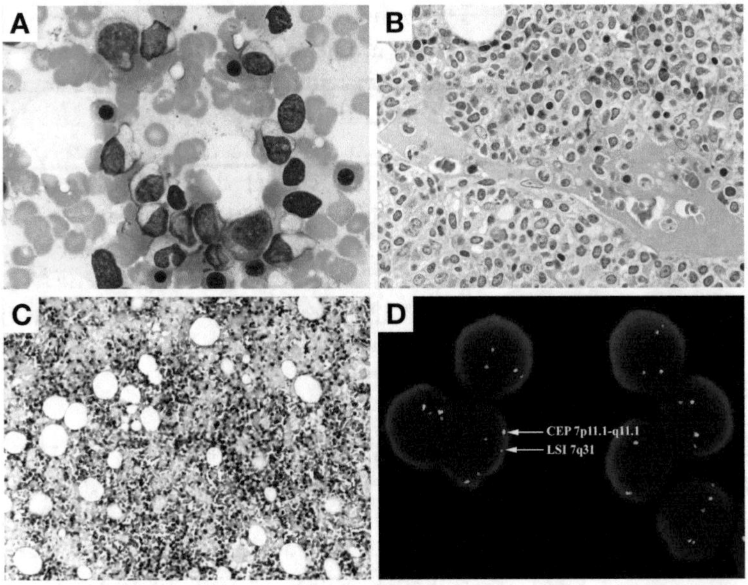

Fig. 3 Hepatosplenic T-cell lymphoma. (**a**) Trephine biopsy imprint showing infiltration by a heterogeneous population of granulated abnormal lymphoid cells. Wright-Giemsa × 1000. The immunophenotype was: CD2+ CD3+ TCR-$\gamma\delta$ + CD1a- CD4- CD8- CD5- CD7- CD16/56- TCR-$\alpha\beta$-. (**b**) Trephine biopsy showing heterotopic abnormal lymphoid cells in bone marrow sinusoids. H&E × 600. (**c**) The abnormal lymphoid cells were EBV+ as demonstrated by in situ hybridization for EBV early RNA (EBER). (**d**) Interphase FISH by LSI 7q31/CEP7 probe (CEP7: green and LSI 7q31: *orange*) showing 201G signal pattern consistent with isochromosome 7q. Conventional cytogenetics showed normal karyotype only

3.8 Other Miscellaneous Abnormalities

Enteropathy-associated T-cell lymphoma is characterized by frequent complex gains of 9q31.3-qter in 70% of cases or by an almost mutually exclusive 2.5 Mb loss of 16q12.1 in 23% of cases [44]. Gain of chromosome 9q is seen in both type 1 and type 2 enteropathy-associated T-cell lymphoma. The chromosme 9q34 region contains two candidate genes *NOTCH1* and *ABL1* that are preferentially amplified [45].

Increasing numbers of novel chromosmomal translocations and other aberrations are discovered in PTCL with the widespread use of genomic profiling by deep sequencing to catch up with the B-cell malignancies, for translation into clinical application supporting disease diagnosis, prognostication, and therapy. For example, the *CTLA4-CD28* gene fusion is recently identified in diverse types of T-cell lymphoma [46] which may not only shed light on T-cell lymphoma pathogenesis but represents a potential target for anti-CTLA4 tumor immunotherapy.

4 Conclusion

Lymphoma genetics has evolved from conventional cytogenetics, FISH and PCR to gene expression profiling, array comparative genomic hybridization, transcriptome analysis, methylation profiling, and deep sequencing for mutational signature. High-throughput sequencing has been applied to the study of common NHL such as DLBCL [47] and CLL [48]. These studies have advanced the field not only in understanding disease pathogenesis and categorization, but contribute to the identification of prognostic markers and potential drug targets. Currently, the clinical application of recurrent chromosomal abnormalities and other genetic markers is focused on prediction of disease behavior, such as detection of *MYC*, *BCL2*, and *BCL6* rearrangements as marker of clinical aggressiveness in DLBCL, or for prognostication purposes such as interphase FISH panel for risk stratification in CLL. The hope for the future is to translate the genomics information into better clinical outcome for lymphoma patients. A successful example is moving from the identification of *BRAF* V600E mutation in HCL through whole exome sequencing [16] to the documented clinical effectiveness of *BRAF* inhibitor vemurafenib in patients with relapsed or refractory HCL [49]. With the availability of novel therapies targeting *BCL2* gene, Bruton tyrosine kinase inhibitor, phosphoinositide 3-kinase inhibitor inhibitor, and others to come, the stage is set for genetics and genomics to play a major contributory role to achieve personalized therapy in lymphoma.

References

1. Swerdlow SH, Campo E, Pileri SA et al (2016) The 2016 revision of the World Health Organization (WHO) classification of lymphoid neoplasms. Blood pii: blood-2016-01-643569
2. Belaud-Rotureau MA, Parrens M, Carrere N et al (2007) Interphase fluorescence in situ hybridization is more sensitive than BIOMED-2 polymerase chain reaction protocol in detecting IGH-BCL2 rearrangement in both fixed and frozen lymph node with follicular lymphoma. Hum Pathol 38(2):365–372
3. Espinet B, Bellosillo B, Melero C et al (2008) FISH is better than BIOMED-2 PCR to detect IgH/BCL2 translocation in follicular lymphoma at diagnosis using paraffin-embedded tissue sections. Leuk Res 32(5):737–742
4. van Dongen JJ, Langerak AW, Bruggemann M et al (2003) Design and standardization of PCR primers and protocols for detection of clonal immunoglobulin and T-cell receptor gene recombinations in suspect lymphoproliferations: report of the BIOMED-2 Concerted Action BMH4-CT98-3936. Leukemia 17(12):2257–2317
5. Dohner H, Stilgenbauer S, Benner A et al (2000) Genomic aberrations and survival in chronic lymphocytic leukemia. N Engl J Med 343(26):1910–1916
6. Mayr C, Speicher MR, Kofler DM et al (2006) Chromosomal translocations are associated with poor prognosis in chronic lymphocytic leukemia. Blood 107(2):742–751
7. Byrd JC, Smith L, Hackbarth ML et al (2003) Interphase cytogenetic abnormalities in chronic lymphocytic leukemia may predict response to rituximab. Cancer Res 63(1): 36–38
8. Garg R, Wierda W, Ferrajoli A et al (2012) The prognostic difference of monoallelic versus biallelic deletion of 13q in chronic lymphocytic leukemia. Cancer 118(14):3531–3537
9. Zenz T, Eichhorst B, Busch R et al (2010) TP53 mutation and survival in chronic lymphocytic leukemia. J Clin Oncol 28(29):4473–4479

10. Lozanski G, Heerema NA, Flinn IW et al (2004) Alemtuzumab is an effective therapy for chronic lymphocytic leukemia with p53 mutations and deletions. Blood 103(9):3278–3281
11. Pflug N, Bahlo J, Shanafelt TD et al (2014) Development of a comprehensive prognostic index for patients with chronic lymphocytic leukemia. Blood 124(1):49–62
12. Guo Y, Karube K, Kawano R et al (2005) Low-grade follicular lymphoma with t(14;18) presents a homogeneous disease entity otherwise the rest comprises minor groups of heterogeneous disease entities with Bcl2 amplification, Bcl6 translocation or other gene aberrances. Leukemia 19(6):1058–1063
13. Katzenberger T, Kalla J, Leich E et al (2009) A distinctive subtype of t(14;18)-negative nodal follicular non-Hodgkin lymphoma characterized by a predominantly diffuse growth pattern and deletions in the chromosomal region 1p36. Blood 113(5):1053–1061
14. Fonseca R, Blood EA, Oken MM et al (2002) Myeloma and the t(11;14)(q13;q32); evidence for a biologically defined unique subset of patients. Blood 99(10):3735–3741
15. Treon SP, Cao Y, Xu L et al (2014) Somatic mutations in MYD88 and CXCR4 are determinants of clinical presentation and overall survival in Waldenstrom macroglobulinemia. Blood 123(18):2791–2796
16. Tiacci E, Trifonov V, Schiavoni G et al (2011) BRAF mutations in hairy-cell leukemia. N Engl J Med 364(24):2305–2315
17. Liu H, Ruskon-Fourmestraux A, Lavergne-Slove A et al (2001) Resistance of t(11;18) positive gastric mucosa-associated lymphoid tissue lymphoma to Helicobacter pylori eradication therapy. Lancet 357(9249):39–40
18. Rosenwald A, Wright G, Chan WC et al (2002) The use of molecular profiling to predict survival after chemotherapy for diffuse large-B-cell lymphoma. N Engl J Med 346(25):1937–1947
19. Meyer PN, Fu K, Greiner TC et al (2011) Immunohistochemical methods for predicting cell of origin and survival in patients with diffuse large B-cell lymphoma treated with rituximab. J Clin Oncol 29(2):200–207
20. Scott DW, Wright GW, Williams PM et al (2014) Determining cell-of-origin subtypes of diffuse large B-cell lymphoma using gene expression in formalin-fixed paraffin-embedded tissue. Blood 123(8):1214–1217
21. Boerma EG, Siebert R, Kluin PM et al (2009) Translocations involving 8q24 in Burkitt lymphoma and other malignant lymphomas: a historical review of cytogenetics in the light of today's knowledge. Leukemia 23(2):225–234
22. So CC, Yung KH, Chu ML et al (2013) Diagnostic challenges in a case of B cell lymphoma unclassifiable with features intermediate between diffuse large B-cell lymphoma and Burkitt lymphoma. Int J Hematol 98(4):478–482
23. Friedberg JW (2012) Double-hit diffuse large B-cell lymphoma. J Clin Oncol 30(28):3439–3443
24. Tzankov A, Xu-Monette ZY, Gerhard M et al (2014) Rearrangements of MYC gene facilitate risk stratification in diffuse large B-cell lymphoma patients treated with rituximab-CHOP. Mod Pathol 27(7):958–971
25. Pedersen MO, Gang AO, Poulsen TS et al (2014) MYC translocation partner gene determines survival of patients with large B-cell lymphoma with MYC- or double-hit MYC/BCL2 translocations. Eur J Haematol 92(1):42–48
26. Horn H, Ziepert M, Becher C et al (2013) MYC status in concert with BCL2 and BCL6 expression predicts outcome in diffuse large B-cell lymphoma. Blood 121(12):2253–2263
27. Hu S, Xu-Monette ZY, Tzankov A et al (2013) MYC/BCL2 protein coexpression contributes to the inferior survival of activated B-cell subtype of diffuse large B-cell lymphoma and demonstrates high-risk gene expression signatures: a report from The International DLBCL Rituximab-CHOP Consortium Program. Blood 121(20):4021–4031
28. Bruggemann M, White H, Gaulard P et al (2007) Powerful strategy for polymerase chain reaction-based clonality assessment in T-cell malignancies. Report of the BIOMED-2 Concerted Action BHM4 CT98-3936. Leukemia 21(2):215–221
29. Pascal V, Schleinitz N, Brunet C et al (2004) Comparative analysis of NK cell subset distribution in normal and lymphoproliferative disease of granular lymphocyte conditions. Eur J Immunol 34(10):2930–2940
30. Morris SW, Kirstein MN, Valentine MB et al (1994) Fusion of a kinase gene, ALK, to a nucleolar protein gene, NPM, in non-Hodgkin's lymphoma. Science 263(5151):1281–1284
31. Savage KJ, Harris NL, Vose JM et al (2008) ALK- anaplastic large-cell lymphoma is clinically and immunophenotypically different from both ALK+ ALCL and peripheral T-cell lymphoma, not otherwise specified: report from the International Peripheral T-Cell Lymphoma Project. Blood 111(12):5496–5504
32. Gesk S, Martin-Subero JI, Harder L et al (2003) Molecular cytogenetic detection of chromosomal breakpoints in T-cell receptor gene loci. Leukemia 17(4):738–745
33. Feldman AL, Law M, Remstein ED et al (2009) Recurrent translocations involving the IRF4 oncogene locus in peripheral T-cell lymphomas. Leukemia 23(3):574–580

34. Wada DA, Law ME, Hsi ED et al (2011) Specificity of IRF4 translocations for primary cutaneous anaplastic large cell lymphoma: a multicenter study of 204 skin biopsies. Mod Pathol 24(4):596–605
35. Feldman AL, Dogan A, Smith DI et al (2011) Discovery of recurrent t(6;7)(p25.3;q32.3) translocations in ALK-negative anaplastic large cell lymphomas by massively parallel genomic sequencing. Blood 117(3):915–919
36. Vasmatzis G, Johnson SH, Knudson RA et al (2012) Genome-wide analysis reveals recurrent structural abnormalities of TP63 and other p53-related genes in peripheral T-cell lymphomas. Blood 120(11):2280–2289
37. Parrilla Castellar ER, Jaffe ES, Said JW et al (2014) ALK-negative anaplastic large cell lymphoma is a genetically heterogeneous disease with widely disparate clinical outcomes. Blood 124(9):1473–1480
38. Streubel B, Vinatzer U, Willheim M et al (2006) Novel t(5;9)(q33;q22) fuses ITK to SYK in unspecified peripheral T-cell lymphoma. Leukemia 20(2):313–318
39. Wlodarska I, Martin-Garcia N, Achten R et al (2002) Fluorescence in situ hybridization study of chromosome 7 aberrations in hepatosplenic T-cell lymphoma: isochromosome 7q as a common abnormality accumulating in forms with features of cytologic progression. Genes Chromosomes Cancer 33(3):243–251
40. Siu LL, Wong KF, Chan JK et al (1999) Comparative genomic hybridization analysis of natural killer cell lymphoma/leukemia. Recognition of consistent patterns of genetic alterations. Am J Pathol 155(5):1419–1425
41. Siu LL, Chan V, Chan JK et al (2000) Consistent patterns of allelic loss in natural killer cell lymphoma. Am J Pathol 157(6):1803–1809
42. Iqbal J, Kucuk C, Deleeuw RJ et al (2009) Genomic analyses reveal global functional alterations that promote tumor growth and novel tumor suppressor genes in natural killer-cell malignancies. Leukemia 23(6):1139–1151
43. Huang Y, de RA, de LL et al (2010) Gene expression profiling identifies emerging oncogenic pathways operating in extranodal NK/T-cell lymphoma, nasal type. Blood 115(6):1226–1237
44. Deleeuw RJ, Zettl A, Klinker E et al (2007) Whole-genome analysis and HLA genotyping of enteropathy-type T-cell lymphoma reveals 2 distinct lymphoma subtypes. Gastroenterology 132(5):1902–1911
45. Cejkova P, Zettl A, Baumgartner AK et al (2005) Amplification of NOTCH1 and ABL1 gene loci is a frequent aberration in enteropathy-type T-cell lymphoma. Virchows Arch 446(4):416–420
46. Yoo HY, Kim P, Kim WS et al. (2016) Frequent CTLA4-CD28 gene fusion in diverse types of T cell lymphoma. Haematologica. pii: haematol.2015.139253
47. Lohr JG, Stojanov P, Lawrence MS et al (2012) Discovery and prioritization of somatic mutations in diffuse large B-cell lymphoma (DLBCL) by whole-exome sequencing. Proc Natl Acad Sci U S A 109(10):3879–3884
48. Wang L, Lawrence MS, Wan Y et al (2011) SF3B1 and other novel cancer genes in chronic lymphocytic leukemia. N Engl J Med 365(26):2497–2506
49. Tiacci E, Park JH, De CL et al (2015) Targeting mutant BRAF in relapsed or refractory hairy-cell leukemia. N Engl J Med 373(18):1733–1747

Chapter 23

Recurrent Cytogenetic Abnormalities in Multiple Myeloma

Nelson Chun Ngai Chan and Natalie Pui Ha Chan

Abstract

Multiple myeloma is a heterogeneous disease. Its chromosomal abnormalities have been extensively studied with a view to accurate prognostication and personalized therapy. Here, we describe the techniques commonly employed for elucidating chromosomal aberrations, prognostic impact of recurrent chromosomal abnormalities, and recently updated risk stratification systems.

Key words Myeloma, Conventional cytogenetics, Interphase FISH, Hyperdiploid, *IGH* translocation, Risk stratification

1 Introduction

Multiple myeloma (MM) or plasma cell myeloma (PCM) is a plasma cell neoplasm characterized by 10% or more clonal plasma cells in bone marrow and presence of myeloma defining events, commonly associated with paraproteinaemia [1]. It has an annual incidence of 6.3 per 100,000 populations in the United States and a median age of 73 at diagnosis [2]. To date, treatment decision is based on symptomatic disease as determined by the presence of one or more myeloma defining events. The current recommended treatment for majority of physically fit patients incorporates novel agents and autologous stem cell transplantation. Despite significant improvement in overall survival, multiple myeloma remains incurable. Furthermore, MM is a heterogeneous disease that demonstrates variable treatment response and survival.

In pursuit for better prognostication with an ultimate goal of developing risk-adapted treatment, various risk stratification systems have evolved. Traditional systems include the Durie Salmon Staging and the International Staging System (ISS). They were largely based on plasma cell burden and the former is criticized for being not validated with current treatment regimes [3]. With the advent of cytogenetics, fluorescence in situ hybridization (FISH)

Thomas S.K. Wan (ed.), *Cancer Cytogenetics: Methods and Protocols*, Methods in Molecular Biology, vol. 1541,
DOI 10.1007/978-1-4939-6703-2_23, © Springer Science+Business Media LLC 2017

and genetic expression profiles, genetic mutations were demonstrated to be significant predictors of survival and treatment response. Mayo Stratification for Myeloma and Risk-adapted Therapy (mSMART 2.0) was validated for risk stratification and suggested a risk-adapted approach regarding choice of treatment (Table 1). In 2015, Palumbo et al. refined the original ISS with addition of chromosomal abnormalities by interphase FISH and developed the simple yet powerful Revised International Staging System (R-ISS) (Table 2).

Table 1
The mSMART 2.0 risk stratification of active multiple myeloma. (Reproduced from [4] with permission from Elsevier)

	Intermediate risk	Standard risk
FISH del 17p	*FISH* t(4;14)	All others cytogenetic abnormalities, including hyperdiploidy
t(14;16)	*Cytogenetic*	*FISH*
t(14;20)	del 13 or Hypodiploidy	t(11;14)
GEP High risk signature	*Plasma Cell Labeling Index ≥3%*	t(6;14)

FISH fluorescence in situ hybridization, *GEP* gene expression profile

Table 2
Revised International Staging System (R-ISS). (reproduced from [5] with permission from American Society of Clinical Oncology)

iFISH	
High risk	Presence of del (17p) and/or translocation t(4;14) and/or translocation t(14;16)
Standard risk	No high-risk chromosomal abnormalities
R-ISS stage	
I	ISS stage I and standard-risk iFISH and normal LDH
II	Not R-ISS I or III
III	ISS stage III and either high risk iFISH or high LDH

iFISH Chromosomal abnormalities by interphase fluorescence in situ hybridization, *LDH*: lactate dehydrogenase

2 Conventional Cytogenetics

Yield of abnormal metaphases with conventional cytogenetics is low, reported to be 20–30% due to low proliferative activity of terminally differentiated plasma cells. Karyotype usually shows normal metaphases of myeloid elements [6]. Nevertheless, yield of abnormal metaphases per se is regarded as an adverse prognostic predictor [7]. Cytogenetic abnormalities with MM are typically complex with frequent numerical and structural aberrations like solid tumors [8]. They are particularly common and complex in plasma cell leukemia [9]. Aneuploidy of multiple myeloma can be divided into hyperdiploid and non-hyperdiploid subtypes.

2.1 Hyperdiploid

Hyperdiploid subtype commonly involves trisomies of chromosomes 3, 5, 7, 9, 11, 15, 19, and 21. It is considered a primary cytogenetic abnormality in MM and generally associated with better prognosis that could at least partially ameliorate impact of adverse cytogenetic abnormalities detected by FISH [10]. Phenotypically, it is associated with IgG isotype, kappa light chain expression, and older patients [11].

2.2 Non-hyperdiploid

Non-hyperdiploid subtype comprises three ploidy groups, including hypodiploidy, pseudodiploidy, and near tertraploidy. Most common monosomies are 13, 14, 16, and 22 [12]. Near tetraploid appears to represent 4 N duplications and most often arises from pseudodiploid or hypodiploid karyotypes [13]. More than 85% of non-hyperdiploid subtype is associated with *IGH* translocations compared with less than 30% in hyperdiploid subtype [12]. Phenotypically, it is associated with IgA isotype, lambda light chain expression, younger patients, and aggressive disease [11].

2.3 Other Chromosomal Aberrations

Cytogenetically detected monosomy 13 and 13q interstitial deletions were high-risk markers in the era without novel agents and autologous stem cell transplantation. 85% are monosomy 13 and 15% are chromosome 13 interstitial deletions [11]. With current treatment regimes, they are considered intermediate-risk cytogenetic abnormalities [14]. Cytogenetically detected t(4;14) and del(17p) are both markers of high-risk disease [3].

3 Fluorescence In Situ Hybridization (FISH)

Compared with conventional cytogenetic study, yield of interphase FISH is independent of plasma cell proliferative activity. Its potential limitation in sensitivity by proportion of plasma cells in bone marrow could be overcome by adequate plasma cell targeting techniques [15]. Translocations can be detected by either break-apart or dual fusion strategy and the latter is favored because of lower false-positive rate [12].

3.1 Plasma Cell Targeting Techniques

Recommended techniques commonly available in routine laboratory setting include magnetic activated cell sorting (MACS) and fluorescence immunophenotyping and interphase cytogenetic as a tool for the investigation of neoplasm (FICTION, *see* Chapter12) [12]. The former has the advantage of ease of setup, low cost and availability of enriched sample for further genetic testing but constrained by requirement of fresh sample. In comparison, FICTION requires additional cytomorphologic selection of plasma cells but assessment is still feasible with advanced age specimen. With adequate optimization and training, both techniques show comparable results. Other plasma cell targeting options include automated image analysis and fluorescence-activated cell sorting (FACS). Both demonstrate good sensitivity with low plasma cell burden but are limited by their cost and availability [15].

3.1.1 Cell Sorting

CD138 is commonly used for cell sorting by MACS and it deteriorates rapidly after separation with bone marrow stroma. Therefore, fresh sample is preferred for processing [15]. Quality check for adequate plasma cell yield can be performed afterward with flow cytometry or morphological assessment. Due to fragility of plasma cells, assessment of yield by flow cytometry is consistently lower than that by morphologic assessment [16].

3.1.2 Cutoff Values

The cutoff values of 10% for dual-fusion or break-apart translocation probes and 20% for numerical abnormalities are recommended [17]. Some laboratories establish local cutoff with normal samples as mean plus three standard deviations. A conservative approach regarding cutoff selection is preferred [17]. Each FISH assay must be validated against positive and negative controls [12].

3.2 Translocations Involving the Immunoglobulin Locus

Among all translocations involving the immunoglobulin locus, the immunoglobulin heavy chain (*IGH*) is implicated in 50–70% and <20% involve the light chain (*IGL*). Majority of *IGL* reported are *IGL-λ* [18]. *IGH* translocations juxtapose *IGH* gene to oncogenes and are considered a primary cytogenetic abnormality in multiple myeloma and occur early in disease process [19].

Common translocation partners include 4p16.3 (*FGFR3/MMSET*), 11q13 (*CCN D1*), 16q23 (*MAF*), and 20q12 (*MAFB*), whose prognostic significance is well characterized. The rest include 6p21 (*CCND3*), and 6p25 (*IRF4/MUM1*). Their prognostic significance is unknown.

3.2.1 Secondary Cytogenetic Abnormalities

Secondary cytogenetic abnormalities are associated with disease progression and acquired later in disease course, they include 17p13 (*TP53*) deletion, chromosomes 1 abnormalities, and 8q24 (*MYC*) translocation [11].

3.2.2 t(4;14)(p16;q32)

The t(4;14) is traditionally considered a marker of high-risk disease. With novel agents and autologous stem cell transplantation, it is now considered a marker of intermediate risk [11]. The t(4;14) is associated with monosomy 13 and interstitial deletion of chromosome 13 [20]. It is cryptic by conventional cytogenetic study [12]. Phenotypically, it is correlated with IgA isotype and lambda light chain expression [21].

Previous studies showed t(4;14) disease consists of two subgroups. The subgroup constituted of lower β2-microglobulin and higher hemoglobin represented a better risk subset with prolonged survival after tandem transplant and benefited from high dose therapy [22]. Similar findings were also demonstrated in another study utilizing a 70-gene expression profile [23].

3.2.3 t(11;14)(q13;q32)

The t(11;14) juxtaposes *IGH* with *CCND1* resulting in upregulation of oncogene *CCND1*. Phenotypically, it is associated with oligosecretory myeloma, lymphoplasmacytic morphology, expression of CD20, and expression of lambda light chain. About 70% of cases show expression of CCND1 by immunohistochemistry. It also constitutes most cases of IgM myeloma and 50% of light chain amyloidosis [3].

In terms of prognosis, it is considered a standard risk marker [12]. Recent analysis by gene expression profiling separated patients into two subgroups. The first group correlated with CD20 expression and demonstrated slower onset of complete remission but significantly longer complete remission. The other group that is negative for CD20 expression is associated with a higher rate, faster but shorter lasting complete remission [24].

3.2.4 t(14;16)(q32;23)

The t(14;16) is a marker of high-risk disease with median survival of 2–3 years despite treatment [25]. It is cryptic by conventional cytogenetics study and associated with chromosome 13 abnormalities [11, 26].

3.2.5 t(14;20)(q32;q12)

The t(14;20) is a marker of high-risk disease with a median survival of 2–3 years despite treatment [25].

3.2.6 Deletion of 17p13

Deletion of 17p13 causes inactivation of tumor suppressor gene *TP53*. It is a marker of high-risk disease with median survival of 2–3 years despite treatment [25]. It is associated with lower complete remission rate, rapid disease progression, advanced disease stages, plasma cell leukemia, and involvement of central nervous system [11]. Cutoff for clinically relevant del(17p) varied across different studies from 40 to 60% of plasma cells [17, 27].

3.2.7 Deletion of 13q14

By FISH, del(13q) is detected in 50% of myeloma patients compared with only 10–20% with conventional cytogenetics [28]. If detected by FISH only, it is less unfavorable, likely attributed to the presence of abnormal metaphases reflecting poor risk disease by conventional cytogenetics [29].

3.2.8 Trisomies

Detection of trisomies by FISH alone does not carry the same good prognostic information as that detected by conventional cytogenetic study [30].

3.2.9 Abnormalities of Chromosome 1

Reports showed 1q gain, 1p deletion, and 1q21 aberrations were correlated with poorer prognosis and disease progression [31]. 1q gain is currently regarded as an intermediate risk marker. However, evidence is not sufficient to recommend routine testing [3].

3.2.10 Myelodysplastic Syndrome Type Chromosomal Aberrations

Chromosomal abnormalities including trisomy 8, deletions of 5q, 7q and 20q were described in patients treated with alkylating agents [32].

3.3 Other Techniques

Other techniques employed for deciphering cytogenetic abnormalities in multiple myeloma include metaphase spectral karyotype imaging (SKY), multicolor FISH (mFISH), and comparative genomic hybridization (CGH). SKY and mFISH both require metaphases to demonstrate cytogenetic abnormalities while CGH cannot detect balanced structural abnormalities [12]. They are invaluable tools in the research setting but are not recommended for routine testing.

3.4 MGUS and Asymptomatic Myeloma

Monoclonal gammopathy of undetermined significance (MGUS) is considered a precursor of MM, characterized by paraproteinaemia, clonal plasma cells less than 10% in bone marrow and absence of myeloma defining events. It has an annual transformation rate to MM at about 1–2% [33].

Asymptomatic myeloma or smoldering myeloma represents the pre-symptomatic phase of MM. It is characterized by 10% or more clonal plasma cells in bone marrow but absence of myeloma defining events. It has an annual transformation rate to symptomatic myeloma at 10% for the first 5 years after diagnosis [34].

The del(17p), t(4;14), and 1q21 gain were associated with higher risk of progression to symptomatic myeloma, while trisomies or other *IGH* translocations have no significant impact on disease progression [35]. Nevertheless, preventive treatment for this group of patients should only be considered in the context of clinical trials [30].

3.5 Testing in Clinical Practice

Conventional cytogenetics can capture clinically relevant aneuploidy and uncommon cytogenetic abnormalities not covered by the FISH probe panel, while FISH has higher sensitivity in detecting cytogenetic abnormalities. In clinical practice, they are complementary and should be performed simultaneously for newly diagnosed MM patients [36]. For patients with relapse or progressive disease and non-high-risk disease at diagnosis, repeat testing for high-risk markers is recommended [3, 11].

The International Myeloma Working Group (IMWG) has recommendations regarding FISH probe combinations. The t(4;14)(p16;q32), t(14;16)(q32;q23), and deletion of 17p13 are considered established markers and essential for routine testing. An expanded panel, which consists of markers with modest effects, can be considered at the institute's discretion and it includes t(11;14)(q13;q32), 13q deletion, 1q amplification, 1p deletion, hyperdiploidy, and other translocations.

3.6 Risk Stratification Systems

Mayo clinic has developed the mSMART 2.0 system for genetic risk stratification and risk-adapted treatment (Table 1). However, cytogenetic abnormality alone is suboptimal in predicting overall survival and risk stratification systems that incorporate multiple predictive factors can further enhance their predictive values [37]. R-ISS incorporating cytogenetic abnormalities by interphase FISH has demonstrated prognostic value independent of patient age and therapy (Table 2).

References

1. Rajkumar SV, Dimopoulos MA, Palumbo A et al (2014) International Myeloma Working Group updated criteria for the diagnosis of multiple myeloma. Lancet Oncol 15(12):e538–e548. doi:10.1016/S1470-2045(14)70442-5
2. Smith A, Howell D, Palmore R et al (2011) Incidence of haematological malignancy by subtype: a report from the Haematological Malignancy Research Network. Br J Cancer 105(11):1684–1692. doi:10.1038/bjc.2011.450
3. Munshi NC, Anderson KC, Bergsagel PL et al (2011) Consensus recommendations for risk stratification in multiple myeloma: report of the International Myeloma Workshop Consensus Panel 2. Blood 117(18):4696–4700. doi:10.1182/blood-2010-10-300970
4. Mikhael JR, Dingli D, Roy V et al (2013) Management of newly diagnosed symptomatic multiple myeloma: updated Mayo Stratification of Myeloma and Risk-Adapted Therapy (mSMART) consensus guidelines 2013. Mayo Clin Proc 88(4):360–376. doi:10.1016/j.mayocp.2013.01.019
5. Palumbo A, Avet-Loiseau H, Olivia S et al (2015) Revised International staging system for multiple myeloma: a report from International Myeloma Working Group. J Clin Oncol 33(26):2863–2869. doi:10.1200/JCO.2015.61.2267
6. Dewald GW, Kyle RA, Hicks GA et al (1985) The clinical significance of cytogenetic studies in 100 patients with multiple myeloma, plasma cell leukemia, or amyloidosis. Blood 66(2):380–390
7. Hose D, Rème T, Hielscher T et al (2011) Proliferation is a central independent prognostic factor and target for personalized and risk-adapted treatment in multiple myeloma. Haematologica 96(1):87–95. doi:10.3324/haematol.2010.030296
8. Pratt G (2002) Molecular aspects of multiple myeloma. Mol Pathol 55(5):273–283
9. Avet-Loiseau H, Daviet A, Brigaudeau C et al (2001) Cytogenetic, interphase, and multicolor fluorescence in situ hybridization analyses in primary plasma cell leukemia: a study of 40 patients at diagnosis, on behalf of the Intergroupe Francophone du Myélome and the Groupe Français de Cytogénétique Hématologique. Blood 97(3):822–825
10. Kumar S, Fonseca R, Ketterling RP et al (2012) Trisomies in multiple myeloma: impact on survival in patients with high-risk cytogenetics. Blood 119(9):2100–2105. doi:10.1182/blood-2011-11-390658
11. International Myeloma Working group (IMWG) (2016) Molecular classification of multiple myeloma. http://myeloma.org. Accessed 4 April 2016
12. Fonseca R, Barlogie B, Bataille R et al (2004) Genetics and cytogenetics of multiple myeloma: a workshop report. Cancer Res 64(4):1546–1558
13. Smadja NV, Bastard C, Brigaudeau C et al (2001) Hypodiploidy is a major prognostic factor in multiple myeloma. Blood 98(7):2229–2238

14. Rajkumar SV (2012) Multiple myeloma: 2012 update on diagnosis, risk-stratification, and management. Am J Hematol 87(1):78–88
15. Hartmann L, Biggerstaff JS, Chapman DB et al (2011) Detection of genomic abnormalities in multiple myeloma: the application of FISH analysis in combination with various plasma cell enrichment techniques. Am J Clin Pathol 136(5):712–720. doi:10.1309/AJCPF7NFLW8UAJEP
16. Paiva B, Almeida J, Pérez-Andrés M et al (2010) Utility of flow cytometry immunophenotyping in multiple myeloma and other clonal plasma cell-related disorders. Cytometry B Clin Cytom 78(4):239–252. doi:10.1002/cyto.b.20512
17. Ross FM, Avet-Loiseau H, Ameya G et al (2012) Report from the European Myeloma Network on interphase FISH in multiple myeloma and related disorders. Haematologica 97(8):1272–1277
18. Fonseca R, Bailey RJ, Ahmann GJ et al (2002) Genomic abnormalities in monoclonal gammopathy of undetermined significance. Blood 100(4):1417–1427
19. Kuehl WM, Bergsagel PL (2002) Multiple myeloma: evolving genetic events and host interactions. Nat Rev Cancer 2(3):175–187
20. Avet-Loiseau H, Facon T, Grosbois B et al (2002) Oncogenesis of multiple myeloma: 14q32 and 13q chromosomal abnormalities are not randomly distributed, but correlate with natural history, immunological features, and clinical presentation. Blood 99(6):2185–2191
21. Moreau P, Facon T, Leleu X et al (2002) Recurrent 14q32 translocations determine the prognosis of multiple myeloma, especially in patients receiving intensive chemotherapy. Blood 100(5):1579–1583
22. Moreau P, Attal M, Garban F et al (2007) Heterogeneity of t(4;14) in multiple myeloma. Long-term follow-up of 100 cases treated with tandem transplantation in IFM99 trials. Leukemia 21(9):2020–2024
23. Shaughnessy JD Jr, Zhan F, Burington BE et al (2007) A validated gene expression model of high-risk multiple myeloma is defined by deregulated expression of genes mapping to chromosome 1. Blood 109(6):2276–2284
24. Nair B, van Rhee F, Shaughnessy JD Jr et al (2010) Superior results of Total Therapy 3 (2003-33) in gene expression profiling-defined low-risk multiple myeloma confirmed in subsequent trial 2006-66 with VRD maintenance. Blood 115(21):4168–4173. doi:10.1182/blood-2009-11-255620
25. Fonseca R, Blood E, Rue M et al (2003) Clinical and biologic implications of recurrent genomic aberrations in myeloma. Blood 101(11):4569–4575
26. Sawyer JR, Lukacs JL, Munshi N et al (1998) Identification of new nonrandom translocations in multiple myeloma with multicolor spectral karyotyping. Blood 92(11):4269–4278
27. Avet-Loiseau H, Leleu X, Roussel M et al (2010) Bortezomib plus dexamethasone induction improves outcome of patients with t(4;14) myeloma but not outcome of patients with del(17p). J Clin Oncol 28(30):4630–4634. doi:10.1200/JCO.2010.28.3945
28. Avet-Louseau H, Daviet A, Sauner S et al (2000) Chromosome 13 abnormalities in multiple myeloma are mostly monosomy 13. Br J Haematol 111(4):1116–1117
29. Chiecchio L, Protheroe RK, Ibrahim AH et al (2006) Deletion of chromosome 13 detected by conventional cytogenetics is a critical prognostic factor in myeloma. Leukemia 20(9):1610–1617
30. Rajan AM, Rajkumar SV (2015) Interpretation of cytogenetic results in multiple myeloma for clinical practice. Blood Cancer J 5(10), e365. doi:10.1038/bcj.2015.92
31. Hebraud B, Leleu X, Lauwers-Cances V et al (2014) Deletion of the 1p32 region is a major independent prognostic factor in young patients with myeloma: the IFM experience on 1195 patients. Leukemia 28(3):675–679
32. Jacobson J, Barlogie B, Shaughnessy J et al (2003) MDS-type abnormalities within myeloma signature karyotype (MM-MDS): only 13% 1-year survival despite tandem transplants. Br J Haematol 122(3):430–440
33. Ola L, Gloria G, Ingemar T et al (2005) Risk of monoclonal gammopathy of undetermined significance (MGUS) and subsequent multiple myeloma among African American and white veterans in the United States. Blood 107(3):904–906
34. Robert K, Ellen R, Terry T et al (2007) Clinical course and prognosis of smoldering (asymptomatic) multiple myeloma. N Engl J Med 356:2582–2590. doi:10.1056/NEJMoa070389
35. Rajkumar SV, Gupta V, Fonseca R et al (2013) Impact of primary molecular cytogenetic abnormalities and risk of progression in smoldering multiple myeloma. Leukemia 27(8):1738–1744. doi:10.1038/leu.2013.86
36. Dimopoulos M, Kyle R, Fermand JP et al (2011) Consensus recommendations for standard investigative workup: report of the International Myeloma Workshop Consensus Panel 3. Blood 117(18):4701–4705. doi:10.1182/blood-2010-10-299529
37. Chng WJ, Dispenzieri A, Chim CS et al (2014) IMWG consensus on risk stratification in multiple myeloma. Leukemia 28(2):269–277. doi:10.1038/leu.2013.247

Chapter 24

Cytogenetic Nomenclature and Reporting

Marian Stevens-Kroef, Annet Simons, Katrina Rack, and Rosalind J. Hastings

Abstract

A standardized nomenclature is critical for the accurate and consistent description of genomic changes as identified by karyotyping, fluorescence in situ hybridization and microarray. The International System for Human Cytogenomic Nomenclature (ISCN) is the central reference for the description of karyotyping, FISH, and microarray results, and provides rules for describing cytogenetic and molecular cytogenetic findings in laboratory reports. These laboratory reports are documents to the referring clinician, and should be clear, accurate and contain all information relevant for good interpretation of the cytogenetic findings. Here, we describe guidelines for cytogenetic nomenclature and laboratory reports for cytogenetic testing applied to tumor samples.

Key words Karyotyping, FISH, Microarray, Nomenclature, Diagnostic reports

1 Introduction

Cytogenetic and molecular genetic analysis of clonal neoplastic disorders is important in the diagnosis, prognosis, risk stratification to aid in the selection of treatment intensity, the identification of patients' eligibility for targeted drugs and/or monitoring response to treatment [1]. Therefore, the interpretation, correct use of nomenclature, and reporting of these data according to international standards is of paramount importance for diagnostic laboratories.

Karyotyping, fluorescence in situ hybridization (FISH), and genomic (SNP-based) microarray are the most commonly used techniques for cytogenetic studies, and their results should be described according to the International System for Human Cytogenomic Nomenclature (ISCN; previously named International System for Human Cytogenetic Nomenclature). It is recommended that the most recent version of ISCN, which is at the moment ISCN 2016 [2], is used.

In recent years, several best practice meetings with experts in the field have been held to discuss reporting of cytogenetic results [3–7]. Based on these meetings, this chapter provides the most

Thomas S.K. Wan (ed.), *Cancer Cytogenetics: Methods and Protocols*, Methods in Molecular Biology, vol. 1541,
DOI 10.1007/978-1-4939-6703-2_24, © Springer Science+Business Media LLC 2017

common ISCN rules regarding karyotyping, FISH and array nomenclature, recommendations for (molecular) cytogenetic interpretation, and general guidelines for the writing of cytogenetic and molecular cytogenetic diagnostic reports in tumors.

2 Nomenclature Regarding Cell Numbers and Clones

1. Karyotype designation should use the correct current version of ISCN nomenclature.
2. The number of cells constituting a clone should be given in square brackets.
3. Constitutional abnormalities are distinguished by the letter c.
4. The slant line is used to separate different clones or subclones. A double slant line is used for transplants where the recipient and donor karyotypes are different.
5. The definition of a cytogenetic abnormal clone is provided by the ISCN. An abnormality is regarded as clonal when it is a gain or a structural abnormality present in at least two cells. Where there is loss of a whole chromosome this has to be observed in at least three cells for proof of clonality. However, two cells with identical losses of one or more chromosomes and the same other numerical or structural aberration(s) may be considered clonal and included in the nomenclature.
6. The finding of a single abnormal metaphase, even if it includes a rearrangement of potential significance, cannot define a clone. However, proof of clonality can be obtained by another method (e.g., FISH or microarray).
7. When the abnormality in a single cell has been found in an initial study in the same patient (e.g., diagnostic and follow-up sample), it may be regarded as a clonal abnormality and should be included in the karyotype.
8. Where there are multiple related clones, the most basic clone (stemline) should be listed first. The order of sidelines should be given in increasing complexity. Note that the abbreviations idem, sl, sdl include the sex-chromosomes, and therefore the sex chromosomes are not described again.
9. Unrelated clones are listed according to their size (largest clone first).
10. In case of a combination of related and unrelated clones, the related clones are listed first (in order of increasing complexity) and then the unrelated clones in order of decreasing frequency.

11. Every effort should be taken to describe the clones and subclones so that clonal evolution is evident. However, in case this is not possible one can use the composite karyotype (cp).
12. The normal diploid clone is always listed last.

3 FISH Nomenclature

1. FISH results can be provided according to the current ISCN or otherwise can be given as summary statement that is succinct and clear.
2. In case FISH results are not provided according to ISCN, one should include a clear FISH result summary. It is essential to indicate whether the FISH result is normal or abnormal, and the number of investigated interphases or metaphases.
3. Only clinically relevant FISH results need to be in the ISCN, normal results for control probes should not be mentioned.
4. For sex chromosome probes, the Y probe is not listed in the ISCN description for female patients.
5. Interphase FISH is indicated by the abbreviation nuc ish (nuclear in situ hybridization).
6. The number of cells scored is placed in square brackets. When both normal and abnormal cells are found, the number of abnormal cells is listed over the total number of cells scored for each abnormal pattern.
7. If multiple probes are used the string of probes should be listed according to chromosome number, e.g., if a *BCR-ABL1* probe is used, in the ISCN result *ABL1* (chromosome 9) is listed before *BCR* (chromosome 22). If multiple FISH hybridizations are performed, e.g., the *BCR-ABL1* and *KMT2A* (*MLL*) probes are used, in the ISCN result *BCR-ABL1* (*ABL1* on chromosome 9) is listed before *KMT2A* (chromosome 11).
8. If both metaphase and interphase FISH are performed, each is reported in the same string, separated by a period.
9. In case both karyotyping and metaphase FISH have been performed, and the FISH further clarifies the karyotype and, in retrospect, the abnormality can be visualized with banding the karyotype may be rewritten. However, if the abnormality is cryptic and cannot be visualized by banding, the abnormality should not be listed in the banded karyotype, e.g., 46,XX,t(12;21)(p13;q22) is not allowed since this translocation is not visible with karyotyping.
10. In order to avoid misinterpretation the term "positive" should not be used when describing FISH results, e.g., for reporting a *BCR-ABL1* FISH result: *BCR-ABL1* rearrangement present/not detected.

4 Microarray Nomenclature

1. Noncomplex microarray results should be reported according to the current ISCN. In highly rearranged microarray profiles of tumor samples the ISCN may be difficult and an alternative unambiguous presentation of array results is acceptable.
2. The genome build should be included for all abnormal results as this is pertinent to the interpretation of array results. This can be omitted in case of a normal array result or whole chromosome abnormalities are reported.
3. In case of a normal array result, the autosomes are listed first, followed by the sex chromosomes.
4. In case of abnormal array result, only the aberrations are listed, the lowest chromosome number first, followed by the sex chromosomes [2]. Note that this is different from description of karyotyping and FISH results where the sex chromosomes are listed first.
5. In order to report only tumor-related abnormalities, and no benign constitutional copy number variants (CNVs), microarray interpretation guidelines have been described previously [7, 8]. According to these guidelines:
   (a) All copy number aberrations >5 megabase (Mb) (resolution of conventional karyotyping) should be interpreted as abnormal. This avoids the reporting of small anomalies with unclear clinical significance which are frequently detected by array and which will not affect risk stratification in the short term.
   (b) Copy number aberrations <5 Mb should be considered aberrant only when they encompass known tumor-related genes that are associated with the referral reason.
   (c) Focal copy number aberrations in T-cell receptor and immunoglobulin genes should be excluded since these lesions generally represent nonmalignant genomic rearrangements occurring during normal T-cell and B-cell development.
   (d) Interpretation of regions of copy-neutral loss of heterozygosity can be challenging. In general, these are only considered tumor-related if these regions are >10 Mb in size or if they extend toward the telomeres of the involved chromosomes.
   (e) In case paired control DNA is not used, alterations that coincide with normal genomic variants are excluded. For this approach the publicly available Database of Genomic Variants (http://dgv.tcag.ca) can be used.

5 Nomenclature Order of Different Tests

If multiple tests are undertaken on the same sample, the order of reporting is: karyotype, metaphase FISH, interphase FISH, microarray. If sequencing-based tests are used, they will be listed last.

6 Cytogenetic Reporting

1. Reports must be clear, concise, accurate, fully interpretative including an explanation of the clinical implications of the results.
2. Patients must be identified on reports by at least two unique patient identifiers (e.g., full name and date of birth). It is recommended that the patient gender is also identified on the report.
3. Inclusion of unique laboratory number is mandatory to ensure that the report unequivocally links to that specific patient.
4. Date of sample collection (if given) and date of receipt in the laboratory must be recorded within the laboratory report.
5. The type and origin of sample, including details whether fresh, fixed, or frozen.
6. The cell source used in case test is performed on selected group of cells, e.g., after CD34 or CD138 cell enrichment.
7. The name and contact details of the requesting physician(s) or authorized persons to whom the report is provided. Also, additional recipients of copy reports must be clearly indicated.
8. The laboratory issuing the report must be clearly identified, with full contact details.
9. The report should carry a title (e.g., results of cytogenetic analysis).
10. Reason for referral, e.g., suspected diagnosis, follow-up after treatment or bone marrow transplantation.
11. Date of final report and (digital) signature of an authorized person.
12. It may, in some circumstances, be useful to issue a report before all studies are complete (e.g., when indicative preliminary results have been obtained but a long delay is expected before the final results will be ready). Preliminary data should be clearly stated in the report.
13. The overall result or conclusion must be clearly visible. In addition, a written description of the result should be provided.

14. A clear statement whether the test result is normal or abnormal.
15. A clear written description of the cytogenetic abnormality and the interpretation of the results of the analysis must be clearly stated. In cases with complex cytogenetic or microarray results only the salient abnormalities need to be discussed.
16. In general, it should be stated whether the karyotype is male or female, unless the X and/or Y-chromosome are involved in an aberrant karyotype or no information is available about X and Y.
17. Clinically significant constitutional abnormalities including recommendations for genetic counseling should be provided where appropriate.
18. The clinical significance of a result, if applicable, consistent with referral reason, or other possible diagnosis.
19. The association with prognosis in case a robust association in large published series of clinical trials (including literature reference) exists.
20. Any technical details relevant to interpretation must be made clear or the report should include a referral that the information is available upon request.
21. Where a cytogenetic abnormality of unknown significance is detected, the term "malignancy" should not be used in reports. Terms such as "clonal disease" or "neoplasm" are recommended instead.
22. The interpretation and reporting of loss of the Y chromosome or trisomy 15 can be problematic. Both features are seen in bone marrow cells of elderly patients with no hematological disease, but may also occur as markers of neoplastic clones [9, 10].
23. When relevant the report should refer to previous genetic test results.
24. Normal karyotypic, FISH, and microarray results must always be regarded with suspicion, since malignant cells may be underrepresented in the tested sample (culture). If appropriate this should be stated in the report.
25. If the proportion of malignant cells in the sample is unknown, this must be qualified to point out the possibility that the malignant clone was not represented in the analysis, i.e., the possibility of a false-negative result. In order to obtain information regarding the percentage of malignant cells, close collaboration with a pathologist or physician is recommended.
26. If commercially available kits, (FISH) probes, software packages (including version), or microarray platforms are used, then the manufacturer, kit number, and version number must be reported.

27. The technical sensitivity and practical resolution of the test must be provided where applicable.
28. The resolution of array platform as well as the practical resolution used for analysis to exclude benign constitutional variants (e.g., copy number aberrations >5 Mb) should be provided.
29. In general, limitations of the test or where the minimal quality or requirements are not achieved, should be stated. Limitations of the microarray test, including cut-off levels for the detection of mosaicism and a statement that the test will not detect point mutations and balanced rearrangements and, for some platforms, polyploidy and copy neutral loss of heterozygosity should be provided.
30. For microarray studies, relevant genes located within the interval of aberrations that are known to be associated with the disorder stated in the referral or have possible prognostic or predictive implications should be reported.
31. Integrated reporting of results for a patient is encouraged. This may be multiple tests within one laboratory or several test results from different laboratory disciplines for one patient event.
32. It is realistic to expect a result within 28 days. However, if the test is known to influence treatment decisions, the laboratory should have a policy for prioritization of samples. Reporting times should be adjusted with local clinicians, e.g., a urgent FISH result of childhood acute leukemia or a t(15;17) should be expected within 48 h.

References

1. Heim S, Mittelman F (eds) (2015) Cancer cytogenetics: chromosomal and molecular genetic aberrations of tumor cells, 4th edn. Wiley-Blackwell, London
2. McGowan-Jordan J, Simons A, Schmid M (eds) (2016) An international system for human cytogenomic nomenclature. S. Karger, Basel. [Reprint of Cytogenet Genome Res 149(1–2)]
3. Hastings RJ, Cavani S, Bricarelli FD, ECA PWG Co-ordinators et al (2007) Cytogenetic Guidelines and Quality Assurance: a common European framework for quality assessment for constitutional and acquired cytogenetic investigations. Eur J Hum Genet 15:525–527
4. Dawson AJ, McGowan-Jordan J, Chernos J et al (2011) Canadian College of Medical Geneticists guidelines for the indications, analysis, and reporting of cancer specimens. Curr Oncol 18:e250–e255
5. Claustres M, Kožich V, Dequeker E et al (2013) European Society of Human Genetics. Recommendations for reporting results of diagnostic genetic testing (biochemical, cytogenetic and molecular genetic). Eur J Hum Genet 22:160–170. doi:10.1038/ejhg.2013.125
6. Hastings RJ, Brown N, Tibiletti MG et al (2016) Guidelines for cytogenetic investigations in tumours. Eur J Hum Genet 24:6–13. doi:10.1038/ejhg.2015.35
7. Schoumans J, Suela J, Hastings R et al (2016) Guidelines for genomic array analysis in acquired haematological neoplastic disorders. Genes Chromosomes Cancer 55:480–491. doi:10.1002/gcc.22350
8. Simons A, Sikkema-Raddatz B, de Leeuw N et al (2012) Genome-wide arrays in routine diagnostics of hematological malignancies. Hum Mutat 33:941–948. doi:10.1038/ejhg.2015.35
9. Hanson CA, Steensma DP, Hodnefield JM et al (2008) Isolated trisomy 15: a clonal chromosome abnormality in bone marrow with doubtful hematologic significance. Am J Clin Pathol 129:478–485
10. Goswami RS, Liang CS, Bueso-Ramos CE et al (2015) Isolated +15 in bone marrow: disease-associated or a benign finding? Leuk Res 39:72–76

Chapter 25

Cytogenetic Resources and Information

Etienne De Braekeleer, Jean-Loup Huret, Hossain Mossafa, and Philippe Dessen

Abstract

The main databases devoted *stricto sensu* to cancer cytogenetics are the "Mitelman Database of Chromosome Aberrations and Gene Fusions in Cancer" (http://cgap.nci.nih.gov/Chromosomes/Mitelman), the "Atlas of Genetics and Cytogenetics in Oncology and Haematology" (http://atlasgeneticsoncology.org), and COSMIC (http://cancer.sanger.ac.uk/cosmic).

However, being a complex multistep process, cancer cytogenetics are broadened to "cytogenomics," with complementary resources on: general databases (nucleic acid and protein sequences databases; cartography browsers: GenBank, RefSeq, UCSC, Ensembl, UniProtKB, and Entrez Gene), cancer genomic portals associated with recent international integrated programs, such as TCGA or ICGC, other fusion genes databases, array CGH databases, copy number variation databases, and mutation databases. Other resources such as the International System for Human Cytogenomic Nomenclature (ISCN), the International Classification of Diseases for Oncology (ICD-O), and the Human Gene Nomenclature Database (HGNC) allow a common language.

Data within the scientific/medical community should be freely available. However, most of the institutional stakeholders are now gradually disengaging, and well-known databases are forced to beg or to disappear (which may happen!)

Key words Cytogenetic, Cancer, Database, Mitelman database, Atlas of Genetics and Cytogenetics in Oncology and Haematology, COSMIC, UCSC, Ensembl, ICD-O, HGNC

1 Introduction

A genetic event is present in each cancer case [1]. Cytogenetics has been a major player in the understanding of cancer genetics, and providing specific keys for diagnostic as well as prognostic assessments, enabling the subclassification of otherwise seemingly identical disease entities [2].

"Cancer Cytogenetics," *stricto sensu*, deals with chromosomes and cancer. "Cytogenomics," as coined by Alain Bernheim [3], means the "genetics—as a whole—of the cell," with complex interconnections and interactions between the various actors. Therefore, the "Cancer Cytogenetics" field should include

Thomas S.K. Wan (ed.), *Cancer Cytogenetics: Methods and Protocols*, Methods in Molecular Biology, vol. 1541,
DOI 10.1007/978-1-4939-6703-2_25,

knowledge of the biology of normal and cancerous cells, gene fusions, mutations or copy number variations, epigenetics, protein domains, signaling pathways, as well as gross and microscopic pathological presentation.

Presently, Internet gives access to a vast and complex network of knowledge that can make it a challenge for you to find specific answer to your questions. Several databases are freely accessible. We will briefly describe the main ones in the following pages. In addition, there are several descriptions of databases (and particularly in cancer) in the special annual "Database issues" of Nucleic Acid Research.

1.1 Brief History

In the 1970s, the introduction of chromosomal banding techniques invented by Caspersson and Zech [4] gave the possibility of identifying individual chromosomes, which were defined by a unique banding pattern. The description of chromosomal rearrangements in leukemias immediately became clearer giving more gravity to the conclusions drawn. This was a new era for cancer cytogenetics with an increasing number of aberrant human malignant and benign karyotypes.

In the 1980s, the advent of molecular genetic techniques gave an opportunity to characterize the chromosomal breakpoints at the molecular level which has consequently highlighted two classes of genes implicated in these karyotypical rearrangements: the oncogenes and the tumor suppressor genes.

The study of fusion genes led to the development of specific drugs targeting chimeric proteins. The tyrosine kinase inhibitor Imatinib, approved in 2001, was the first drug that was specifically designed to target the chimeric protein BCR-ABL1 in chronic myelogenous leukemia (CML) [5, 6] by blocking its kinase activity. This drug dramatically improved the lifespan and quality of life of patients bearing CML.

1.2 Catalog of Chromosome Aberrations in Cancer

In 1983, Felix Mitelman published a colossal catalogue of all the known chromosomal rearrangements. In 2000, the catalogue became accessible for the public under the name of "Mitelman Database of Chromosome Aberrations in Cancer" on the Internet, making it freely accessible.

1.3 Atlas of Genetics and Cytogenetics in Oncology and Haematology

How did the idea of the Atlas appear? Prognosis of a leukemia depends on the genes involved and treatments depends on the severity of the disease. However, thousands of genes were found to be implicated in cancer. The conclusion was that huge databases were needed to collect and summarize data to produce meta-analyses. The Atlas was established in 1997 to answer that call to contribute to "meta-medicine," meaning the mediation between the knowledge and the knowledge users in medicine.

2 General Resources

2.1 General Databases

2.1.1 Gene Nomenclature: HGNC (http://www.genenames.org/)

The HUGO Gene Nomenclature Committee (HGNC) is the authority that assigns standardized nomenclature to human genes. HGNC is responsible for approving unique symbols and names for human loci, including protein coding genes, ncRNA genes, and pseudogenes to allow unambiguous scientific communication. The database contains 39,000 approved symbols [7].

2.1.2 An International System for Human Cytogenomic Nomenclature (ISCN)

ISCN is the language used to describe abnormal karyotypes. Periodic revisions and updates occurred and ISCN has become ever more complicated [8]. A new version is being released by the end of 2016 [9] but will not be freely available on the web.

2.1.3 International Classification of Diseases for Oncology (ICD-O) (http://www.who.int/classifications/icd/adaptations/oncology/en/)

A common language must be found for reasons of interoperability of different databases. The ICD-O code (International Classification of Diseases—Oncology) has been established by the World Health Organization) WHO/OMS. It contains an International Classification of Diseases for Oncology, Third Edition (ICD-O-3) for coding the site (topography) and the histology (morphology) providing a topographical (organ) identifier, and the basic and detailed pathology.

However, such classification of tumors is not used by all databases (e.g., the Mitelman database or the Catalogue of Somatic Mutations in Cancer (COSMIC) database have their own classifications, with no apparent matching). This is a real obstacle for the integration of data by new resources.

2.1.4 Nucleic Acid Databases

The first DNA sequence database gave way to the creation of the public GenBank (http://www.ncbi.nlm.nih.gov/genbank/) [10] in 1982. As of February 2016, GenBank has 190,250,235 loci, 207,018,196,067 bases, from 190,250,235 reported sequences.

The need to have (in parallel to the genome projects) the best representation of genomic and transcript sequences has instigated the development of consensus databases (as Reference Sequences (RefSeq), UC Santa Cruz Genomics Institute (UCSC), Ensembl).

Several databases of consensus nucleic sequences provide detailed structures of genes and isoforms. All this information can easily be visualized in different browsers (UCSC, Ensembl) or described in detail on the Entrez Gene (*see* Subheading 2.2.1). RefSeq (http://www.ncbi.nlm.nih.gov/refseq/) maintains and curates a database of annotated genomic, transcript, and protein consensus sequence records. RefSeq represents sequences of more than 55,000 organisms. Ensembl (http://www.ensembl.org/) produces automatic annotation on selected eukaryotic genomes [7]. The UCSC Genome Browser database (*see* Subheading 2.3.1) is a large collection containing 160 genome assemblies representing 91 species [11].

2.1.5 Protein Sequence Databases

In parallel to the nucleic databases, a curated protein database, SwissProt, was developed by Amos Bairoch. This was extended by the UniProt Knowledgebase (UniProtKB). In addition to the amino acid sequence, protein name, and description with domains, it provides brief annotation information (Fig. 1). UniProtKB (http://www.uniprot.org/) consists of two sections: "TrEMBL," computationally analyzed, and "Swiss-Prot," manually annotated, with information extracted from the literature and

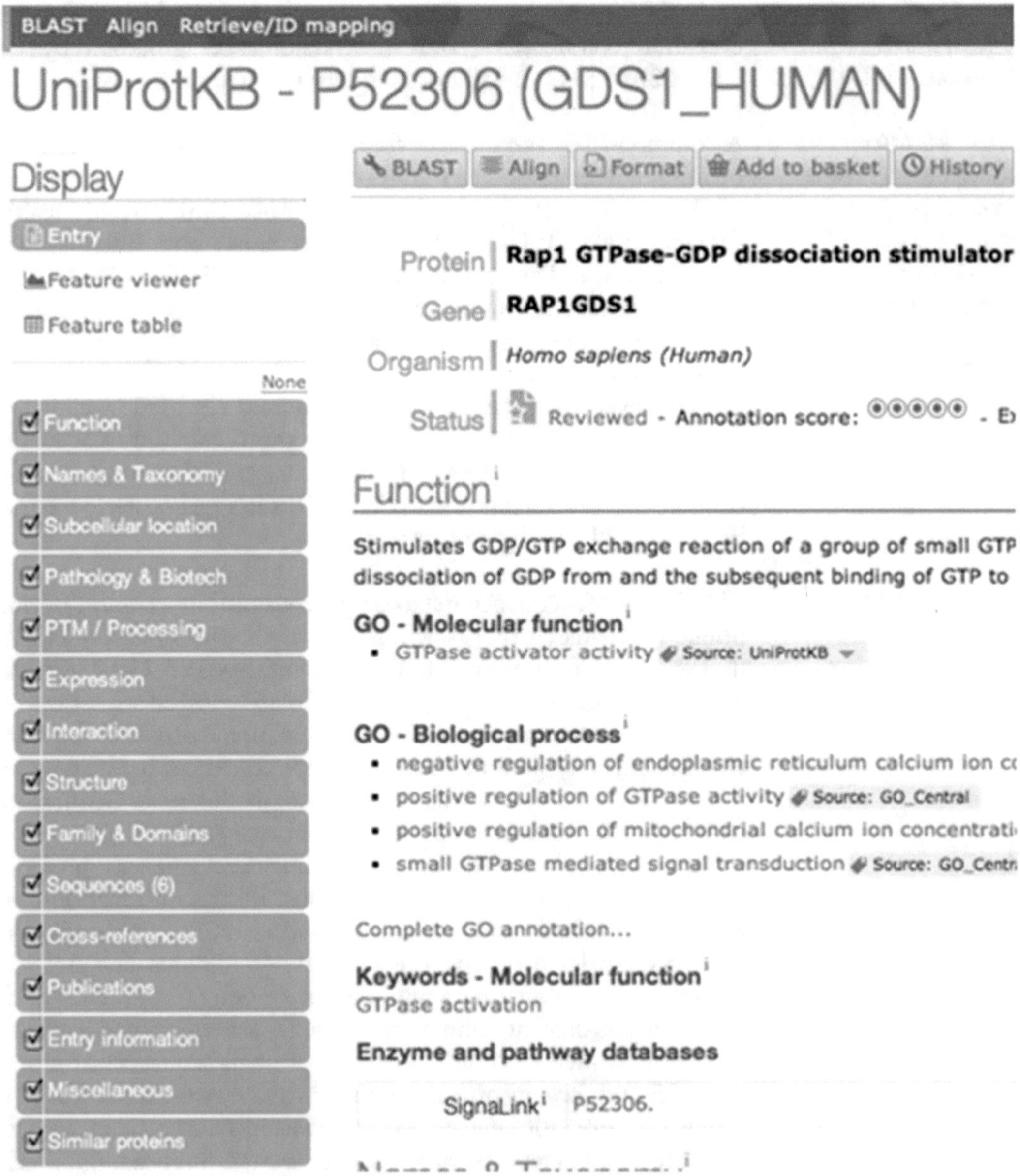

Fig. 1 *RAP1GDS1* at UniProtKB (http://www.uniprot.org/uniprot/P52306)

curator-evaluated computational analysis. The number of proteins entered in UniProtKB/Swiss-Prot has risen to 550,960 for the SwissProt part and 63,686,057 for the nonreviewed part for TrEMBL [12].

Other complementary resources on human proteins are neXt-Prot (http://www.nextprot.org/db/) [13], PhosphoSitePlus [14], PROSITE [15], Pfam [16], and InterPro [17]. Description of proteins with domains and iconography, expression and localization, function, homologs, can also be found in the Atlas of Genetics and Cytogenetics in Oncology and Haematology (*see* Subheading 3.2) (Fig. 2).

2.2 Cards

2.2.1 Entrez Gene (http://www.ncbi.nlm.nih.gov/gene/)

Entrez is a primary text search and retrieval system of the NCBI that integrates the PubMed database of biomedical literature with other literature and molecular databases including DNA and protein sequence, structure, gene, genome, genetic variation, and gene expression. Entrez Gene, dedicated to genes, integrates

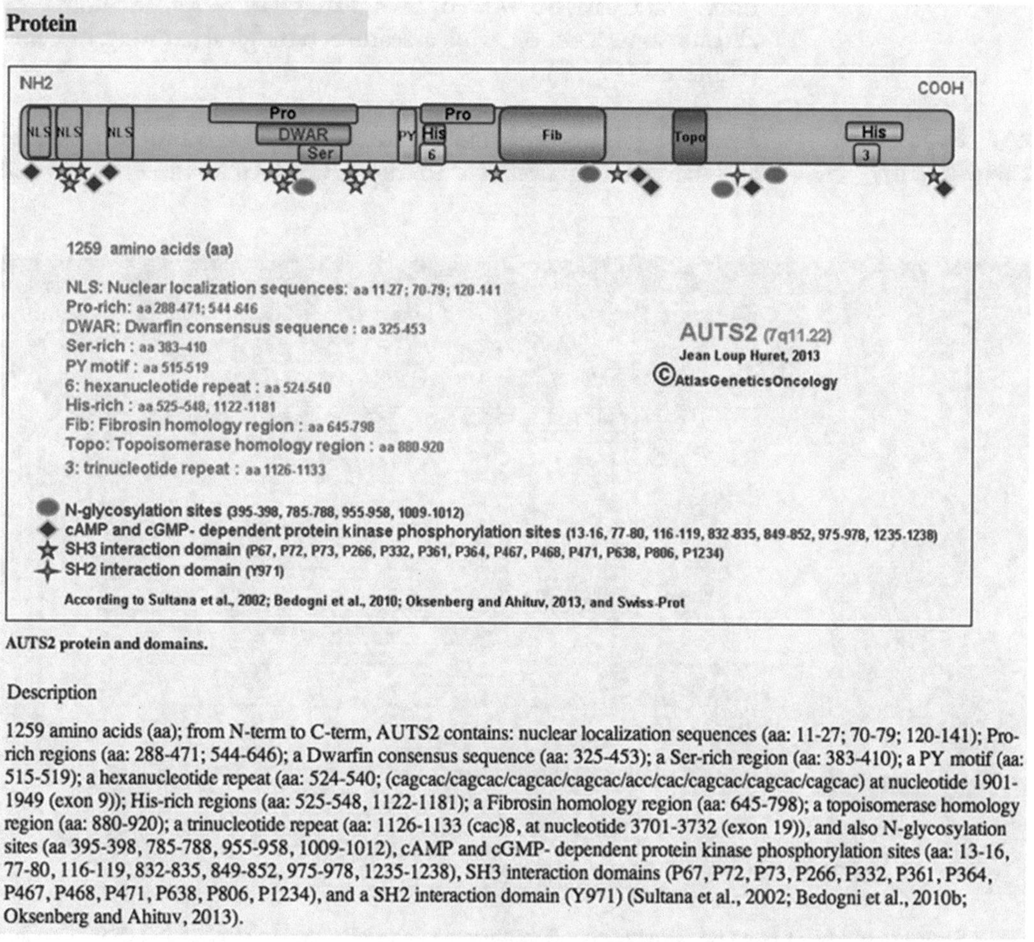

Fig. 2 *AUTS2* at Atlas: domains of the protein (http://atlasgeneticsoncology.org/Genes/AUTS2ID51794ch7q11.html)

nomenclature, Reference Sequences (RefSeqs), maps, pathways, variations, and phenotypes. For humans, Entrez Gene catalogs 59,941 genes.

2.2.2 Genecards (http://www.genecards.org/)

Genecards is a searchable, integrative database that integrates gene data from about 125 web sources, including genomic, transcriptomic, proteomic, genetic, clinical and functional information.

2.3 Genome Cartography

The localization of genes within the genome has always been a practical way to present genomic information.

2.3.1 UCSC (http://genome.ucsc.edu/) and UCSC-Cancer (https://genome-cancer.ucsc.edu/)

The UCSC Genome Browser website contains the reference sequence for a large collection of genomes. The Genome Browser zooms and scrolls over chromosomes, showing the work of annotators worldwide. "Blat" quickly maps your sequence to the genome. The UCSC Cancer Browser (https://genome-cancer.ucsc.edu/proj/site/help/) allows researchers to interactively explore cancer genomics data and its associated clinical information. Data can be viewed in a variety of ways, including by chromosome location, clinical feature, biological pathway, or genes of interest (Fig. 3).

2.3.2 Ensembl (http://www.ensembl.org)

Ensembl generates genomic datasets. It acts as a hub of reference and baseline data similar to the UCSC Genome Browser and

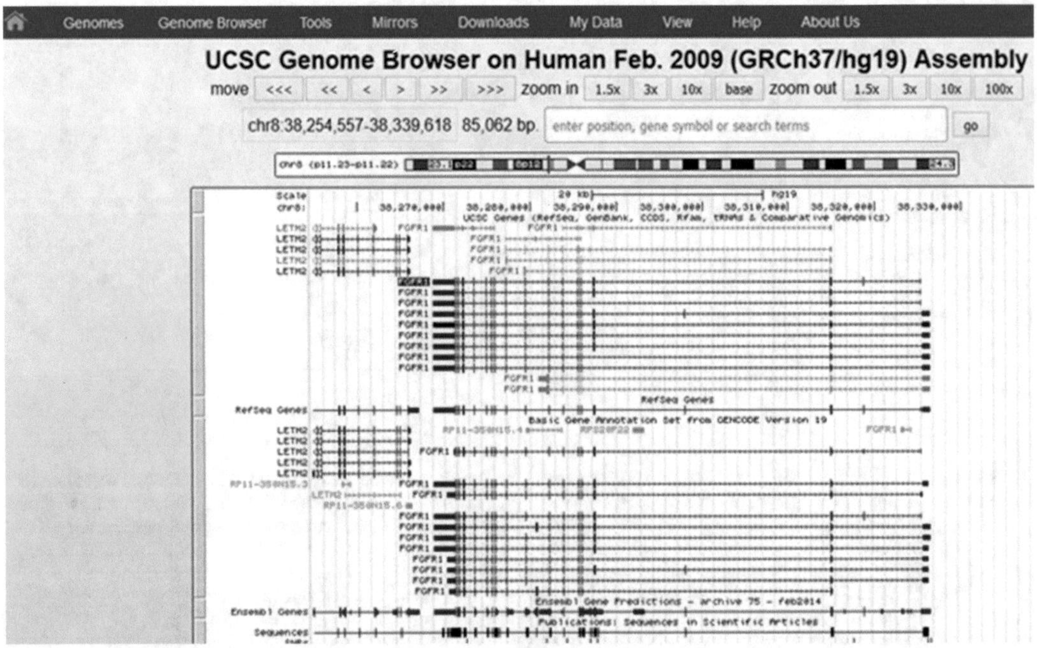

Fig. 3 Structure of FGFR1 gene on chromosome 8, represented as exons and introns on the UCSC Genome Browser, with different isoforms, depending on the origin of the annotation (RefSeq, UCSC, GenCode) (http://genome.ucsc.edu)

RefSeq. Ensembl is updated four to five times per year. For human data, Ensembl provides two sets of data based on the hg19 genome build (February 2009) which has been updated by the data set based on the December 2013, Homo sapiens high coverage assembly GRCh38 from the Genome Reference Consortium (http://www.ensembl.org/Homo_sapiens/Info/Index).

2.4 Portals

2.4.1 TCGA (http://cancergenome.nih.gov/)

TCGA (The Cancer Genome Atlas) is a project to catalogue genetic mutations responsible for cancer, using genome sequencing and bioinformatics. TCGA applies high-throughput genome analysis to progress our ability to diagnose, treat, and prevent cancer. The project scheduled 500 patient samples and used different techniques to analyze them: gene expression profiling, copy number variation profiling, SNP genotyping, genome-wide DNA methylation profiling, microRNA profiling, and exon sequencing of at least 1200 genes (Fig. 4). In phase II, TCGA is performing whole exon sequencing and whole genome sequencing, characterizing 33 cancer types including 10 rare cancers.

2.4.2 ICGC (https://icgc.org/)

ICGC (The International Cancer Genome Consortium) has been organized to launch and coordinate a large number of research projects that have the common aim of comprehensively elucidating the genomic changes present in many forms of cancers (Fig. 5). The primary goals of the ICGC are to generate comprehensive catalogs of genomic abnormalities (somatic mutations, abnormal

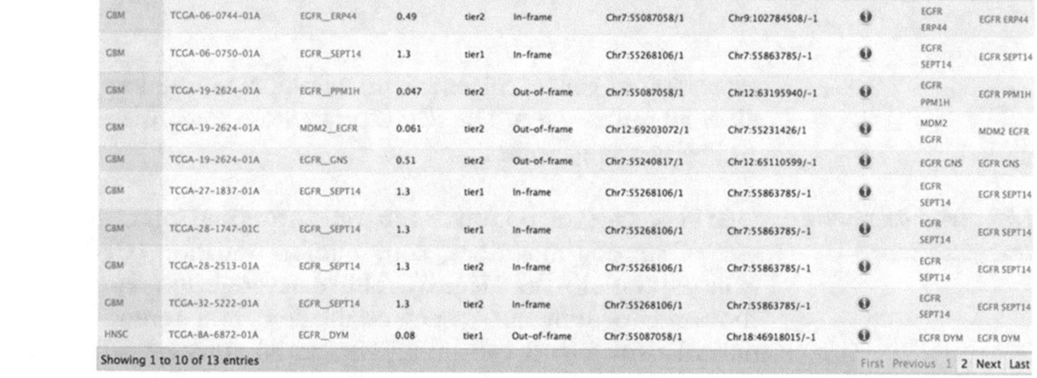

THE UNIVERSITY OF TEXAS MD Anderson Cancer Center

TCGA Fusion gene Data Portal

Landscape of cancer-associated fusions using the Pipeline for RNA sequencing Data Analysis

Introduction | By Gene | By Fusion | By Sample | By Cancer Type | Contact Us

Gene-Centric Fusions Results

Gene Name: EGFR Query eg:EGFR

Gene constituting a part of fusion can be individually queried by Gene Symbol here.

Show 10 entries Search:

Cancer	TCGA SampleId	FusionPair	E-value	Tier	Frame	5' Gene Junction	3' Gene Junction	Details	CNV	Somatic Muts
GBM	TCGA-06-0744-01A	EGFR__ERP44	0.49	tier2	In-frame	Chr7:55087058/1	Chr9:102784508/-1		EGFR ERP44	EGFR ERP44
GBM	TCGA-06-0750-01A	EGFR__SEPT14	1.3	tier1	In-frame	Chr7:55268106/1	Chr7:55863785/-1		EGFR SEPT14	EGFR SEPT14
GBM	TCGA-19-2624-01A	EGFR__PPM1H	0.047	tier2	Out-of-frame	Chr7:55087058/1	Chr12:63195940/-1		EGFR PPM1H	EGFR PPM1H
GBM	TCGA-19-2624-01A	MDM2__EGFR	0.061	tier2	Out-of-frame	Chr12:69203072/1	Chr7:55231426/1		MDM2 EGFR	MDM2 EGFR
GBM	TCGA-19-2624-01A	EGFR__GNS	0.51	tier2	Out-of-frame	Chr7:55240817/1	Chr12:65110599/-1		EGFR GNS	EGFR GNS
GBM	TCGA-27-1837-01A	EGFR__SEPT14	1.3	tier1	In-frame	Chr7:55268106/1	Chr7:55863785/-1		EGFR SEPT14	EGFR SEPT14
GBM	TCGA-28-1747-01C	EGFR__SEPT14	1.3	tier1	In-frame	Chr7:55268106/1	Chr7:55863785/-1		EGFR SEPT14	EGFR SEPT14
GBM	TCGA-28-2513-01A	EGFR__SEPT14	1.3	tier2	In-frame	Chr7:55268106/1	Chr7:55863785/-1		EGFR SEPT14	EGFR SEPT14
GBM	TCGA-32-5222-01A	EGFR__SEPT14	1.3	tier2	In-frame	Chr7:55268106/1	Chr7:55863785/-1		EGFR SEPT14	EGFR SEPT14
HNSC	TCGA-BA-6872-01A	EGFR__DYM	0.08	tier1	Out-of-frame	Chr7:55087058/1	Chr18:46918015/-1		EGFR DYM	EGFR DYM

Showing 1 to 10 of 13 entries First Previous 1 2 Next Last

Fig. 4 Example of search of fusion with *EGFR* (http://54.84.12.177/PanCanFusV2/) in TCGA (TCGA Fusion gene Data Portal, http://54.84.12.177/PanCanFusV2/)

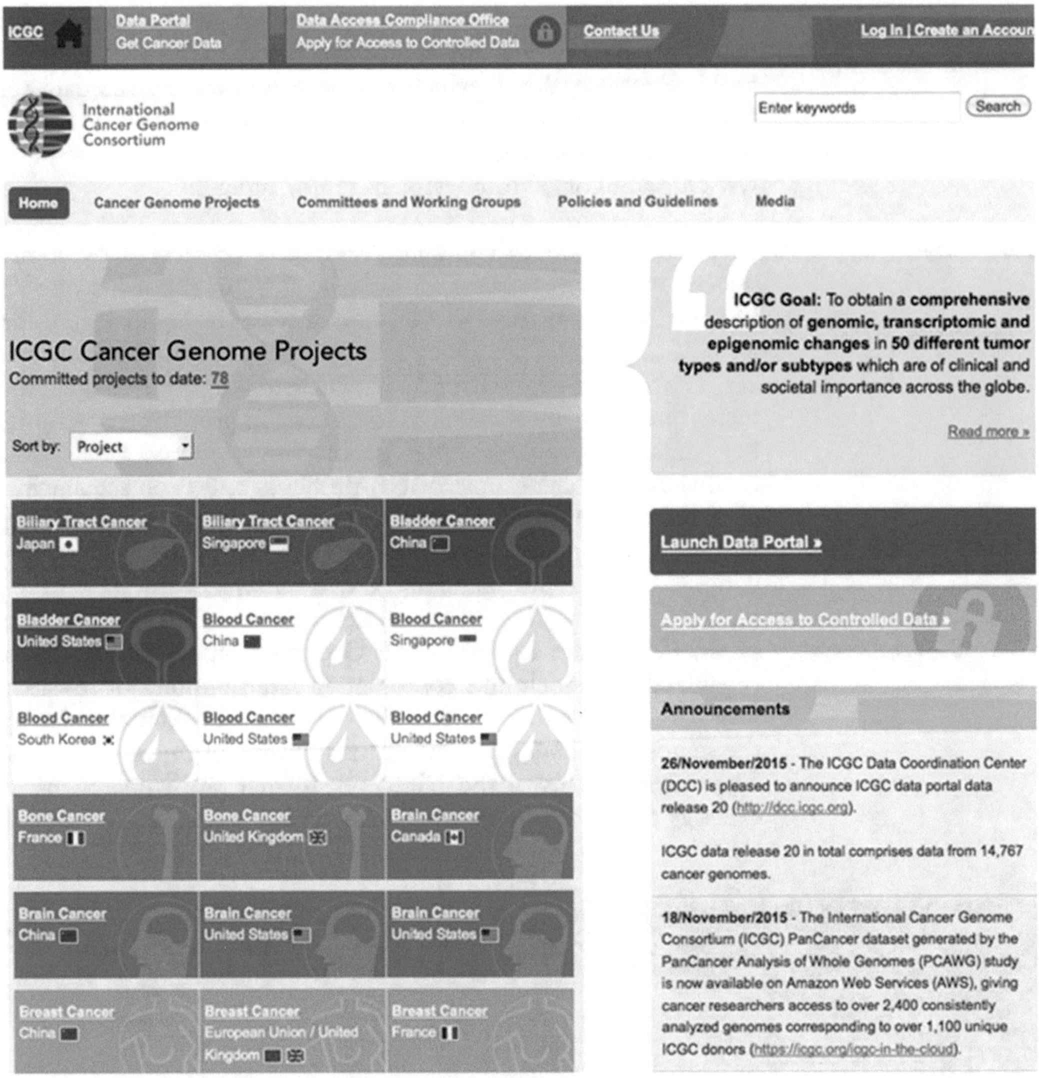

Fig. 5 ICGC International Cancer Genome consortium: Home page (https://icgc.org/)

expression of genes, epigenetic modifications) in tumors from 50 different cancer types. The ICGC data release comprises data from 14,767 cancer genomes.

2.4.3 OASIS (http://www.oasis-genomics.org/)

OASIS provides an option to run exploratory and integrative analyses of somatic mutations, copy number variation (CNV), and gene expression data (Fig. 6). This data originates from several thousands of different tissues originating from tumor samples, normal tissues, and cell lines. The portal contains 30 datasets (mainly from TCGA), with access to mutations, CNV, expression (microarrays), and expression (RNA-Seq).

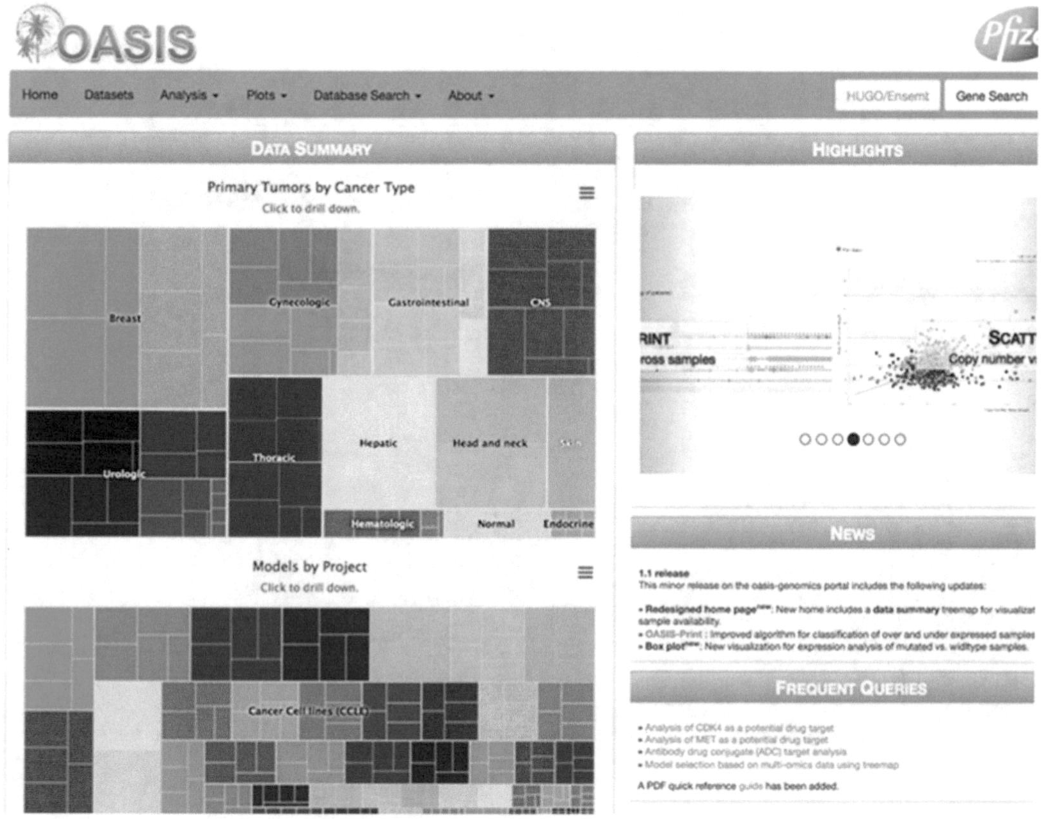

Fig. 6 OASIS Portal developed by Pfizer. Home page with access to data on primary tumors by Cancer Type or by Cancer cell Lines (http://www.oasis-genomics.org/)

2.4.4 Firebrowse (http://firebrowse.org/)

This portal developed at the Broad Institute presents 38 cancer cohorts and 14,729 samples, mainly from the TCGA program, and has an option to browse reports, clinical analysis, copy number, mutation, and expression (Fig. 7).

3 Chromosome Rearrangements/Fusion Gene Resources

Besides the main cytogenetics of cancer resources "Mitelman database" and the "Atlas of Genetics and Cytogenetics in Oncology and Haematology," some other resources provide primer sequences to verify the existence of the fusion genes [18–20]. Finally, it needs to be noted that fusion genes are not present only in neoplasms, but also in normal tissues [21].

3.1 Mitelman Database

With the support of the National Cancer Institute (NCI), the "Catalog of Chromosome Aberrations in Cancer" database became available online and publicly accessible in 2000 (Fig. 8). The database was last updated in February 2016, with a total number of cases amounting to 66,479, implicating 10,277 gene fusions [22].

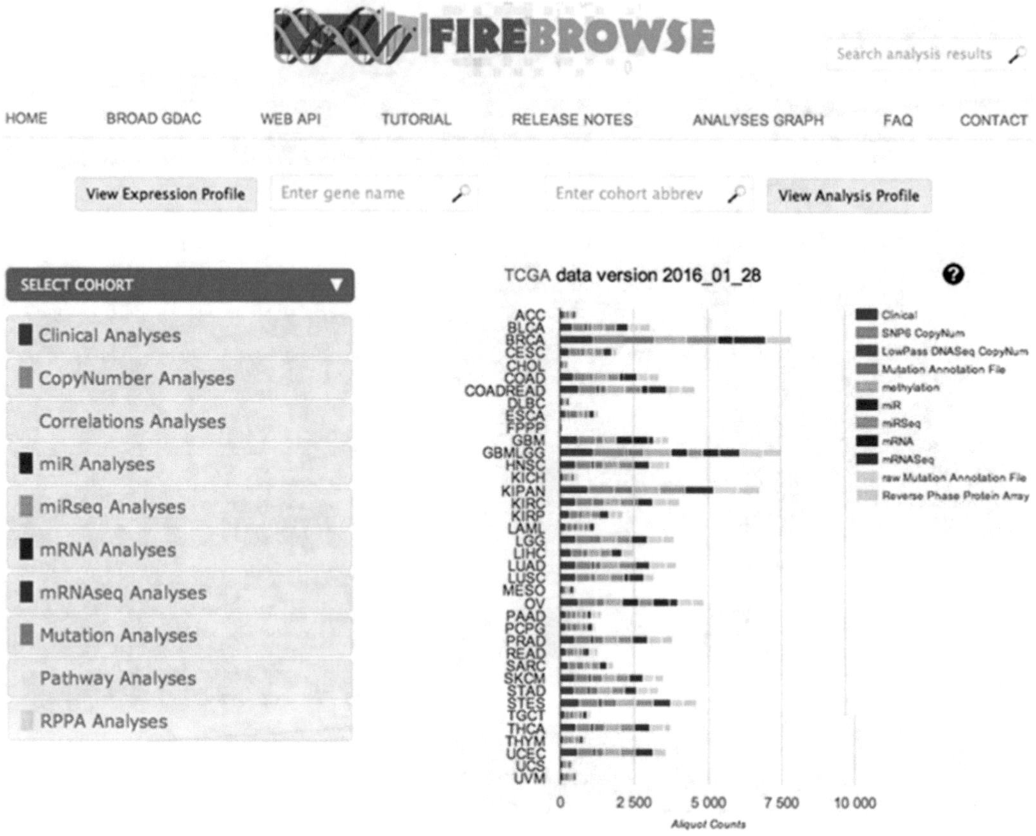

Fig. 7 Differents types of data in each dataset analyzed by GDAC Broad FireBrowse (http://firebrowse.org/)

The data is manually culled from the literature and subsequently organized into distinct sub-databases: The "Cases Quick Searcher" and the "Cases Full Searcher" contain the data related to chromosomal aberrations in individual cases, with the specific tumor characteristics. The "Molecular Biology Associations Searcher" collects cases according to the gene rearrangements, with a mention to tumor histologies. It is accessed by a "Gene List." The "Clinical Associations Searcher" is based on tumor characteristics, related to chromosomal aberrations and/or gene rearrangements. It is based on a "Topography List" stating the site of the tumor, coupled with a "Morphology List," according to histology subtypes of the tumor. Other sub-databases are: "Recurrent Chromosome Aberrations Searcher," which provides a way to search chromosome abnormalities that are recurrent, and the "Reference Searcher," which queries the bibliographic references. Each sub-database indicates relevant references with PMID numbers with hyperlinks to PubMed.

This free access database shows raw data; it is (almost) complete, showing roughly 99% of the various published rearrangements, and highly reliable (each case is manually culled by

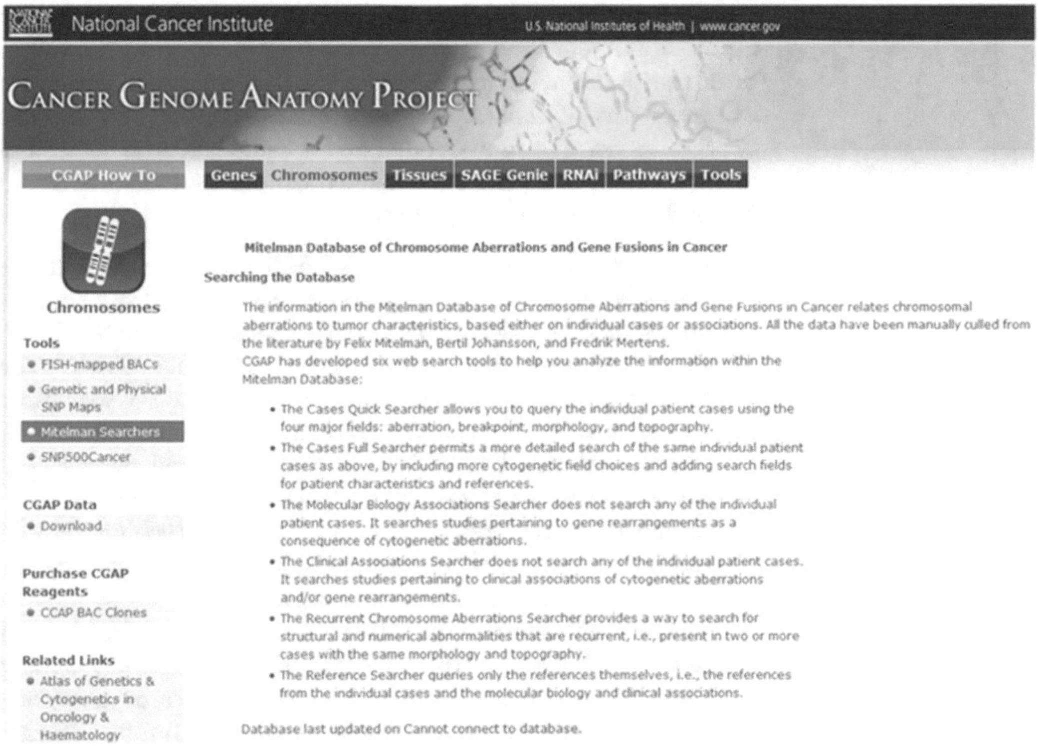

Fig. 8 Mitelman database: "Cases Quick Searcher," "Molecular Biology Associations Searcher," and "Clinical Associations Searcher" (http://cgap.nci.nih.gov/Chromosomes/AllAboutMitelman)

prominent experts). The Mitelman catalog and database has been and still remains an indispensable companion to cancer cytogeneticists. Without the Mitelman database the overall progress of cancer cytogenetics would have been much slower.

3.2 Atlas of Genetics and Cytogenetics in Oncology and Haematology

The Atlas of Genetics and Cytogenetics in Oncology and Haematology [23, 24] (http://atlasgeneticsoncology.org) is a peer-reviewed online journal (ISSN: 1768-3262), encyclopaedia, and database with free access on the Internet. It is an integrated structure comprising the following topics: genes, cytogenetics and clinical entities in cancer, and cancer-prone diseases. The Atlas combines various types of knowledge on one site: genes, gene rearrangements, cytogenetics, protein domains, function, cell biology, pathways. It also includes clinical genetics section, listing cancer-prone hereditary conditions and diseases, focusing on cancers, but also listing other medical conditions. This unifies cancer genetic information, while data found elsewhere is dispersed between several sites. The Atlas is the only cancer genetics database that quotes the prognosis. The iconography in the Atlas is diverse (medical imaging, pathology, chromosomes, 3-dimensional structure of proteins, genetic maps, etc.).

The objectives of the project is the transfer of scientific innovation toward research itself and moreover, towards patient care (translational health research), medical treatment assistance in rare forms of cancer, efficiency savings in the fight against cancer, decrease in fundamental and applied research, as well as medical costs, toward a personalized cancer medicine. It is also a tool for researchers in genomics.

1. Content: The Atlas contains 45,500 pages (30,519 documents, with 32,554 images) from 3216 authors from roughly 50 countries (in decreasing order: France, USA, Italy, United Kingdom, Germany, Japan, Spain, Canada, China, The Netherlands, etc.). The Atlas is mainly composed of structured review articles or "cards" (original monographs written by invited authors), but it also contains traditional overviews, a portal toward websites and databases devoted to cancer and/or genetics, case reports in hematology, and teaching items in various languages. It is a pooling of knowledge regarding the biology of normal and cancerous cells.

   There are annotated cards/review articles on 1460 genes (e.g., *TP53* http://atlasgeneticsoncology.org/Genes/P53ID88.html), and 27,800 nonannotated cards on genes, 600 annotated leukemias (Fig. 9), 210 solid tumors, 115 cancer prone diseases, and 110 deep insight.

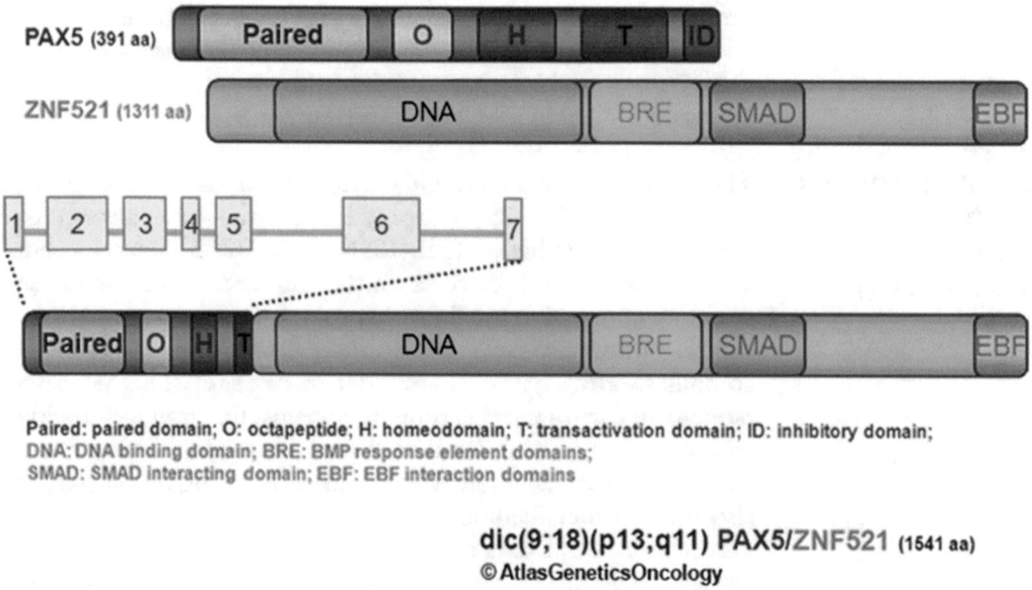

Fig. 9 dic(9;18)(p13;q11) *PAX5/ZNF521* at Atlas (http://atlasgeneticsoncology.org/Anomalies/dic0918p13q11ID1556.html)

The Atlas items are usually searched by chromosome or using the search box for genes or chromosome abnormalities, in dedicated pages for solid tumors or for cancer-prone diseases. However, a "Search by Chromosome band" has recently been developed: it is a synthesis of all fusion gene resources for each chromosome band, which represent 435 pages presenting the chromosomal abnormalities and genes implicated, with data collected from databases and the literature and links to the original web sites (e.g., http://atlasgeneticsoncology.org/Bands/1p36.html).

2. Annotations/Meta-analyses: This database gives annotated data with meta-analyses (e.g., survival curves in the t(3;21)(q26;q22) *RUNX1-MECOM* (http://atlasgeneticsoncology.org/Anomalies/t0321ID1009.html)), which are calculated from the cases available in the literature; type of data is not available elsewhere. Also, the detailed description of the gene *AUTS2* domains (Fig. 2) is the result of an elaborate annotation of data collected from various research papers that cannot be found elsewhere.
3. Diagnosis and treatment: The Atlas contributes to the cytogenetic diagnosis and may guide treatment decision making, particularly regarding rare diseases (numerous, rare diseases are frequently encountered). Under the section "Genes," an extraction can be made of 600 genes implicated in colorectal cancer, 732 in breast cancer, and 480 genes in prostate cancer (e.g., *see* paragraph "Other genes implicated" at: http://atlasgeneticsoncology.org/Tumors/breastID5018.html). This, together with cell biology development, demonstrates that the encyclopaedic content in the Atlas and other similar data sources is a potential basis for developing personalized medicine for cancer. ICD-O3 nomenclature: Nosology and phylum of solid tumors and hematological malignancies can be found in the Atlas at http://atlasgeneticsoncology.org/Tumors/Solid_Nosology.html and http://atlasgeneticsoncology.org/Anomalies/ICD-O_Hematology.html.
4. Cell biology and physio-pathology: Information in the Atlas is a defined resource in cell biology and physio-pathology that is collected in specific pages (e.g., angiogenesis: http://atlasgeneticsoncology.org/Categories/Angiogenesis.html).
5. Links: There are more than 17,000 internal hyperlinks in the Atlas. The expertised gene cards are completed by external links to a large number of up-to-date databases covering complementary aspects. The external links are selected for their cancer relevance.
6. Educational tools: The Atlas has also developed educational genetic tools in English, Spanish, and French (e.g., http://atlasgeneticsoncology.org/GeneticFr.html). Together with the aforementioned data for professionals, this denotes continuing medical education.

7. Electronic journal: An open access electronic journal/pdf version of the Atlas has been developed by Institute for Scientific and Technical Information (INIST) of the French National Centre for Scientific Research (CNRS). Archives available consist of a quarterly journal since 1997, which became a bimonthly journal in 2008 and a monthly journal in 2009, comprising 2500 articles in more than 120 volumes, constituting a 10,000 pages collection, available at http://irevues.inist.fr/atlasgeneticsoncology.

   On the other hand, the Atlas as an encyclopedia with 45,000 pages of reference work, remains incomplete and partially dated. As a product of collaborative work, the usefulness of the Atlas is dependent on colleague participation in updating and completing it.

3.3 COSMIC (http://cancer.sanger.ac.uk/cosmic)

COSMIC is a catalog of somatic mutations in cancer. It roughly includes all abnormalities, from single nucleotide variations to chromosome rearrangements/fusion genes. COSMIC is designed to store and display somatic mutation information with related details and contains information about human cancers. For fusion genes, COSMIC describes 17,245 fusions, with 283 fusion genes that are curated, and 1271 different pairs when taking inferred breakpoints into account (Fig. 10). These fusions are part of a global database of somatic mutations in cancer.

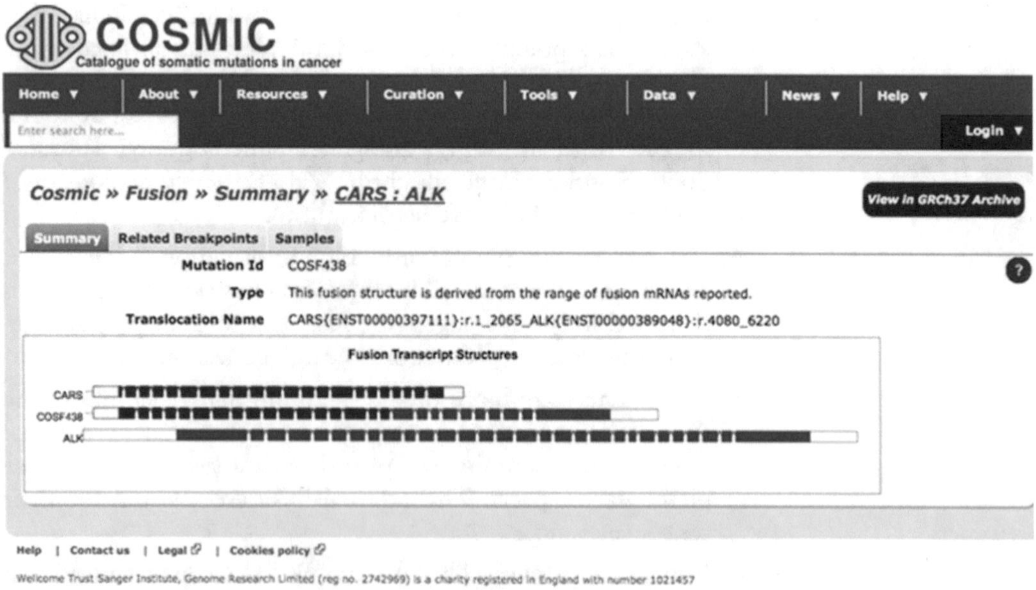

Fig. 10 Example of gene fusion (*CARS/ALK*) on the COSMIC browser (http://cancer.sanger.ac.uk/cosmic/fusion/summary?id=438)

3.4 ChimerDB 2.0 (http://biome.ewha.ac.kr:8080/FusionGene/)

The ChimerDB 2.0 is a knowledgebase for fusion genes, with PubMed references and some information about the structure of chimeric genes [25].

3.5 TICdb (http://www.unav.es/genetica/TICdb/)

TICdb is a database of *T*ranslocation breakpoints *I*n *C*ancer [26]. It contains 1313 fusion sequences found in human tumors, involving 420 different genes. For every fusion, TICdb will return the HGNC names of both partner genes and the original reference, as well as the fusion sequence at the nucleotide level.

3.6 ChiTARS (http://chitars.bioinfo.cnio.es/)

ChiTARS is a database of chimeric transcripts (20,750 chimeric human transcripts) obtained by analysis of EST or RNA sequencing as a part of experimental validation [27].

3.7 TCGA Fusion Gene Data Portal (http://54.84.12.177/PanCanFusV2/)

TCGA fusion gene data portal presents an analysis across 20 tumor types of the TCGA program, with 10,431 fusions in 2961 tumors with fusions (a mean of 3.5 fusions per sample) [28].

3.8 FusionCancer (http://donglab.ecnu.edu.cn/databases/FusionCancer/) [29]

This database of fusion genes in human cancers has its origin in the analysis of RNA-seq data in the Sequence Read Archive (SRA) in 15 cancer types. It contains 11,839 fusions, with structured information of cancer types, SRA breakpoint accession numbers, and chimeric sequences.

3.9 OMIM (http://www.omim.org/)

Victor A. McKusick originally published his catalog "Mendelian Inheritance in Man: Catalogs of Autosomal Dominant, Autosomal Recessive and X-linked Phenotypes" in 1966. "Online Mendelian Inheritance in Man" (OMIM, http://omim.org/) was later published online. There are 23,460 entries: 15,237 gene descriptions, 4705 phenotypes with known molecular basis, and 1626 phenotypes with unknown molecular basis. The OMIM catalog contains 1523 entries for "fusion gene" [30].

3.10 Other Resources

1. Books: The fourth edition (2015) of "Cancer Cytogenetics: Chromosomal and Molecular Genetic Aberrations of Tumor Cells," by Sverre Heim and Felix Mitelman, contains 648 pages. It is a prominent textbook.
2. Iconography: some useful iconography of chromosome rearrangements by the UWCS laboratory, University of Wisconsin, can be found at http://www.slh.wisc.edu/clinical/cytogenetics/cancer/.

   The use of the Atlas, together with the Mitelman, is essential for chromosome rearrangement analysis in hospital practice, particularly for comparing the case study iconography with partial karyotypes available in the Atlas. COSMIC is often used concurrently.

4 Data for Spectral Karyotyping (SKY) and Fluorescence In Situ Hybridization (FISH)

FISH technique enables identification of chromosomal structures to be identified using specific probes. BAC clones provide valuable tools for mapping studies because they contain large inserts of human DNA and can be fluorescently labeled to allow localization of genes and identification of regions involved in cancer chromosomal aberrations. The Cancer Chromosome Aberration Project (CCAP) has generated a set of BAC clones that have been mapped cytogenetically by FISH and physically by STSs to the human genome. The BAC data is integrated into various databases to provide related clinical, histopathologic, genetic, and genomic information (http://cgap.nci.nih.gov/Chromosomes/CCAPBACClones) as well as chromosomal information (e.g., http://cgap.nci.nih.gov/Chromosomes/BACCloneMap?CHR=6). The Human BAC Array (http://mkweb.bcgsc.ca/bacarray/) is constructed using 32,855 clones. The set provides coverage of 98 % of the human May 2005 BAC fingerprint map. All BAC can be located on the UCSC genome browser when BAC end pairs track is selected.

More recently, several commercial companies have developed more specific catalogs of FISH clones as oligonucleotides probes.

A SKY/multiplex FISH (M-FISH) and comparative genomic hybridization (CGH) database provides a public platform for investigators to share and compare their molecular cytogenetic data (http://www.ncbi.nlm.nih.gov/sky/).

5 CGH Resources

CGH (with latest technology of oligonucleotide probes) is the main approach for copy number of (part of) chromosomes, associated with nonequilibrium abnormalities. Numerous designs have been made [from pan-genomic to abnormality specific (custom design)]. For example, the GEO server for instance (Gene Expression Omnibus) has 432 CGH platforms (with 233 as human) and 71 SNP (with 46 for human).

5.1 GEO (http://www.ncbi.nlm.nih.gov/geo/)

This database stores curated gene expression Datasets, as well as original series and platform records in their repository. Mainly used for gene expression, GEO has a limited space dedicated to CGH datasets (1358 experiments for human neoplasms).

5.2 Array Express (http://www.ebi.ac.uk/arrayexpress/)

Array Express, a similar archive of functional genomics data, stores data from high-throughput functional genomics experiments, and provides these data for reuse for the research community [31].

5.3 ArrayMap (http://www.arraymap.org)

ArrayMap (Fig. 11) is a database that provides meta-analysis on 65,042 genomic copy number arrays, in 986 experimental series and on 333 array platforms [32]. The main interest of these resources (originating mostly from GEO datasets) is the fine classification with the ICD-O3 nomenclature.

5.4 Other Sites

Several other sites present reanalyzed data (public or local) with different analytic approaches and provide facilities for exploring abnormalities in different tumor types: Tumorscape (http://www.broadinstitute.org/tcga/home), MetaCGH (http://compbio.med.harvard.edu/metacgh/), CaSNP (http://cistrome.org/CaSNP/), and cancer cell line projects.

6 Mutations

It is important to distinguish between polymorphisms due to single nucleotide (SNP) as the variability within a population and mutations acquired in a neoplastic process.

COSMIC stores 3,942,175 mutations on 1,192,776 samples collected from 22,844 papers. HGMD (The Human Gene Mutation Database, http://www.hgmd.cf.ac.uk/ac/index.php) represents an attempt to collate gene lesions responsible for human-inherited disease [33]. HGMD has two types of access: a free public one with limited data and a professional one requiring a license. LOVD (http://www.lovd.nl/3.0/home) provides a tool for gene-centered collection and display of DNA variations, and also patient-centered data storage and NGS data storage (92,241 entries in all) [34]. The TCGA cBIoPortal for Cancer Genomics (http://www.cbioportal.org/) provides visualization, analysis, and download of 126 cancer genomics data sets. For each dataset the portal presents numerous diagrams for mutations, copy number variations, and survival analysis. It also provides help in analyzing a list of predefined genes [35]. ICGC Data Portal (https://dcc.icgc.org/): the Pancancer Analysis of Whole Genomes (PCAWG) study is an international collaboration identifying common patterns of mutations in more than 2800 cancer whole genomes. It contains descriptions of 36,985,985 mutations in 57,773 genes and 17,867 donors within 66 projects in 21 primary sites [36]. OASIS Portal presents data from 30 datasets with 6817 mutations, 11,222 CNVs and expression (8178 RNA Seq and 4889 microarrays). BioMuta v2 (https://hive.biochemistry.gwu.edu/tools/biomuta/) is a curated single-nucleotide variation (SNV) and disease association database. The database has 5,233,790 SNV for 41 cancer types and displays position of mutation and frequency of each cancer type [37]. Other mutation databases are DoCM (http://docm.genome.wustl.edu/), CIViC

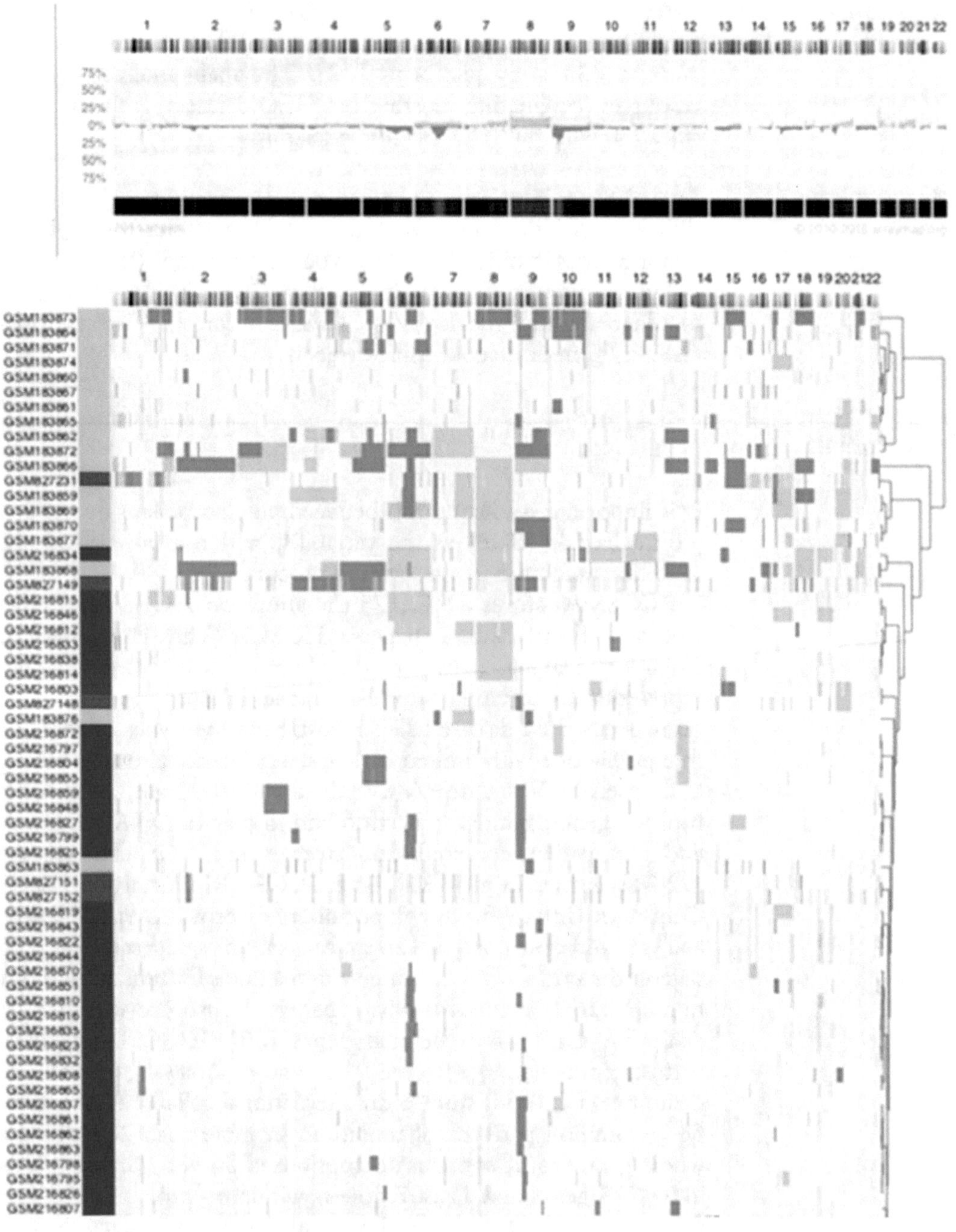

Fig. 11 ArrayMap (http://www.arraymap.org/): Selection of 104 samples of precursor T-cell lymphoblastic leukemia (ICD-O 9817/3) from a general query on leukemia and processing with the default parameters to obtain a CGH profile. Upper part: mean copy number profile (gain in yellow, loss in blue). Lower part: "heatmap" of gain and loss for all the samples on the entire genome showing the variability of CGH profiles of the different sample in the dataset

(https://civic.genome.wustl.edu/#/home), and ExAC (http://exac.broadinstitute.org), a coalition of investigators seeking to aggregate and harmonize exome sequencing data from a variety of large-scale sequencing projects, and to make summary data available for the wider scientific community. The data set provided on this website spans 60,706 unrelated individuals sequenced as part of various disease-specific and population genetic studies.

7 Discussion

We have briefly described the various databases that are useful for clinicians and students in finding answers to their questions.

Only a handful of databases or portals take the cytogenetic information into consideration, although being one of the first check points confirming a cell transformation into a cancerous cell. Over the years (1960–2016), chimeric genes/fusion proteins have been discovered mainly by cytogenetic means. This has led to the wider understanding of major cancerogenetic processes, and, later on, to the concept of treatment targets. Cytogenetics or, rather, cytogenomics of cancer is therefore a major contributor for the concept of "personalized medicine for cancer."

The use of databases condenses the complex information and provides links to other databases for even more specialized information. Databases will need to integrate even more information in the forthcoming years and become more interoperable with other databases. This reinforces the idea of having a common nomenclature and language in this specific field. Resources such as the International System for Human Cytogenomic Nomenclature (ISCN), the International Classification of Diseases for Oncology (ICD-O), and the Human Gene Nomenclature Database (HGNC) are indispensable tools allowing a common language, to generate a common framework of harmonized approaches to enable data-sharing ("Interoperability"), to manage genomic and clinical data, and to present of genotype-phenotype associations better.

Data should remain freely available (concept of "open data": "open source," "open hardware," "open content," and "open access"). However, keeping the data freely accessible remains a daily struggle. Even a free database has a cost, and a business model remains to be established. Although the economic investment from the public sector would be not only beneficial for the whole mankind, but also economically profitable in the end, most of the institutional stakeholders are now gradually disengaging, and well-known databases are forced to beg for funds or to disappear. This disappearance would be a regrettable drawback for the scientific and medical community—yet it may happen!

References

1. Stratton MR, Campbell PJ, Stratton MR (2009) The cancer genome. Nature 458(7239):719–724
2. Mertens F, Johansson B, Fioretos T et al (2015) The emerging complexity of gene fusions in cancer. Nat Rev Cancer 15(6):371–381
3. Bernheim A, Huret JL, Guillaud-Bataille M et al (2004) Cytogenetics, cytogenomics and cancer: 2004 update. Bull Cancer 91(1):29–43
4. Caspersson T, Zech L, Caspersson T (1970) Fluorescent labeling of chromosomal DNA: superiority of quinacrine mustard to quinacrine. Science 170(3959):762
5. Druker BJ, Sawyers CL, Kantarjian H et al (2001) Activity of a specific inhibitor of the BCR-ABL tyrosine kinase in the blast crisis of chronic myeloid leukemia and acute lymphoblastic leukemia with the Philadelphia chromosome. N Engl J Med 344(14):1038–1042
6. Druker BJ, Talpaz M, Resta DJ et al (2001) Efficacy and safety of a specific inhibitor of the BCR-ABL tyrosine kinase in chronic myeloid leukemia. N Engl J Med 344(14):1031–1037
7. Gray KA, Yates B, Seal RL et al (2015) Genenames. org, the HGNC resources in 2015. Nucleic Acids Res 43(Database issue):D1079–1085
8. Shaffer LG, McGowen-Jordan J, Schmid M (eds) (2013) ISCN an International System for Human Cytogenetic Nomenclature. S. Karger, Basel
9. McGowan-Jordan J, Simons A, Schmid M (eds) (2016) ISCN 2016 An International System for Cytogenomic Nomenclature. S. Karger, Basel. [Reprint of Cytogenet Genome Res 149(1-2)].
10. Burks C, Fickett JW, Goad WB et al (1985) The GenBank nucleic acid sequence database. Comput Appl Biosci 1(4):225–233
11. Rosenbloom KR, Armstrong J, Barber GP et al (2015) The UCSC Genome Browser database: 2015 update. Nucleic Acids Res 43(Database issue):D670–D681
12. Pundir S, Magrane M, Martin MJ et al (2015) Searching and navigating UniProt databases. Curr Protoc Bioinform 50:1.27.1–10. doi:10.1002/0471250953.bi0127s50
13. Gaudet P, Michel PA, Zahn-Zabal M et al (2015) The neXtProt knowledgebase on human proteins: current status. Nucleic Acids Res 43(Database issue):D764–D770
14. Hornbeck PV, Zhang B, Murray B et al (2015) PhosphoSitePlus, 2014: mutations, PTMs and recalibrations. Nucleic Acids Res 43(Database issue):D512–D520
15. Sigrist CJ, de Castro E, Cerutti L et al (2013) New and continuing developments at PROSITE. Nucleic Acids Res 41(Database issue):D344–D347
16. Finn RD, Coggill P, Eberhardt RY et al (2016) The Pfam protein families database: towards a more sustainable future. Nucleic Acids Res 44(D1):D279–D285
17. Mitchell A, Chang HY, Daugherty L et al (2015) The InterPro protein families database: the classification resource after 15 years. Nucleic Acids Res 43(Database issue):D213–D221
18. Løvf M, Thomassen GO, Bakken AC et al (2011) Fusion gene microarray reveals cancer type-specificity among fusion genes. Genes Chromosomes Cancer 50(5):348–357
19. Skotheim RI, Thomassen GO, Eken M et al (2009) A universal assay for detection of oncogenic fusion transcripts by oligo microarray analysis. Mol Cancer 8:5. doi:10.1186/1476-4598-8-5
20. Urakami K, Shimoda Y, Ohshima K et al (2016) Next generation sequencing approach for detecting 491 fusion genes from human cancer. Biomed Res 37(1):51–62
21. Babiceanu M, Qin F, Xie Z et al (2016) Recurrent chimeric fusion RNAs in non-cancer tissues and cells. Nucleic Acids Res 44(6):2859–2872
22. Mitelman F, Johansson B, Mertens F (eds.) (2016) Mitelman Database of Chromosome Aberrations and Gene Fusions in Cancer,. http://cgap.nci.nih.gov/Chromosomes/Mitelman.
23. Huret JL, Ahmad M, Arsaban M et al (2013) Atlas of genetics and cytogenetics in oncology and haematology in 2013. Nucleic Acids Res 41(Database issue):D920–D924
24. Dorkeld F, Bernheim A, Dessen P et al (1999) A database on cytogenetics in haematology and oncology. Nucleic Acids Res 27(1):353–354
25. Kim P, Yoon S, Kim N et al (2010) ChimerDB 2.0: a knowledgebase for fusion genes updated. Nucleic Acids Res 38(Database issue):D81–D85. doi:10.1093/nar/gkp982, Epub 2009 Nov 11
26. Novo FJ, de Mendíbil IO, Novo FJ (2007) TICdb: a collection of gene-mapped translocation breakpoints in cancer. BMC Genomics 8:33. doi:10.1186/1471-2164-8-33
27. Frenkel-Morgenstern M, Gorohovski A, Vucenovic D et al (2015) ChiTaRS 2.1:–an improved database of the chimeric transcripts and RNA-seq data with novel sense-antisense

chimeric RNA transcripts. Nucleic Acids Res 43(Database issue):D68–D75

28. Yoshihara K, Wang Q, Torres-Garcia W et al (2015) The landscape and therapeutic relevance of cancer-associated transcript fusions. Oncogene 34(37):4845–4854
29. Wang Y, Wu N, Liu J et al (2015) FusionCancer: a database of cancer fusion genes derived from RNA-seq data. Diagn Pathol 10:131. doi:10.1186/s13000-015-0310-4
30. Amberger JS, Bocchini CA, Schiettecatte F et al (2015) OMIM an online catalog of human genes and genetic disorders. Nucleic Acids Res 43(Database issue):D789–D798
31. Petryszak R, Keays M, Tang YA et al (2016) Expression Atlas update--an integrated database of gene and protein expression in humans, animals and plants. Nucleic Acids Res 44(D1):D746–D752
32. Cai H, Gupta S, Rath P et al (2015) arrayMap 2014: an updated cancer genome resource. Nucleic Acids Res 43(Database issue): D825–D830
33. Cooper DN, Krawczak M (1996) Human Gene Mutation Database. Hum Genet 98(5):629
34. Fokkema IF, Taschner PE, Schaafsma GC et al (2011) LOVD v. 2.0 the next generation in gene variant databases. Hum Mutat 32(5):557–563
35. Deng M, Brägelmann J, Schultze JL et al (2016) Web-TCGA: an online platform for integrated analysis of molecular cancer data sets. BMC Bioinformatics 17:72. doi:10.1186/s12859-016-0917-9
36. Zhang J, Baran J, Cros A et al (2011) International Cancer Genome Consortium Data Portal – a one-stop shop for cancer genomics data. Database (Oxford). doi:10.1093/database/bar026
37. Wu TJ, Shamsaddini A, Pan Y et al (2014) A framework for organizing cancer-related variations from existing databases, publications and NGS data using a High-performance Integrated Virtual Environment (HIVE). Database (Oxford). doi:10.1093/database/bau022

Index

Thomas S.K. Wan (ed.), *Cancer Cytogenetics: Methods and Protocols*, Methods in Molecular Biology, vol. 1541, DOI 10.1007/978-1-4939-6703-2, © Springer Science+Business Media LLC 2017

F

G

Q

S

T

U

W

X

Printed in the United States
By Bookmasters